Registered
Dietitian Exam
SECRETS

Study Guide
Your Key to Exam Success

Dietitian Test Review for the
Registered Dietitian Exam

Published by
Mometrix Test Preparation
Dietitian Exam Secrets Test Prep Team

Written and edited by the Dietitian Exam Secrets Test Prep Staff

Printed in the United States of America

This paper meets the requirements of ANSI/NISO Z39.48-1992 (Permanence of Paper).

Mometrix offers volume discount pricing to institutions. For more information or a price quote, please contact our sales department at sales@mometrix.com or 888-248-1219.

ISBN 13: 978-1-61072-803-4
ISBN 10: 1-61072-803-3

Dear Future Exam Success Story:

Congratulations on your purchase of our study guide. Our goal in writing our study guide was to cover the content on the test, as well as provide insight into typical test taking mistakes and how to overcome them.

Standardized tests are a key component of being successful, which only increases the importance of doing well in the high-pressure high-stakes environment of test day. How well you do on this test will have a significant impact on your future- and we have the research and practical advice to help you execute on test day.

The product you're reading now is designed to exploit weaknesses in the test itself, and help you avoid the most common errors test takers frequently make.

How to use this study guide

We don't want to waste your time. Our study guide is fast-paced and fluff-free. We suggest going through it a number of times, as repetition is an important part of learning new information and concepts.

First, read through the study guide completely to get a feel for the content and organization. Read the general success strategies first, and then proceed to the content sections. Each tip has been carefully selected for its effectiveness.

Second, read through the study guide again, and take notes in the margins and highlight those sections where you may have a particular weakness.

Finally, bring the manual with you on test day and study it before the exam begins.

Your success is our success

We would be delighted to hear about your success. Send us an email and tell us your story. Thanks for your business and we wish you continued success-

Sincerely,

Mometrix Test Preparation Team

Need more help? Check out our flashcards at: http://MometrixFlashcards.com/RD

TABLE OF CONTENTS

Top 20 Test Taking Tips

1. Carefully follow all the test registration procedures
2. Know the test directions, duration, topics, question types, how many questions
3. Setup a flexible study schedule at least 3-4 weeks before test day
4. Study during the time of day you are most alert, relaxed, and stress free
5. Maximize your learning style; visual learner use visual study aids, auditory learner use auditory study aids
6. Focus on your weakest knowledge base
7. Find a study partner to review with and help clarify questions
8. Practice, practice, practice
9. Get a good night's sleep; don't try to cram the night before the test
10. Eat a well balanced meal
11. Know the exact physical location of the testing site; drive the route to the site prior to test day
12. Bring a set of ear plugs; the testing center could be noisy
13. Wear comfortable, loose fitting, layered clothing to the testing center; prepare for it to be either cold or hot during the test
14. Bring at least 2 current forms of ID to the testing center
15. Arrive to the test early; be prepared to wait and be patient
16. Eliminate the obviously wrong answer choices, then guess the first remaining choice
17. Pace yourself; don't rush, but keep working and move on if you get stuck
18. Maintain a positive attitude even if the test is going poorly
19. Keep your first answer unless you are positive it is wrong
20. Check your work, don't make a careless mistake

Content of the Exam

Principles of Dietetics

Food Science and Nutrient Composition of Foods

Fruits and vegetables

Pigments
- Chlorophyll: Green. When an acid is added to chlorophyll, the pigment changes to an olive green pigment. This pigment is called pheophytin. For example, if you are cooking and you add green beans to tomato sauce, the green beans will turn olive green. When an alkaline solution is added to chlorophyll, the resulting product is chlorophyllin, which has a bright green pigment.
- Carotenoids: Yellow/orange. This pigment shows little change in an acid or an alkaline solution. Lycopene is a carotenoid that is responsible for giving tomato products and watermelon their red color.
- Anthocyanins: Red, blue, and purple. When an acid is added to this pigment, it changes to bright red. When this pigment is added to an alkaline solution, it turns a bluish color.
- Anthoxanthins or flavones: White. This pigment is colorless in acid solutions and yellow when added to alkaline solutions. For example, onions turn yellow when cooked in an aluminum pan.

Changes that occur in plant pigments during the preparation of fruits and vegetables can increase or decrease the nutrient content and appeal of these foods.

Chlorophyll is the energy-synthesizing molecule that gives plants their characteristic green color. The magnesium atom in chlorophyll is replaced with a hydrogen atom in the presence of acid, forming pheophytin and resulting in a drab olive color. Conversely, chlorophyll turns bright green in the presence of an alkaline solution.

Carotenoids are usually yellow, orange, or red, and include the well-known nutrient carotene, an important vitamin A precursor. Carotenes are insoluble in water, and they are also stable in an acid or alkaline solution, so cooking does little to reduce the bright color.

Flavonoids include the red and blue anthocyanins found in blueberries, which serve as an antioxidant in the diet. These water-soluble pigments turn bright red in the presence of acid, and take on a more bluish hue in the presence of alkaline solutions.

Osmosis and diffusion
Osmosis is the process by which water enters or leaves a cell to establish equilibrium between the contents of the cell and its environment (e.g., water moves into vegetables such as lettuce or celery to keep them crisp).

$$H_2O \longrightarrow \ominus \longrightarrow H_2O$$

Diffusion is the process by which a molecules spread from higher concentrations to lower concentrations. It is called equilibrium when the molecules are even (e.g., dissolving sugar in water, or dehydration, which is the process of replacing the water of a vegetable with a concentrated salt solution).

- 3 -

Grading process

The United States Department of Agriculture (USDA) has developed official grade standards for fruits and vegetables that are based on quality, firmness, color, shape, and lack of defects.

Canned fruits or vegetables are graded according to the following:
- Grade A (Fancy): desserts, salads.
- Grade B (Choice): processed fruits or vegetables.
- Grade C (Standard): puddings and pies.

Fresh produce is graded by using the following terms:
- Fancy
- Extra #1
- No. 1
- Combination
- No. 2.

Ripening process

The hormone ethylene is largely responsible for the ripening process in fruits. This gas passes through the air from one fruit to another and acts like an invisible signal to other fruits to begin to ripen and decay. The gas is produced in higher amounts by some fruits, such as apples, bananas, peaches, and pears, while other fruits, such as grapes, strawberries, and citrus fruits produce less of the gas. The gas is produced in higher amounts in reaction to certain environmental stresses, such as high temperatures and wounding. Growers have been able to use their knowledge of ethylene to their advantage, so that ethylene conditions in the warehouse may be perfectly controlled to determine the time at which peak ripeness occurs.

Consumers can control the ripening effects of ethylene at home by storing most produce in the refrigerator and placing unripe produce on the counter to achieve peak flavor.

Meat, poultry and fish

USDA inspection and grading

USDA inspection is mandatory if meat is sold across state lines. The Wholesome Meat Act of 1967 required that all states have inspection programs equal to that of the federal government. Inspection ensures that the animal was healthy and slaughtered under sanitary condition. The Food Safety and Inspection Service (FSIS) is a branch of the USDA that inspects meat for safe processing, labeling, and packaging according to the Federal Meat Inspection Act. A USDA seal ensures that the meat is WHOLESOME, properly labeled, and not adulterated in any way. Quality is NOT determined, only wholesomeness. The inspection process uses random sampling to uncover hidden dangers such as pathogens or chemical contamination, and meat that passes the testing process receives a round purple stamp.

USDA grading indicates quality of the meat product. The USDA's Agricultural Marketing Service is the agency responsible for grading meat and poultry. It is based on maturity of the animal, marbling of fat, color, and texture. Grades include prime, choice, select, and standard. Poultry is graded using the following: Grade A, B, or C.

Seafood inspection

The FDA is the governing body that oversees seafood products to ensure safety through its Hazard Analysis Critical Points Control Program. Rather than focusing on the finished seafood product to identify safety issues, this program seeks to identify and prevent problems that could cause illness in seafood. The US Department of Commerce also runs a voluntary, fee-for-service program via the National Oceanic and Atmospheric Administration. This program goes beyond the basic safety assurances of the FDA program to further examine seafood for wholesomeness and quality. If the product meets the guidelines set forth by the USDC for quality, the manufacturer is permitted to label the product as "grade A," indicating that the highest level of quality has been met. Unlike other food products inspected by the government for quality, there are no lesser grades for seafood.

Color

Two pigments are primarily responsible for the color variations we see in meat and poultry: myoglobin and oxymyoglobin. Myoglobin produces the reddish-purple color seen in beef. When meat tissues are exposed to oxygen, myoglobin produces oxymyoglobin, the pigment that gives meat a bright red color. Therefore, meat products that are vacuum-sealed, and thus protected from oxygen exposure, will have a purplish-red appearance, while those meat products displayed in the butcher's case will have the bright red appearance characteristic of oxymyoglobin formation.

Color is not a reliable indicator of the freshness of meat or doneness in cooking. Using an instant read thermometer to ensure cooking temperatures have reached 160°F throughout ensures the destruction of pathogens.

Poultry can vary in appearance from white to yellowish-white to bluish white, depending on the feed used, age of the bird, and activity level of the bird. As with beef, color is not an indicator of doneness, and cooked temperatures of 165°F should determine cooking times rather than reliance on color.

Aging process

A sequence of events occurs after the slaughter of an animal as muscle turns into meat. Blood is removed from the carcass of the animal, which means that nutrients and oxygen is no longer being delivered to the muscle. Furthermore, waste products are no longer removed from the muscle. This lack of oxygen means that only anaerobic metabolism can take place. Lactic acid is a byproduct of this metabolism, and remains in the muscles. This leads to a drop in the pH of the animal. When the animal expires, its immune system no longer functions, making the carcass susceptible to pathogens. The color of the meat changes from bright red to purplish-red due to a lack of oxygen. Beef is aged for about 7 days after slaughter to increase flavor and tenderness. Enzymes act on the muscle during this time to break down collagen and muscle fibers.

Structure

Meat is made up of muscle, connective tissue, fat, and bone.
- Connective tissue is made of up collagen and elastin. Collagen softens when cooking and turns to gelatin when heated. Elastin is resistant to heat.
- Fat: "Marbling" is the fat distribution in the muscle, while the "finish" is the amount of fat cover on the carcass.
- Bone shape identifies the cut of the meat. Round bone is leg; T-bone is back and ribs.

Nutrient Composition

12% to 23% of meat is protein, and there are minimal carbohydrates. Vitamins/Minerals = thiamin, niacin, riboflavin, iron, copper, and trace minerals. Fish has fewer calories and fat than meat.

Tenderizing methods
- Mechanical Tenderizer includes grinding, scoring, and cubing.
- Chemical Tenderizers include papaya, pineapple, and fig. Acidic chemicals and salt increase the water holding capacity.

Cooking methods

Dry heat methods for preparing meat commonly include frying, broiling, grilling, and roasting. Cuts of meat close to the rib or loin have less connective tissue (collagen), and are the most suitable for these cooking methods. The USDA recommends that while hamburger products should be cooked to a temperature of 165°F, whole muscle meats may be cooked to 145°F if rare beef is desired.

Moist heat cooking is a good way to utilize less expensive, tougher cuts of meat that come from the chuck or round. Weight bearing muscles contain more collagen, and older animals contain more collagen. Slow cooking methods of applying moist heat take advantage of the fact that collagen is soluble in water.

Methods such as stewing, simmering, braising, and steaming allow the collagen to gelatinize, tenderizing the meat.

Eggs

The grading of eggs is governed by USDA standards, although it is not mandatory. The grades encompass both interior and exterior quality, and eggs may be assigned a grade of AA, A, or B. Grade AA eggs have the most superior quality, with firm yolks that stand up tall and thick whites that cling to the yolk area. Grade A eggs are most commonly found in the grocery store, and most consumers would not be able to discern a difference between A and AA eggs. Grade B eggs, although suitable for eating, are usually shipped to food manufacturers for use in recipes. The yolks appear flattened out and the whites are thin.

Eggs are grouped for sale according to size, so that the weight of a dozen eggs meets the standard for that size. The following 6 size equivalents are offered for sale: peewee (15 oz), small (18 oz), medium (21 oz), large (24 oz), extra-large (27 oz), and jumbo (30 oz). The standard size for recipe use is large.

Nutritive value

Eggs are considered a nutrient-dense food, as they supply a large amount of nutrition in relation to the calories they contain. One large whole egg can provide over 10% of the daily recommended value of protein, including all of the amino acids essential to the body.

The egg white, or albumen, is a high-quality, fat-free source of protein in the eggs. The white also contains about half of the vitamin and mineral content of the egg, making it a good source of niacin, riboflavin, potassium, and magnesium.

The egg yolk contains all of the egg's fat, vitamin A, vitamin D, vitamin E, iron and zinc. The yolk is also the source of cholesterol in the egg, so egg yolks may be restricted for those on a low-cholesterol diet. 80 calories, 6 g protein, 5 g fat.

Structure

Porous shell that is used for gas and moisture exchange. The air space at the large end of the egg becomes larger as the egg ages.

Baked goods

Starches

Gelatinization: The gelatinization of starch plays an important role in achieving the desired thickness and texture in many foods, including puddings, gravy, and sauces. Starch is a compound made up of amylose and amylopectin, which remain linked together in cold water. When the temperature of the water begins to rise, the intermolecular bond between the amylose and amylopectin is disrupted and water begins to penetrate the bonds. When the crystal structure is completely disrupted, gelatinization is complete. This results in a suspension that lends viscosity, binding power, and adhesive properties to the final food product. The temperature at which this occurs depends on the type of starch and the presence of other substances such as fats, proteins, sugars, or acid.

Retrogradation: Starch is composed of amylose and amylopectin, and those starches with a higher proportion of amylose are more prone to retrogradation. More waxy starches containing high amylopectin amounts, such as corn and rice, do not experience this problem. When starch is exposed to water and heat the molecules swell and viscosity is increased; this is part of the gelatinization process. When the gel cools, the starch may lose some of its ability to hold water, water is forced out of the gel, and syneresis or weeping of fluid can occur. The crystalline structure of the gel breaks down and the hydrogen bonds in the amylose recrystallize in a more orderly way. This results in a grainy product or a sauce that has a viscous layer surrounded by a puddle of water due to syneresis. Freezing exacerbates retrogradation and choosing waxy starch ingredients prevents the problem.

Leavening methods

Regardless of the method of leavening used in bakery products, the goal is the same: to produce carbon dioxide gas. Mechanical leavening takes place when air is incorporated into the batter or dough as a result of the mixing technique used. Egg whites are one of the primary mechanical leavening agents, as egg whites foam when beaten or whipped, trapping air bubbles in the batter. The proteins in the foam coagulate and stabilize in the presence of cooking temperatures. Steam can also contribute to volume in some products.

Chemical leavening agents include baking soda and baking powder. Baking soda needs to come into contact with moisture and an acidic ingredient to be activated. Baking powder only needs moisture to release its leavening power.

Yeast is considered a biological leavening product, as it is a live organism. The leavening occurs when the organism feeds off of the sugar or flour in the presence of moisture in the product and produces carbon dioxide and ethanol.

Wheat flour
- Graham, whole wheat flour: Uses the entire grain and spoils fast because of the fat in the germ.
- Bread (hard wheat) flour: Contains strong gluten and has the most protein (11.8%).
- All-purpose flour: This type of flour is a blend of hard and soft wheats. It contains less gluten. It has 10.5% protein. This flour is the best for making cakes.

- Pastry flour: This type of flour is soft wheat weak gluten. It has even less protein than all-purpose.
- Cake flour: This type of flour is also soft wheat and has the least and weakest gluten. However, it has more starch.

The more protein and gluten in the flour = a stronger flour.

Gluten development: Many different flours are used in baking, but only wheat flour has enough of the protein gluten to contribute to structural changes in the final product. When gluten comes into contact with moisture, the proteins adhere to water and form a web-like structure that exhibits elastic qualities. Mechanical manipulation such as kneading, beating, or stirring enhances gluten's ability to bind with water. After the gluten has reached the desired stage of development, the net-like structure functions to hold gas bubbles in the batter or dough, which makes gluten an important leavening agent. When the product encounters the heat of the oven, the moisture evaporates and the previously elastic gluten structure becomes rigid, yielding a baked good whose volume is stable. Different types of wheat flour have different gluten levels, and the choice of flour one uses depends of the desired texture of the final product. For example, more tender products such as cakes call for flour with lower gluten content.

Dairy products

Milk
- Homogenized milk: Milk that has been heat-treated and processed to break up the fat globules and distribute them evenly throughout the milk.
- Evaporated milk: A form of condensed milk made from homogenized milk. Cow's milk consists of roughly 3.5% milkfat, 8.5% non-fat solids, and 88% water. Evaporated milk has about 60% of its water removed by evaporation. Evaporated milk is brown in color because of the caramelization of lactose when it is canned.
- Sweetened condensed milk: A form of evaporated milk. Sixty percent of the water is removed from whole milk through heating, and then sugar is added to the milk.
- Cultured buttermilk: A type of fermented milk. The formation of buttermilk is based on the fermentation by bacteria, which turns skimmed milk sugar (lactose) into lactic acid. As lactic acid is formed, the pH of the milk drops and it gets tart. *If you ever want to replace regular milk with buttermilk in a recipe, it is important that you also increase the baking soda.
- Filled milk: Skim milk that has vegetable oil and water added to it.

Cheese
The making of cheese involves separating the curd from the whey in milk or cream, consolidating the curd, and usually ripening the final product. Coagulation disrupts the casein protein in the milk, causing a gel to form. Coagulation is facilitated by using enzymes, acid, or a combination of heat and acid. After the gel has been allowed to firm, the curds are cut into pieces, which begin to expel the liquid whey. Cooking helps to separate the whey from the curd, and also determines the final moisture content and pH level of the cheese. Most cheeses undergo a ripening process to achieve the desired body, texture, and flavor. Ripening agents cause the protein, fat, and lactose to break down. Common agents used include introduced molds, enzymes, rennet, and lipase. The ripening stage can take weeks, months, or even years, depending on the type of cheese.

Dairy processing techniques

Pasteurization is one of the most important steps in the production of milk products. The rationale for pasteurization is twofold: to destroy pathogens harmful to humans, and to extend shelf life by destroying bacteria that cause spoilage. The extent of pathogen destruction depends on the temperature and the length of exposure to the heat.

Ultra-high temperature processing (UHT) takes this notion one step further by using temperatures in excess of boiling to render the product sterile. This results in a product with a shelf life of 6 months or longer, but the "cooked milk flavor" is a downside.

Homogenization acts as a mechanical emulsifying process, suspending the fatty globules of whole milk in the water layer. Without this, the fat would rise to the top as cream. The fat globules are forced through an extruder to break them into smaller particles, and this smaller surface area allows the emulsion to stabilize.

Maillard reaction

The Maillard reaction, named for the chemist who studied it in the 1900s, is a nonenzymatic browning process that contributes to the flavor, color, and nutrient quality of many foods. The reaction occurs when virtually any food is heated, as it requires the presence of amino acids and sugars found in many foods. The 2 substrates undergo a 3-step process. If there is a high concentration of sugar and amino acid, the brown pigment will form at lower temperatures, but if a low concentration of sugars and amino acids is present, high temperatures are necessary to produce the browning. The resulting caramel flavors and aromas are desirable in most products, but the reaction can produce undesirable results as well, such as discoloration in dried milk or the excessive darkening that occurs in burnt food. Although the biochemical reaction is basically the same from one food to the next, a myriad of flavors and aromas can result, depending on variations in temperature, water content, type of sugar and amino acid, and other factors.

Bowes & Church's Food Values of Pertion Commonly Used

One of the most comprehensive print versions of nutrient composition tables is Bowes & Church's Food Values of Portions Commonly Used, by Jean A. T. Pennington, Ph.D.

Some 8,500 foods are listed according to food group with analysis results for 30 nutrients, but they are not in "Nutrition Facts" label format.

Food additives

Safety

GRAS list: GRAS means generally recognized as safe. This list was developed in 1958 to categorize food additives generally thought to be safe for consumption. Congress felt that food manufacturers should not have to prove the safety of substances they already added to foods; instead this was deemed to be the responsibility of the FDA. Many chemicals on the GRAS list have not been rigorously tested because of the expense. Instead, these additives are generally thought to be safe because of their long history of safe use.

Delaney clause: The Delaney clause was added to the 1958 Pure Food and Drug Act in the United States to ensure that food additives known to be carcinogenic to humans or animals would not be used in food, regardless of the margin of safety.

No observable effect: The no observable effect level corresponds to the highest dose of a food additive that can be found to produce no adverse health effects in animals. This number is then used to establish a margin of safety for the use of the additive in human foodstuffs.

Types of additives
1. **Preserves:** This group includes agents to stop, or completely destroy, microbic reaction, such as sodium nitrates and ascorbic acid.
2. **Antioxidation:** includes materials used to prevent, or delay, rancidity, which results from the fat reacting with air, and to protect dissolved vitamins in fat from oxidation.
3. **Coloring agents:** includes all natural and artificial colors added to food to give it distinctive look, making it attractive to consumers.
4. **Sweeteners:** such as sugar alternatives, which are widely used now.
5. **Flavorings**
6. **Emulsifiers and stabilizers:** The materials that assist and enable mixing of oils and greases with water, adding a creamy and rich texture to food, such as ice cream.

Preservatives: There are many types of preservatives, and their role includes preventing rancidity, inhibiting microbial growth, and preventing oxidation of foods. Nitrates and nitrites are commonly found in processed meats as a *C. botulinum* inhibitor. Other common preservatives include ascorbic acid, calcium propionate, sodium benzoate, and vitamin C.

Antioxidants: Antioxidants such as BHA, BHT, and vitamin E function to maintain the freshness of foods by preventing fats from turning rancid and preventing discoloration.

Color additives: A color additive is any dye, pigment, or substance that, when added or applied to a food, drug, or cosmetic, or to the human body, is capable (alone or through reactions with other substances) of imparting color. FDA is responsible for regulating all color additives to ensure that foods containing color additives are safe to eat, contain only approved ingredients, and are accurately labeled. Color additives are used in foods for many reasons:
1. To offset color loss due to exposure to light, air, temperature extremes, moisture, and storage conditions.
2. To correct natural variations in color.
3. To enhance colors that occur naturally.
4. To provide color to colorless and "fun" foods.

FDA's permitted colors are classified as subject to certification or exempt from certification, both of which are subject to rigorous safety standards prior to their approval and listing for use in foods. Certified colors are synthetically produced (or human made) and used widely because they impart an intense, uniform color, are less expensive, and blend more easily to create a variety of hues. There are nine certified color additives approved for use in the United States. Certified food colors generally do not add undesirable flavors to foods.

*Approved color additives:*FD&C Blue Nos. 1 and 2, FD&C Green No. 3, FD&C Red Nos. 3 and 40, FD&C Yellow Nos. 5 and 6, Orange B, Citrus Red No. 2, annatto extract, beta-carotene, grape skin extract, cochineal extract or carmine, paprika oleoresin, caramel color, fruit and vegetable juices, saffron. (Note: Exempt color additives are not required to be declared by name on labels but may be declared simply as colorings or color added.)

Common sweeteners: Sucrose (sugar), glucose, fructose, sorbitol, mannitol, corn syrup, high fructose corn syrup, saccharin, aspartame, sucralose, acesulfame potassium (acesulfame-K), neotame.

Emulsifiers: Emulsifiers allow smooth mixing of ingredients and prevent separation. They keep emulsified products stable, reduce stickiness, control crystallization, keep ingredients dispersed, and help products dissolve more easily. Emulsifiers are commonly used in salad dressings, peanut butter, chocolate, margarine, and frozen desserts. Emulsifiers include: soy lecithin, mono- and diglycerides, egg yolks, polysorbates, sorbitan monostearate.

Fat replacers: Olestra, cellulose gel, carrageenan, polydextrose, modified food starch, microparticulated egg white protein, guar gum, xanthan gum, whey protein concentrate.

pH Control Agents and Acidulants:
- Control acidity and alkalinity, prevent spoilage.
- Beverages, frozen desserts, chocolate, low-acid canned foods, baking powder.
- Lactic acid, citric acid, ammonium hydroxide.

Firming agent: Firming agents are used to maintain crispness and firmness in processed fruits and vegetables. Common agents are calcium chloride and calcium lactate.

Humectants: Humectants are used to retain moisture in items such as shredded coconut, marshmallows, soft candies, and confections. Common humectants are glycerin and sorbitol.

Anti-Caking Agents: Anti-caking agents keep powdered foods free-flowing and prevent moisture absorption. These agents are used in items like salt, baking powder, and confectioner's sugar. Common anti-caking agents include calcium silicate, iron ammonium citrate, and silicon dioxide.

pH Control Agents and Acidulants: These agents control acidity and alkalinity, as well as prevent spoilage. Beverages, frozen desserts, chocolate, low-acid canned foods, and baking powder commonly contain such agents. The items commonly used are lactic acid, citric acid, and ammonium hydroxide.

Common preservatives

Ascorbic acid, citric acid, sodium benzoate, calcium propionate, sodium erythorbate, sodium nitrite, calcium sorbate, potassium sorbate, BHA, BHT, EDTA, tocopherols (vitamin E).

Common sweetners

Sucrose (sugar), glucose, fructose, sorbitol, mannitol, corn syrup, high fructose corn syrup, saccharin, aspartame, sucralose, acesulfame potassium (acesulfame-K), neotame.

Humectants

Retain moisture
Shredded coconut, marshmallows, soft candies, confections
Glycerin, sorbitol

Stabilizers, Thickners, Binders, and Texturizers

Stabilizers and Thickeners, Binders, Texturizers
Produce uniform texture, improve "mouth-feel"
Frozen desserts, dairy products, cakes, pudding and gelatin mixes, dressings, jams and jellies, sauces
Gelatin, pectin, guar gum, carrageenan, xanthan gum, whey

Engineered foods

Engineered foods are products that are manufactured from ingredients in such a way as to resemble another product in taste, texture, and appearance. Engineered foods are desirable to populations who cannot or will not consume a particular product, for example, the meat analogs designed to replace animal protein for vegetarians. Engineered foods can also be designed to have a higher nutritive quality than the product they replaced. Meat analogs are usually lower in fat, are cholesterol free, and can be fortified with B vitamins to make them similar to meat as a nutrient source. Engineered foods can be convenient and economical, as in the case of seafood analogs. Instead of crabmeat, which may be unavailable in certain regions or seasons, seafood analogs composed of fish, soy protein, and natural flavorings can be substituted. The analog product is typically less expensive as well.

Daily Reference Values (DRVs)

(Based on 2,000 calories a day for adults and children older than 4 years only)
Food Component/DRV
Fat/65 grams (g)
Saturated fatty acids/20 g
Cholesterol/300 milligrams (mg)
Total carbohydrate/300 g
Fiber/25 g
Sodium/2,400 mg
Potassium/3,500 mg
Protein**/50 g
**DRV for protein does not apply to certain populations; Reference Daily Intake (RDI) for protein has been established for these groups: children 1 to 4 years: 16 g; infants younger than 1 year: 14 g; pregnant women: 60 g; breastfeeding mothers: 65 g.

High-Potassium Foods

Apricots, avocados, bananas, beets
Brussel sprouts, cantaloupe, clams, dates
Figs, kiwi fruit, lima beans, melons
Milk, nectarines, orange juice, oranges
Peanuts, pears (fresh), potatoes, prune juice
Prunes, raisins, sardines, spinach
Tomatoes, winter squash, yogurt

Functions of acids in food

The pH scales ranges from 1, which is the strongest acid, to 14, which indicates a strong base or alkalinity. The acidity of produce determines what canning method should be used in order to destroy the bacteria responsible for some foodborne illnesses. Fruits, tomatoes, and vegetables processed in vinegar are generally acidic enough to be processed without the aid of pressure. Although molds and yeasts can flourish in acidic conditions, bacteria growth is not fostered. Most other vegetables hover in the neutral zone on the pH scale, and must be processed under pressure to kill bacteria.

Acid is responsible for some of the color changes observed in vegetables in the cooking process. When hydrogen ions are liberated from acid during cooking, chlorophyll is transformed into pheophytin, which is drab olive in color. This can be prevented by reducing cook times.

Cream of tartar is an acid that contributes to a desirable baked product by stabilizing the foam in meringues and angel food cake.

Enzymes

Enzymes naturally present in fruits and vegetables are proteins that facilitate biochemical reactions. Enzyme activity can continue to occur even after the cellular tissue is dead, producing changes in foods that are not harmful, but are nonetheless undesirable. Because enzymes are proteins, they can be denatured by the application of heat and acid. Enzymes are responsible for the oxidative browning commonly seen in cut fruits such as apples and bananas. The application of acid, in the form of lemon juice or ascorbic acid preservative powders, will halt enzyme action and delay this browning. Enzymatic browning may be desirable in the drying of fruit, as it lends characteristic color and flavor.

When preparing fruits and vegetables for preservation by freezing, it is common to scald or blanch the produce briefly in boiling water or steam to stop the action of enzymes.

Hydrogenation of fats

Hydrogenation contributes to the stability and shelf life of products such as pastries, chips, crackers, frosting, and candies. It prevents the fat in the product from weeping oils, so that the frosting on the cookie remains palatable, and it keeps fats solid, which would otherwise liquefy at room temperatures, such as margarine.

The process of hydrogenation involves converting unsaturated fatty acids to saturated fatty acids by adding hydrogen to the carbons in the fatty acid chain by using high temperatures, a metal catalyst, or hydrogen gas applied under pressure. The result is a structure different from the naturally occurring kinked shape that results from hydrogens on the same side at the double bond. Synthetically hydrogenated fats are called trans fatty acids because the hydrogen molecules are attached to the fatty acid chain in alternating 180 degree fashion, straightening the natural curve of the chain.

- 13 -

Foodborne infections

<u>Salmonella</u>
A variety of Salmonella bacteria cause thousands of cases of food poisoning in the United States each year. Illness comes from consuming the live bacteria, which are toxic. The bacteria thrive in animal and human feces and enter the food chain through dirty cutting boards, infected water, contaminated meat, broken or cracked eggs, or actual bits of feces in foodstuffs. The symptoms are similar to those of *S. aureus*, but take longer to develop, up to 72 hours. Symptoms are flu-like and include nausea and vomiting, headache, diarrhea, and abdominal cramps. Salmonella infection can be avoided by refrigerating eggs, meat, and poultry products at the proper temperatures. Care should be taken to sanitize food preparation surfaces after contact with raw meats or eggs to avoid cross-contamination. Consuming undercooked eggs, meat, and poultry puts one at risk for Salmonella, but thorough cooking kills the bacteria.

<u>Streptococcus</u>
Some strains of *Streptococcus* bacteria are associated with foodborne illness, and symptoms include abdominal cramps, diarrhea, and sometimes vomiting. The bacteria thrive at temperatures between 50° and 120°F, and are destroyed by cooking temperatures.

<u>Listeria monocytogenes</u>
The source of infection with *L. monocytogenes* can be difficult to pinpoint, as the onset of symptoms may not occur until several days or even a few weeks after ingesting the contaminated food.

Symptoms may include fever, headache, or vomiting, but susceptible individuals such as pregnant women, infants, and those with suppressed immune function may suffer more severe symptoms or even death. The bacteria are much more resilient than other foodborne pathogens and can resist heat, temperatures below 40°F, and acidity.

Common sources include unpasteurized dairy products, such as semi-soft cheeses. Deli meats and hot dogs have also been implicated, and pregnant women are advised to heat these products to 160°F and steaming before consumption. Individuals at high risk should avoid consuming semi-soft cheeses (for example, brie) and other unpasteurized dairy products or products made with raw milk.

<u>Campylobacter jejuni</u>
Campylobacter microbes grow slowly and are found in meats, poultry, and dairy products. Symptoms do not present until 3 to 5 days after ingestion of the contaminated food, and include abdominal pain, diarrhea, fever, and headache. The microbe is very sensitive to heat, so proper cooking methods prevent illness.

<u>Shigella</u>
Shigella bacteria are present in feces and may be transmitted to food when proper handwashing techniques are not observed. The foods most commonly contaminated include cold salads prepared with meat or mayonnaise and raw vegetables. The symptoms appear within 12 to 48 hours after ingesting contaminated food and include bloody diarrhea, fever, and abdominal cramps.

<u>Staphylococcus aureus</u>
S. aureus is a commonly occurring bacterium that lives in nasal passages and in cuts on the skin. Infection with the toxin can be avoided when proper food-handling practices are observed. Foods should be refrigerated promptly and at the proper temperature. Observe good hand-washing

practices, and keep cuts and abrasions bandaged. *S. aureus* produces toxins when contaminated foods are left at room temperature for prolonged periods. Common culprits include protein-rich foods such as meats, poultry, eggs, mayonnaise-based salads, and cream-filled pastry products. Symptoms mimic the flu, but are rarely fatal, and can include diarrhea, vomiting, and abdominal cramps. The illness comes on quickly, within a few hours after eating, and can last 24 to 48 hours.

Clostridium botulinum

C. botulinum is a rare but deadly microbe commonly occurring in the soil and probably in most foodstuffs. However, the bacteria thrive in an anaerobic environment, and botulism cases in the United States are rare.

Common sources of botulism poisoning include canned products, especially home-canned products with low acidity, such as meat, corn, beans, and asparagus. Commercially canned products can harbor the toxin as well, and cans should be inspected for bulging, rust, or milky fluid. Any canned foods bearing signs of spoilage should be discarded, as one bite-sized portion can harbor enough toxins to be fatal.

Symptoms include vomiting, dizziness, and respiratory failure. Treatment is possible with a quick diagnosis, but recovery may take weeks. Botulism poisoning can also occur in infants younger than 1 year of age who ingest honey, as their stomach acidity is not strong enough to kill the spores sometimes found in honey. Following proper home-canning procedures advocated by the USDA can reduce the risk of this rare foodborne illness.

Clostridium perfringens

C. perfringens is an anaerobic bacterium common throughout the environment. Symptoms are seen within 8 to 24 hours of consuming contaminated food, and include diarrhea, nausea, and cramping, but usually not vomiting. The bacteria are resistant to heat and thrive in the deep-dish style pans used in cafeterias because of the anaerobic environment of these dishes. Dividing leftover portions into smaller dishes prevents infection by exposing the food to oxygen and promoting rapid chilling.

Bacillus cereus

Bacillus cereus is a bacterium commonly found in the soil that produces a diarrhea-causing form of illness and an illness associated with nausea and vomiting. Cereals and products prepared with starch or noodles are associated with the emetic form of illness. Protein foods and vegetables are associated with the diarrhea-causing form of illness. Observing proper cooking and refrigeration temperatures prevents *B. cereus* from thriving.

Norwalk virus

The Norwalk virus is found in contaminated water, and affects shellfish and salads most frequently. Symptoms include nausea, vomiting, diarrhea, headache, and fever 1 to 2 days after exposure. Proper handwashing prevents spread of the virus.

Vibrio vulnificus

Vibrio vulnificus is a bacterium found in seafood and shellfish. Consuming raw or undercooked seafood and shellfish puts individuals at high risk for contracting this illness. Onset of symptoms varies from several hours to several days after consumption of contaminated food. Symptoms include diarrhea, sometimes bloody; vomiting; abdominal cramps; and sometimes skin lesions.

Nutrition and Supporting Sciences

Anabolism and catabolism

Anabolism is also referred to as "building up." This phase of metabolism involves reactions in which small molecules are put together to build larger ones. Example: Glucose molecules join together to make glycogen chains. Amino acids can be linked together to make proteins. All of these reactions require work and energy.

Catabolism is the breakdown of body compounds. Catabolic reactions take large molecules and break them down into smaller molecules. Catabolic reactions use and release energy. Example: The breakdown of glycogen to glucose, triglycerides to fatty acids and glycerol, or protein to amino acids.

Energy expenditure

The 3 components of energy expenditure include basal metabolism, physical activity, and the thermic effect of food (TEF).

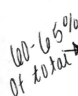

Basal Metabolism

Basal Metabolism is the largest component (60% to 65%). It is the energy needed to maintain life when the body is at rest in a fasting state. This is also called basal energy expenditure (BEE) or resting energy expenditure (REE). BEE or REE is measured as basal metabolic rate (BMR). BMR is measured in the morning or after a 12-hour fast. BMR can be affected by a person's sex (women have a lower BMR than men), age (the highest BMR is for ages 0 to 2 years; BMR decreases with age), and body composition. BMR is higher in periods of growth, during pregnancy, and in some diseases such as cancer and hypertension.

Basal metabolism represents the minimum energy expenditure it takes to keep a body at rest alive, so that heartbeat, breathing, temperature maintenance, and other essential functions are maintained. About 40% of the roughly 1,400 calories a day needed for survival are used by the brain and liver, 20% by lean muscle mass, and the rest by fat tissue. Lean muscle mass is one of the primary factors in determining one's basal metabolic rate (BMR), so males usually have a higher BMR because of their muscle mass. Aging is associated with a decline in BMR, especially if muscle mass decreases. Physical activity can counteract this through maintaining lean body mass. Febrile patients, trauma patients, and pregnant women have an increased basal metabolism. A low caloric intake can decrease the BMR by as much as 10% to 20% a day, which presents a challenge to individuals following weight-loss plans.

Physical activity

Physical activity is the most variable component of energy expenditure. It depends on muscle mass, body weight, and activity.

Thermic effect of food

TEF is proportional to the food energy taken in and is usually 10% of energy intake. It estimates how much energy is required to digest, absorb, transport, metabolize, and store ingested nutrients.

Calorimetry

Direct calorimetry and indirect calorimetry are the 2 ways to measure human energy expenditure.

- Direct calorimetry: Direct calorimetry monitors the amount of heat produced by an organism inside a respiration chamber. This method is limited by its high costs and complex engineering.
- Indirect calorimetry: Indirect calorimetry estimates energy expenditure by measuring the oxygen consumed and carbon dioxide produced using a portable machine. The Respiratory Quotient (RQ) is defined as the following formula:
RQ = Moles Carbon dioxide expired / moles Oxygen consumed
The RQ depends on the fuel mixture that is being metabolized. If you are metabolizing carbohydrates, the RQ will be 1.
RQ = Protein alone: 0.82
     Fat alone: 0.7
     Mixed intake: 0.85
To lower the RQ, you have to increase the fat intake. The RQ will help determine which nutrients are being burned for energy.

Carbohydrates

Carbohydrates (CHO) are compounds composed of carbon, hydrogen, and oxygen.

Simple carbohydrates
Simple carbohydrates include monosaccharides and disaccharides.
- Monosaccharides are glucose, fructose, and galactose.
- Disaccharides are sucrose, maltose, and lactose.
* Fructose is the sweetest CHO, while lactose is the least sweet.

[handwritten: glu + glu = sucrose / glu + fruct = maltose / glu + gala = lactose]

Complex carbohydrates
Complex carbohydrates are called polysaccharides and include starch, cellulose, pectin (found in fruits), glycogen (major storage form of glucose), and dextrin (intermediate products of starch breakdown).

Sources
Sources of carbohydrate are flour, fruits, starchy vegetables, cereals, and milk products. The main function of carbohydrates is to provide energy, but they also spare protein by allowing the protein to be used for tissue synthesis. Carbohydrates also help regulate fat metabolism. Diet requirement: 50% to 60% of total calories.

Dietary carbohydrate
- Dietary carbohydrate = 4 kcal/g; IV dextrose = 3.4 kcal/g.
- 45% to 65% of total caloric intake. Minimal requirement = 1 mg/kg/min (may be met by dextrose 5% IVF).
- CHO intake should not exceed 5 to 7 mg/kg/min (or 7 to 8 g/kg/d). Limit to 4 mg/kg/min in ICU.
- Complications from excessive CHO intake: hyperglycemia, hypercapnia, and hypertriglyceridemia.

Protein

Protein is made up of carbon, hydrogen, oxygen, and nitrogen arranged into amino acids. Some amino acids contain sulfur (cysteine, cystine, and methionine). Amino Acids consist of an amine group (base) and a carboxyl group (acid). Proteins are essential, complete, or incomplete. The 9 essential (the body does not make these) amino acids are isoleucine, leusine, lysine, methionine, phenylaline, threonine, valine, tryptophan, and histidine. Complete proteins are proteins that have all 9 essential amino acids. High Biological Value proteins are complete proteins. Incomplete proteins are lacking 1 or more essential amino acids.

Sources
Meat, poultry, fish, milk, eggs, and legumes.

Functions
Maintains growth, synthesis of tissues, regulation of body processes, and some energy (nitrogen must be taken away).

Diet requirement:
10% to 15% of total calories.

Protein quality
Biologic value: The biological value (BV) of a protein is a measure of how easily food protein can be turned into body tissues. If all of the essential amino acids are present, the food is said to have a high biological value. If the amino acid pattern in the food closely matches the amino acid in the body, then the food protein can more easily be turned into body tissues. Proteins from eggs, meat, and dairy products have a high BV.

Net protein utilization: Protein quality can also be discussed in terms of how digestible it is. This value is called net protein utilization (NPU). Most proteins are entirely digested and absorbed, so the NPU will closely resemble the BV.

Protein Digestibility Corrected Amino Acid Score: The Protein Digestibility Corrected Amino Acid Score (PDCAAS) has been adopted by the World Health Organization as the preferred method for determining protein value. This method compares the amino acids in the food being tested against a standard amino acid profile. The most highly ranked proteins yield all of the essential amino acids after digestion.

Protein metabolism
Proteins fulfill a major structural role in the body in the building and maintenance of tissues. They also play a role in the formation of hormones, enzymes, and antibodies. Proteins consist of an amino group and a carboxyl group joined to a carbon atom. The basic protein structure has a free carboxyl group at one end and a free amino group at the other. More amino acids can join at either end to form different proteins. When proteins are used for energy, the liver detaches the amino groups and the carbon skeletons converted into glucose, ketone bodies, or other substances that can enter the citric acid cycle and produce ATP. Before protein can be used as a structural component in the body, all of the essential amino acids must be available. The body can then form the specific proteins it needs under the control of DNA, with energy from ATP driving the process.

Fat

Fat (lipid) is composed of carbon, hydrogen, and oxygen. Triglyceride is the major form of fat when it comes from food and the major storage form of fat in the body. Every triglyceride is made up of 1 glycerol and 3 fatty acids. Fatty acids are hydrocarbon carbon chains with a carboxyl group on one end and a methyl group at the other end. Fatty acids may also be saturated or unsaturated.

- Saturated fatty acids have no double bonds and all carbons are filled with hydrogen.
- Unsaturated fatty acids have 1 or more double bonds.

Sources
Butter, oils, nuts, bacon.

Functions
Insulation and padding of vital organs, energy.

Diet requirement
Less than 30% of total calories.

Dietary fat
Dietary fat = 9 kcal/g
Dietary fat, or fat from food, is important for health and normal growth and development of the body. Dietary fat has many different functions in the body, including the following:

- Providing long-lasting energy.
- Creating a feeling of fullness after eating.
- Helping make hormones.
- Forming part of the brain and nervous system.
- Forming cell membranes for every cell in the body.
- Carrying vitamins throughout the body.
- Helping regulate body temperature and maintaining warmth.
- Providing 2 essential fatty acids, called linoleic acid and linolenic acid, which the body cannot make by itself.

Fat metabolism
For normal fat metabolism, the body needs enough carbohydrates to complete oxidation of fat. Fatty acids need carbohydrates to get to acetyl-CoA, and then carbohydrates are needed to get from acetyl-CoA to the Krebs cycle. Carbohydrates are needed again to produce adenosine triphosphate (ATP), CO_2, and water. If the body does not have adequate carbohydrates, fat oxidation cannot be completed, and it causes an increase in ketone bodies (example: uncontrolled diabetes). Fewer than 800 calories of CHO/day are not enough to metabolize fat.

Fiber ↳ 130 g/day

Fat → acetyl-CoA → Krebs → ATP + H_2O + CO_2
        *require CHO

Insoluble Fiber
Insoluble dietary fiber is a natural laxative and includes cellulose and lignin, which occur in whole grains (especially wheat bran), and hemicellulose (partly soluble) found in whole grains, nuts, seeds, fruits, and vegetables.

Soluble Fiber

Water soluble dietary fiber binds with and removes certain things in the gut. Types of soluble fiber include pectin, which occurs in fruits (apples, strawberries, citrus fruits); beta-glucans, found in oats, barley and rye; gums, found in beans, cereals (barley, oats, rice), seeds, and seaweed; and arabinose, found in legumes/pulses. Soluble fiber can be further classified into fermentable and nonfermentable types. Fermentable soluble fiber helps to feed our intestinal bacteria, the "healthy" bacteria that help us digest and absorb nutrition from food.

Many fiber-rich foods, especially plant-foods, contain both soluble and insoluble fiber in varying proportions. But one type of fiber usually dominates.

Vitamins

Fat-Soluble Vitamins

Fat-soluble vitamins are absorbed, together with fat from the intestine, into the circulation. Any disease or disorder that affects the absorption of fat, such as celiac disease, could lead to a deficiency of these vitamins. Once absorbed into the circulation, these vitamins are carried to the liver where they are stored. Vitamins A, D, E, and K make up the fat-soluble vitamins. Vitamins A, D, and K are stored in the liver and vitamin E is distributed throughout the body's fatty tissues.

The importance of vitamin A in the visual cycle is well-documented. One form of vitamin A combines with a protein in the eye to form rhodopsin, which is essential to night vision. The eyes also need vitamin A to maintain mucus-forming cells that lubricate the surface. Vitamin A also helps in immune function, reproductive health, and cell development.

Vitamin D, which is also considered a hormone, is essential to the regulation of calcium and bone development. Vitamin D helps the absorption of calcium in the intestine, causes the kidneys to reabsorb calcium, and controls the deposition of calcium in bones.

Vitamin E, which includes a family of compounds called the tocopherols and tocotrienols, acts as one of the body's antioxidants. Vitamin E buffers the assault of free radicals on the body by acting as an electron donor, causing a more stable compound to form.

Vitamin K is essential for the normal function of the body's blood-clotting mechanism. Vitamin K is necessary for the synthesis of several of the body's blood-clotting factors, including prothrombin.

Water-Soluble Vitamins

Water-soluble vitamins, such as vitamin C and the B vitamins, are stored in the body for only a brief period of time and are then excreted by the kidneys. The one exception to this is vitamin B_{12}, which is stored in the liver. Vitamin C (ascorbic acid) and the B complex group make up the 9 water-soluble vitamins. The B-complex group comprises the following vitamins: B_6 (pyridoxine), B_1 (thiamine), B_2 (riboflavin), B_{12} (niacin, pantothenic acid, biotin, folic acid, and cobalamin).

Vitamin A

Vitamin A is fat-soluble. Vitamin A contains a class of plant pigments called carotenoids, including a provitamin called carotene (precursor).
- Sources: Dark green leafy vegetables, cantaloupe, fish, liver, carrots, fortified milk, apricots, sweet potatoes.
- Function: Vitamin A plays an essential role in vision, growth, and the development and maintenance of epithelial tissue (skin), immune function, and reproduction.

- Deficiency: The most common deficiency is nyctalopia (night blindness). This is completely reversible in early stages of the deficiency.

Vitamin E

- Vitamin E is fat-soluble. Tocopherol is a form of the fat-soluble antioxidant vitamin E.
- Sources: Vegetable oils, whole grains, green vegetables.
- Function: it is the most important lipid-soluble antioxidant in the cell.
- Deficiency: Hemolytic anemia.

Vitamin D

Vitamin D is fat-soluble. Cholesterol is the precursor to vitamin D. 7-dehydrocholesterol is converted to vitamin D_3 cholecalciferol.

- Sources: Sunlight, egg yolk, and fortified milk,
- Function: Vitamin D has essential metabolic roles in the maintenance of calcium and phosphorus; it is also essential to bone development. Vitamin D helps the absorption of calcium in the intestine, causes the kidneys to reabsorb calcium, and controls the deposition of calcium in bones.
- Deficiency: Leads to rickets (soft bones) and osteomalacia (adult rickets).

Vitamin K

Vitamin K is fat-soluble. This vitamin is synthesized by bacteria in the lower intestinal tract. It can be affected by mineral oil, antibiotics, and anticoagulates.

- Sources: The best sources are kale and spinach. Other sources include broccoli and some vegetable oils.
- Function: Essential for the functioning of several proteins involved in blood clotting; it forms prothrombin in the liver, and it is also given to patients before surgery.
- Deficiency: Slow clotting of blood followed by a hemorrhage.

Vitamin B_1

Vitamin B_1 (thiamine) is water-soluble.

- Sources: Grains, pork, liver, egg yolk, wheat germ, nuts, and red meat.
- Function: It plays essential metabolic roles in carbohydrate metabolism and neural function. A diet with increased carbohydrates requires more thiamin.
- Deficiency: Leads to muscle weakness, fatigue, irritability, and loss of memory. It can lead to an increase in plasma pyruvate.
- Severe deficiency can lead to beriberi (Wernicke-Korsakoff syndrome). Also associated with alcoholism.

Vitamin B_2

Vitamin B_2 (riboflavin) is water-soluble, and it is lost in UV light.

- Sources: animal protein (liver, kidney, milk, and meat).
- Function: Intracellular metabolism.
- Deficiency: Leads to painful tongue and fissures in the corners of the mouth, chapped lips.

Niacin

Niacin is a water-soluble vitamin necessary for many aspects of health, growth, and reproduction. It is part of the vitamin B complex. The precursor for niacin is tryptophan. Large doses of niacin can cause liver damage, peptic ulcers, and skin rashes.

- Sources: Dairy products, poultry, fish, lean meats, nuts, and eggs. Legumes and enriched breads and cereals also supply some niacin.
- Functions: Metabolism of carbohydrate, protein, and fat.
- Deficiency: Leads to pellagra. Symptoms include inflamed skin, digestive problems, and mental impairment.

Vitamin B_6

Vitamin B_6 (pyridoxine) is water-soluble. Vitamins B_{12}, B_6, and B_9 (folic acid) work closely together to control blood levels of the amino acid homocysteine. Elevated levels of this substance appear to be linked to heart disease. Plus, vitamin B_6 is essential for normal brain development and function, participating in the process of making important brain chemicals called neurotransmitters. Pyridoxine is an especially important vitamin for maintaining healthy nerve and muscle cells, and it aids in the production of DNA and RNA, the body's genetic material. It is necessary for proper absorption of vitamin B_{12} and for the production of red blood cells and cells of the immune system. An increase in protein causes an increase in pyridoxine.

- Sources: Meat, wheat, corn, yeast, pork, and liver.
- Deficiency: Leads to muscle weakness, nervousness, irritability, depression, difficulty concentrating, and short-term memory loss.

Folate

Folate (folic acid) is water-soluble. It works along with vitamin B_{12} and vitamin C to help the body digest and utilize proteins and to synthesize new proteins when they are needed. It is necessary for the production of red blood cells and for the synthesis of DNA (which controls heredity and is used to guide the cell in its daily activities). Folic acid also helps with tissue growth and cell function. In addition, it helps to increase appetite when needed and stimulates the formation of digestive acids. PABA is the precursor.

- Sources: Beans and legumes, citrus fruits and juices, wheat bran and other whole grains, dark green leafy vegetables, poultry, pork, shellfish, liver.
- Deficiency: Leads to megaloblastic anemia and neural tube defects.

Vitamin B_{12}

Vitamin B_{12} is water-soluble. This vitamin is stored in the liver. It is bound by the intrinsic factor in gastric juice. Cyanocobalamin is the commercially available form of vitamin B_{12}.

- Sources: animal proteins (liver, red meat, dairy products).
- Functions: Essential for manufacturing of genetic material in cells. Involved in the production of erythrocytes.
- Deficiency: Leads to pernicious anemia after the removal of the ileum or a gastrectomy (due to the lack of intrinsic factor). Deficiency is usually disease-related. A dietary deficiency is rare. Schilling test can identify deficiency.

Pantothenic Acid

Pantothenic acid (vitamin B_5) is water-soluble. A B-complex vitamin that plays an essential role in the synthesis and oxidation of fatty acids. It is synthesized by intestinal bacteria. It is unstable to heat, acid, and certain salts (most easily destroyed).

- Sources: Present in all plant and animal foods. Eggs, kidney, liver, salmon, and yeast are the best sources.
- Function: As a part of coenzyme A, it functions in the synthesis and breakdown of many vital body functions. Essential in the intermediary metabolism of carbohydrate, fat, and protein.
- Deficiency: decreased appetite.

Biotin

Biotin is synthesized by intestinal bacteria. It is an essential component in enzymes and functions in the synthesis and breakdown of fatty acids and amino acids. Biotin is inactivated by avidin (protein in raw egg whites). Sources: egg yolk, liver, mushrooms, yeast, milk, and meat.

Ascorbic Acid

Vitamin C is water-soluble. It is biosynthesized from glucose. This vitamin is easily destroyed by heat, alkali, and oxidation.

- Sources: citrus fruits, tomato, melon, peppers, dark green and yellow vegetables.
- Functions: Major function is collagen production; maintains intracellular substance. Important in immune responses, wound healing, and allergic reactions. It also increases absorption of iron.
- Deficiency: scurvy.

Myo-inositol

Myo-inositol is a vitamin-like factor that plays important metabolic roles as a constituent of phospholipids and a mediator of cellular responses to external stimuli. It binds calcium, zinc, and iron. It is related to sugar because it looks like glucose. It is found in plants as phytic acid. Sources: Outer husks of cereal grains, leafy green vegetables.

Minerals

Calcium

Calcium is the most abundant mineral in the body. Bones and teeth store 99% of calcium in the body. Ionic calcium in body fluids is essential for ion transport across cell membranes. Calcium may also be bound to protein, citrate, or inorganic acids. It is regulated by the parathyroid hormones. Vitamin D aids absorption while oxalates and phytates interfere with absorption. Calcium is vital to muscle contraction, allowing protein in the muscles to interact during contraction. Abnormal calcium metabolism can prevent the muscles from relaxing, a condition called tetany. Calcium functions in the transmission of nerve signals by permitting the flow of ions in and out of cells, and also by helping to release neurotransmitters. Finally, calcium plays a role in metabolism by regulating various enzymes, including those that manufacture glycogen.

- Sources: dairy products, leafy vegetables, legumes.
- Functions: blood clotting and cardiac function.
- Deficiency: Leads to rickets with hypocalcemic tetany (irregular muscle contractions). Long-term deficiency is one of the factors responsible for the development of osteoporosis later in life.

All cells need calcium to function, and over 99% of calcium in the body works to form and maintain bones and teeth. The role that calcium plays in cellular function is so important that insufficient intake of the mineral will result in decreased bone mass, or osteopenia. Calcium allows for normal blood clotting, acting as a catalyst to the clotting factor prothrombin. Calcium is vital to muscle contraction, allowing protein in the muscles to interact during contraction. Abnormal calcium metabolism can prevent the muscles from relaxing, a condition called tetany. Calcium functions in the transmission of nerve signals by permitting the flow of ions in and out of cells, and also by helping to release neurotransmitters. Finally, calcium plays a role in metabolism by regulating various enzymes, including those that manufacture glycogen.

Phosphorus
Phosphorus is part of DNA; it is a component of every cell.
- Sources: cheese, milk, egg yolk, meat, fish, poultry, whole-grain cereals, legumes, and nuts.
- Function: Transports fat, through the lymph. It is also important to pH regulation.
- Deficiency: Phosphorus deficiency is not likely if protein and calcium are adequate.

Magnesium
70% of magnesium is located in the bones. The rest is located in the cells. It is a part of chlorophyll.
- Sources: Found in most foods. A diet with high protein, calcium, and vitamin D requires an increase in magnesium.
- Function: Involved in protein synthesis.
- Deficiency: Dietary deficiency is unlikely, but it is sometimes associated with surgery, alcoholism, loss of body fluids, or renal disease.

Iron
About 70% of iron is in hemoglobin and about 25% is stored in the liver, spleen, and bone.
- Forms of iron in the body include:
  - Ferritin is the stored form of iron and the best lab value when assessing iron status.
  - Ferric is the food form of iron.
  - Ferrous is the best-absorbed form of iron.
  - Transferrin is the form of iron that is transported in the body.
- Sources: liver, meat, egg yolk, fish, whole and enriched grains, dark green vegetables.
- Function: Iron is important in oxygen transfer.
- Deficiency: Leads to anemia. Spoon-shaped nails are a sign of deficiency. Meat, fish, poultry, vitamin C, and calcium aid iron absorption. Eggs, cow's milk, and cheese do NOT help with absorption.

Zinc
Zinc is present in almost all tissues. Most zinc is found in the liver, voluntary muscle, and bone.
- Sources: animal proteins (liver, meat, eggs, shellfish, milk).
- Functions: Insulin can enhance insulin action and it increases taste acuity.
- Deficiency: There is no evidence of deficiency.

Sodium
Sodium is the major cation of extracellular fluid. Only a small amount is actually found inside cells. Sodium restriction may be necessary for individuals with cardiovascular or renal disorders.
- Function: It regulates body fluid osmolarity, acid/base balance, and body fluid volume.
- Dietary inadequacy is unlikely because almost all food contains sodium.

Glutamine

Glutamine is the most abundant amino acid (building block of protein) in the bloodstream. It is considered a "conditionally essential amino acid" because it can be manufactured in the body, but under extreme physical stress the demand for glutamine exceeds the body's ability to synthesize it. Most glutamine in the body is stored in muscles followed by the lungs, where much of the glutamine is manufactured.

Glutamine is important for removing excess ammonia (a common waste product in the body). In the process of picking up ammonia, glutamine donates it when needed to make other amino acids, as well as sugar, and the antioxidant glutathione. Several types of important immune cells rely on glutamine for energy; without it, the immune system would be impaired. Glutamine also appears to be necessary for normal brain function and digestion. Adequate amounts of glutamine are generally obtained through diet alone because the body is also able to make glutamine on its own. Certain medical conditions, including injuries, surgery, infections, and prolonged stress, can deplete glutamine levels, however. When the body is stressed (such as from injuries, infections, burns, trauma, or surgical procedures), steroid hormones such as cortisol are released into the bloodstream. Elevated cortisol levels can deplete glutamine stores in the body.

Aldosterone

The mineralocorticoids get their name from their effect on mineral metabolism. The most important of them is the steroid aldosterone. Aldosterone acts on the kidney promoting the reabsorption of sodium ions ($Na+$) into the blood. Water follows the salt and this helps maintain normal blood pressure. Aldosterone also acts on sweat glands to reduce the loss of sodium in perspiration; acts on taste cells to increase the sensitivity of the taste buds to sources of sodium. The secretion of aldosterone is stimulated by:
- A drop in the level of sodium ions in the blood.
- A rise in the level of potassium ions in the blood.

AII

AII has several very important functions:
- Constricts resistance vessels (via AII receptors), thereby increasing systemic vascular resistance and arterial pressure.
- Acts upon the adrenal cortex to release aldosterone, which in turn acts upon the kidneys to increase sodium and fluid retention.
- Stimulates the release of vasopressin (antidiuretic hormone [ADH]) from the posterior pituitary, which acts upon the kidneys to increase fluid retention.
- Stimulates thirst centers within the brain.
- Facilitates norepinephrine release from sympathetic nerve endings and inhibits norepinephrine reuptake by nerve endings, thereby enhancing sympathetic adrenergic function.
- Stimulates cardiac hypertrophy and vascular hypertrophy.

Renin-angiotensin system

The renin-angiotensin system plays an important role in regulating blood volume, arterial pressure, and cardiac and vascular function. While the pathways for the renin-angiotensin system have been found in a number of tissues, the most important site for renin release is the kidney. Sympathetic stimulation (acting via beta-1-adrenoceptors), renal artery hypotension, and decreased sodium delivery to the distal tubules stimulate the release of renin by the kidney.

Renin is an enzyme that acts upon a circulating substrate, angiotensinogen, that undergoes proteolytic cleavage to from the decapeptide angiotensin I. Vascular endothelium, particularly in the lungs, has an enzyme, angiotensin-converting enzyme (ACE), that cleaves off 2 amino acids to form the octapeptide, angiotensin II (AII).

Parathyroid hormone

The parathyroid glands are small bodies near the thyroid gland. They secrete PTH. The secretion of this hormone is regulated by the serum calcium level: if the serum calcium level falls, the parathyroid secretes the hormone; if the serum calcium level is high, PTH production is inhibited.

PTH serves 2 functions:
- PTH promotes the normal bone resorption process and is adversely affected by calcitonin.
- PTH also stimulates the excretion of phosphates by the kidneys; this inhibition of phosphate resorption in turn enables calcium resorption.

PTH also decreases kidney reabsorption of phosphate and stimulates (osteoblasts and osteoclasts).

Serum Creatinine, Glomerular Filtration Rate (GFR), andBlood Urea Nitrogen (BUN)

Serum Creatinine: Creatinine is a waste product in the blood that comes from muscle activity. It is normally removed from the blood by the kidneys, but when kidney function slows down, the creatinine level rises.

Glomerular Filtration Rate (GFR): GFR tells how much kidney function a patient has. It may be estimated from the blood level of creatinine. If the GFR falls below 30, the patient will need to see a kidney disease specialist; GFR below 15 indicates a need for treatment.

Blood Urea Nitrogen (BUN): Urea nitrogen is a normal waste product in the blood that comes from the breakdown of protein from the foods we eat and from the body metabolism. It is normally removed from the blood by the kidneys, but when kidney function slows down, the BUN level rises. BUN can also rise if the patient eats more protein, and it can fall if the patient eats less protein.

Dumping syndrome

Dumping syndrome is a response to the presence of excess amounts of undigested food in the jejunum. When patients have a large amount of the stomach surgically removed and resume a normal diet, the food can pass in large amounts into the jejunum instead of the normal process of gradually passing in small amounts. When the ingested food is broken down rapidly, the contents of the intestine can become hypertonic. The body seeks to achieve osmotic balance by drawing water from the plasma to dilute the contents, leading to decrease in blood volume. This causes sweating, weakness, and rapid heart beat. The digested carbohydrates then rapidly enter the blood stream and cause elevated blood glucose, which triggers overproduction of insulin and subsequent hypoglycemia.

Simple carbohydrates, which are hydrolyzed quickly, should be limited. Proteins and fats are better tolerated. Patients with severe dumping may only take liquids between meals, to avoid overwhelming the jejunum.

Drug and nutrient interactions

Therapeutic Class/Drug/Nutrient Interaction
Antidepressants/Imipramine
May induce riboflavin deficiency; increased appetite.

Antihypertensives/Hydralazine
Pyridoxine antagonist; increased urinary excretion of manganese and pyridoxine.

Antimalarials/Pyrimethamine, Sulfadoxine
Folate antagonists.

Antineoplastics/Methotrexate
Folate antagonist; may impair fat, calcium, cobalamin, lactose, folate, and carotene absorption.

Therapeutic Class/Drug/Nutrient Interaction

Diuretics/Furosemide, Thiazides, Spironolactone
Increased urinary potassium, sodium, chloride, magnesium, zinc, and iodine excretion; reduced calcium excretion leading to hypercalcemia and hypophosphatemia with thiazides, increased calcium excretion with furosemide; increased urinary sodium and chloride; reduced urinary potassium excretion.

Hypocholesterolemic Agents/Cholestyramine, Colestipol
Reduced absorption of fat, fat-soluble vitamins, calcium, cobalamin, folate.

Antidiuretic hormone

Antidiuretic hormone, also known as vasopressin, is a 9 amino acid peptide secreted from the posterior pituitary. Within hypothalamic neurons, the hormone is packaged in secretory vesicles with a carrier protein called neurophysin, and both are released upon hormone secretion. The single most important effect of antidiuretic hormone is to conserve body water by reducing the output of urine. A diuretic is an agent that increases the rate of urine formation. Injection of small amounts of antidiuretic hormone into a person or animal results in antidiuresis or decreased formation of urine, and the hormone was named for this effect. Antidiuretic hormone binds to receptors in the distal or collecting tubules of the kidney and promotes reabsorption of water back into the circulation. In the absence of antidiuretic hormone, the kidney tubules are virtually impermeable to water, and it flows out as urine. Antidiuretic hormone stimulates water reabsorption by stimulating insertion of "water channels" or aquaporins into the membranes of kidney tubules. These channels transport solute-free water through tubular cells and back into blood, leading to a decrease in plasma osmolarity and an increase osmolarity of urine. Decreased blood volume can cause secretion of vasopressin.

Lipoproteins

There are 5 major types of lipoproteins in the human body. Lipoproteins are classified, as follows, according to their density.

Chylomicrons
These are normally found in the blood only after a person has eaten foods containing fats. They contain about 7% cholesterol. Chylomicrons transport fats and cholesterol from the intestine into the liver, then into the bloodstream. They are metabolized in the process of carrying food energy to muscle and fat cells. Chylomicrons are created in the intestine from dietary fat.

Very low-density lipoproteins (VLDL)
These lipoproteins carry mostly triglycerides, but they also contain 16% to 22% cholesterol. VLDLs are made in the liver and eventually become intermediate-density lipoprotein (IDL) particles after they have lost their triglyceride content.

Intermediate-density lipoproteins (IDL)
IDLs are short-lived lipoproteins containing about 30% cholesterol that are converted in the liver to low-density lipoproteins (LDLs). LDL precursor.

Low-density lipoproteins (LDL)
LDL molecules carry cholesterol from the liver to other body tissues. They contain about 50% cholesterol. Extra LDLs are absorbed by the liver and their cholesterol is excreted into the bile. LDL particles are involved in the formation of plaques (abnormal deposits of cholesterol) in the walls of the coronary arteries. LDL is known as "bad cholesterol."

High-density lipoproteins (HDL)
HDL molecules are made in the intestines and the liver. HDLs are about 50% protein and 19% cholesterol. They help to remove cholesterol from artery walls. Lifestyle changes, including exercising, keeping weight within recommended limits, and giving up smoking can increase the body's levels of HDL cholesterol. HDL is known as "good cholesterol."

Omega-3 fatty acids

Omega-3 fatty acids are considered essential fatty acids, which means that they are essential to human health but cannot be manufactured by the body. For this reason, omega-3 fatty acids must be obtained from food. Omega-3 fatty acids can be found in fish and certain plant oils. There are 3 major types of omega-3 fatty acids that are ingested in foods and used by the body: alpha-linolenic acid (ALA), eicosapentaenoic acid (EPA), and docosahexaenoic acid (DHA). Once eaten, the body converts ALA to EPA and DHA, the 2 types of omega-3 fatty acids more readily used by the body. Extensive research indicates that omega-3 fatty acids reduce inflammation and help prevent certain chronic diseases such as heart disease and arthritis. These essential fatty acids are highly concentrated in the brain and appear to be particularly important for cognitive and behavioral function. In fact, infants who do not get enough omega-3 fatty acids from their mothers during pregnancy are at risk for developing vision and nerve problems. Omega-3 fatty acids help reduce inflammation and most omega-6 fatty acids tend to promote inflammation.

Brekadown of fats

Fats in the diet are an important part of the body's energy source, even when carbohydrates are present. The liver is the center of lipid metabolism, serving several important functions: to make triglycerides from carbohydrates and proteins, to make other lipids such as cholesterol the body needs from triglycerides, to desaturate fatty acids so that they can be stored in adipose cells, and to break down triglycerides for use as energy. Most fats in the diet are absorbed through the small intestine and enter the lymphatic system. They then travel to the liver and are stored, used immediately for energy, or broken down. Lipoprotein lipase is the enzyme responsible for breaking down triglycerides into fatty acids small enough to pass into human fat cells. Fatty acids are oxidized in the liver to ultimately form acetyl-CoA, which then enters the citric acid cycle with oxaloacetic acid to yield ATP for energy.

liver fat met-

Cholesterol lab values

Optimal LDL cholesterol: less than 100 mg/dL and total cholesterol less than 160 mg/dL.

Desirable LDL cholesterol: 100-129 mg/dL; total cholesterol 160-199mg/dL.

Borderline high risk: LDL cholesterol 130-159 mg/dL; total cholesterol 200 to 239 mg/dL.

High risk: LDL cholesterol greater than 160 mg/dL; total cholesterol greater than or at 240 mg/dL.

Coenzyme Q10

Coenzyme Q10 (CoQ10) is a compound found naturally in the energy-producing center of the cell known as the mitochondria. CoQ10 is involved in the making of an important molecule known as ATP. ATP serves as the cell's major energy source and drives a number of biological processes, including muscle contraction and the production of protein. CoQ10 also works as an antioxidant. Antioxidants are substances that scavenge free radicals, damaging compounds in the body that alter cell membranes, tamper with DNA, and even cause cell death. Free radicals occur naturally in the body, but environmental toxins (including ultraviolet light, radiation, cigarette smoking, and air pollution) can also increase the number of these damaging particles.

Free radicals are believed to contribute to the aging process as well as the development of a number of health problems, including heart disease and cancer. Antioxidants such as CoQ10 can neutralize free radicals and may reduce or even help prevent some of the damage they cause. CoQ10 boosts energy, enhances the immune system, and acts as an antioxidant. A growing body of research suggests that using coenzyme Q10 supplements alone or in combination with other drug therapies and nutritional supplements may help prevent or treat some conditions.

Electrolytes

Electrolytes are substances that, when dissolved in water, dissociate into ions. These ions are positively charged (cations) and negatively charged (anions). Electrolytes include inorganic salts of sodium and potassium as well as other complex organic molecules. Sodium is the major cation in extracellular fluid (outside the cell). Potassium is the major cation of intracellular fluid (inside the cell). Sodium and Potassium both function in acid/base balance, and osmotic pressure. 40% of sodium is in sodium chloride.

Water

<u>Total body water</u>
Total body water (TBW) = Intracellular fluid (ICF) + Extracellular fluid (ECF).

<u>Intracellular water</u> (ICW):
This is water that is contained within the cell.

<u>Extracellular water</u> (EWC):
This accounts for 20% of body weight and includes the water in plasma, lymph, spinal fluid, and secretions, as well as the intercellular water between and around the cells.

<u>Insensible water loss</u>:
This is water that is lost imperceptively, such as when air is expired from the lungs or when water vapor escapes in the skin's surface. The body loses 0.8 to 1.2 liters of water per day from this. It depends on gestational age (more preterm: more IWL) and it depends on postnatal age (skin thickens with age: older is better --> less IWL). Also consider losses of other fluids such as stool (diarrhea/ostomy), NG/OG drainage, CSF (ventricular drainage).

Insensible water loss (IWL)
"Insensible" water loss is water loss that is not obvious through skin (2/3) or respiratory tract (1/3).

Depends on gestational age (more preterm: more IWL).

Depends on postnatal age (skin thickens with age: older is better --> less IWL).

Also consider losses of other fluids such as stool (diarrhea/ostomy), NG/OG drainage, CSF (ventricular drainage).

<u>Sensible water loss</u>:
This is water that is lost through your sweat, urine, or feces.

Acid/Base Balance

Acid/base balance is the state of equilibrium of hydrogen ion concentration in the body. A low pH is associated with an acidic state called acidosis. A high pH value is associated with an alkaline state called alkalosis. The normal pH range is 7.35 to 7.45. A blood pH lower than 6.8 or higher than 7.8 is not compatible with life. Acid/base balance is controlled in the body through 3 lines of defense: the buffer system, respiratory system, and the kidneys. Buffer is a mixture of acid and base components that protects against either a strong acid or a strong base. The main buffer in the body is carbonic acid (H_2CO_3).

The lungs and the kidneys work together to maintain a normal pH of 7.4. If there is change in either side of buffer, there will be a compensatory change in the other side to restore balance. The lungs regulate carbonic acid while the kidneys regulate bicarbonate (base).

Severe diarrhea can cause acidosis by causing the body to excrete too much sodium bicarbonate from the body. Diabetics can be at risk for acidosis when fatty acids are mobilized at a rate that the citric acid cycle cannot manage. The result is a build up of acetone and ketone acids in the body that can dangerously elevate the body's acidity.

Alkalosis is the build up of too much base or the loss of hydrogen ions or acid from the body. Metabolic alkalosis can be caused by the loss of chloride through excessive vomiting. Hypokalemic alkalosis can be a risk for hypertensive patients taking diuretics, which can adversely affect the kidney's ability to metabolize potassium.

Dehydration

Dehydration is caused by a lack of water intake, an excessive loss of water, or high solute load. Most lab values will be increased with dehydration, but other signs of dehydration include fever, sweating, hyperventilation, rapid weight loss, decreased urine output, poor skin turgor, or an increase in solutes (serum uric acid lab value). The best lab assessment for determining fluid balance and dehydration status is serum sodium. Serum sodium should be looked at first. If the serum sodium is out of range (normal values, 136 to 145 mEq/L), this indicates fluid imbalance, which therefore affects other lab values. If serum sodium is in normal range, fluid balance is normal. The best way to treat dehydration is to give the patient water by mouth or dextrose 5% solution in water.

Proximal Convoluted Tubule

A large amount of nutrients and water is filtered from the blood in the glomerulus. It is necessary to reabsorb most of the nutrients and water but leave waste in the tubule. Selective reabsorption occurs in the proximal convoluted tubule. Glucose, vitamins, important ions, and most amino acids are reabsorbed from the tubule back into the capillaries near the proximal convoluted tubule. These molecules are moved into the peritubular capillaries by active transport, a process that requires energy. Cells of the proximal convoluted tubule have numerous microvilli and mitochondria that provide surface area and energy. When the concentration of some substances in the blood reaches a certain level, the substance is not reabsorbed; it remains in the urine. This prevents the composition of the blood from fluctuating. This process regulates the levels of glucose and inorganic ions such as sodium, potassium, bicarbonate phosphate, and chloride. Urea remains in the tubules. Without reabsorption, death would result from dehydration and starvation.

Early Distal Convoluted Tubule and Collecting Tubule

The early distal convoluted tubule:
Reabsorption of sodium ions
Reabsorption of Ca2+
Reabsorption of Cl-

Collecting Tubules:
Reabsorption of sodium ions
Secretion of hydrogen ions (for blood pH homeostasis)
Secretion of potassium ions
Reabsorption of H20-regulated by vasopressin
Both the distal convoluted tubule (DCT) and the collecting duct are involved in reabsorption of water.

Acidosis and Alkalosis

The blood pH is kept fairly constant and slightly alkaline at 7.35 to 7.45. This balance is carefully regulated by the lungs, kidneys, and blood proteins. If too much acid accumulates in the body or too much bicarbonate, or base, is lost, acidosis can result.

Severe diarrhea can cause acidosis by causing the body to excrete too much sodium bicarbonate from the body. Diabetics can be at risk for acidosis when fatty acids are mobilized at a rate that the citric acid cycle cannot manage. The result is a build up of acetone and ketone acids in the body that can dangerously elevate the body's acidity.

Alkalosis is the build up of too much base or the loss of hydrogen ions or acid from the body. Metabolic alkalosis can be caused by the loss of chloride through excessive vomiting. Hypokalemic alkalosis can be a risk for hypertensive patients taking diuretics, which can adversely affect the kidney's ability to metabolize potassium.

Metabolic Alkalosis

Metabolic alkalosis is the abnormal accumulation of bicarbonate (base), or excessive acid loss or loss of extracellular fluid. Volume depletion is a common cause. Alkalosis means an increase in HCO_3.
- Profile: H+ decreased with increased pH.
- Compensation: ventilation decreases to retain more CO_2 to make more carbonic acid (to decrease pH).

Example:
A patient with the following lab values has metabolic alkalosis:
pH = 7.48
HCO_3 = 31
pCO_2 = 42
The pH is high, the HCO_3 is high, and the lungs (pCO_2) are normal. The kidneys are retaining base, so the lungs have to compensate by retaining CO_2 to lower pH.

Metabolic Acidosis

Metabolic acidosis is when the kidneys produce too much hydrogen or retain too much hydrogen, which leads to an increase in carbonic acid production, or the kidneys may excrete too much base.
- Profile: increased H+ with a decreased pH.
- Compensation: respiration increases, so the lungs excrete more CO_2 to decrease carbonic acid. Causes: uncontrolled diabetes, starvation, high-fat or low-CHO diet. Most metabolic disorders are mainly due to kidney disease.

Example:
A patient with the following lab values is considered to be in metabolic acidosis.
pH = 6.94
15 = HCO_3
pCO_2 = 40
The pH is low, the HCO_3 is low, and the pH is normal.

Respiratory Alkalosis

Respiratory Alkalosis: increased ventilation and elimination of CO_2. Secondary to pneumonia, hypoxia, interstitial lung disease.
- Compensation: the kidneys will excrete bicarbonate (base) to lower pH

Example:
pH = 7.5
HCO_3 = 24
pCO_2 = 27
The pH is high and the HCO_3 is normal, but the pCO_2 is low

Respiratory Acidosis

Respiratory acidosis is inadequate gas exchange in the lungs with CO_2 retention and increased carbonic acid. It can be caused by airway obstruction, emphysema, pneumonia, or respiratory depression/failure. Even though the respiratory system is compromised, buffers and kidneys compensate by retaining bicarbonate (base) and excreting H+. Treatment involves restoration of airways and normal respiration.

Example:
pH = 7.4
HCO_3 = 25
PCO_2 = 56
The pH is low, HCO_3 is normal, and a high pCO_2.

Blood compostion

Blood is the medium in which dissolved gases, nutrients, hormones, and waste products are transported. Blood, along with the heart and the blood vessels (e.g., veins and arteries), comprises the circulatory system of the body.

Blood is composed of a straw-colored liquid called plasma that contains suspended cells. The different specialized cells found in blood are:
Red blood cells
White blood cells
Platelets

Approximately 90% of plasma is water, blood's solvent, with the rest composed of dissolved substances, primarily proteins (e.g., albumin, globulin, fibrinogen). Plasma typically accounts for 55% by volume of blood and of the remaining 45% the greatest contribution is from the red blood cells.

Approximately 8% of total body weight is blood.

Renal Plasma Flow

To measure RPF accurately, the concentration of PAH in the renal venous plasma (RVp) must also be known: RPF = V (Up-RVp)/(Pp-RVp). This requires catheterization of the renal vein, a feasible but not a common procedure.

Note that RBF can be calculated from RPF by the equation RBF = RPF/(1 - hematocrit).

CHF

Inability of heart to pump adequate amount of blood to adequately maintain systemic circulation.

Volume overload, pressure overload, decreased contractility, high cardiac output demands

Generally results from cardiac defects that cause increased volume or increased pressure on ventricles (coarctation of aorta, myocardial failure, disease of organs especially lungs). Eventually, the right side has trouble pumping blood forward to lungs, dilates, and hypertrophies, and signs of right-sided failure are seen.

Cor pulmonale = CHF from obstructive lung disease (CF or bronchopulmonary dysplasia). Low-sodium diet recommended for patients with CHF. Possible fluid restrictions.

Arterial Blood Gases

Arterial Blood Gases (ABG): Measures status of body's respiratory environment via blood; also an indicator of acid/base balance.
ph = 7.35 to 7.45
$PaCO_2$ = 35 to 45
PaO_2 = 80 to 100
HCO_3 = 24 to 28

Hyperventilation: the increased rate and depth of breathing.

Hypoxia: an abnormal deficiency of oxygen in arterial blood.

Respiratory rate: the rate of breathing at rest, about 14 breaths per minute.

Glucose

Glucose is stored in the liver and muscle as glycogen. When blood sugar levels fall, the liver glycogen is converted into glucose and released in the blood stream. Muscle cells use the glucose only during times of exercise.
- Energy: Glucose is used in the body cells as energy. Glucose is broken down into smaller fragments that yield energy when broken down into carbon dioxide and water.
- Protein: 58% of protein is converted to glucose.
- Fat: 10% of glucose is converted to fat.

Insulin and glucagon

Insulin and glucagons are 2 hormones that regulate blood glucose homeostasis. Insulin is produced by the beta cells of the pancreas. The primary function is to control transport of glucose from the bloodstream to the cell. It also fosters glycogenesis (formation of glycogen) and lipogenesis (fat formation). Glucagon is made from the alpha cells of the pancreas and secreted in response to low blood glucose concentration. It brings the glucose out of storage when necessary. Glucagon helps raise blood sugar and release glucose into the blood stream.

Epinephrine

Epinephrine is a hormone of the adrenal gland (adrenal medulla). It is important in stress response and it stimulates the liver and muscle to release glucose from glycogen.

Glycolysis pathway

The function of the glycolysis pathway is to break down glucose. Not only does the process break down single sugars for the body to use as energy, it also provides the building blocks the body needs to help form essential compounds such as glycerol for triglyceride formation.

Glucose is stored as glycogen in the liver and muscle cells, and the net result of the glycolytic pathway is to take this 6-carbon form of glucose and break it down into 2 molecules of pyruvate. During this process each molecule of glucose has the potential to create 36 to 38 ATP molecules, either by yielding nicotinamide adenine dinucleotide (NADH), a potential form of energy, or ATP, a source of energy the body can use immediately.

Blood sugar control

Blood sugar is regulated primarily by the endocrine pancreas through the action of insulin and glucagon, which exert opposing influences in the body. Insulin is released by the beta cells of the pancreas in response to the presence of elevated blood sugar after eating. Insulin increases the synthesis of glycogen in the liver and also stimulates glucose to move from the bloodstream into muscle and fat cells, thereby lowering blood sugar levels and promoting glucose storage.

A few hours after eating, when glucose levels begin to fall, glucagon is produced by alpha cells in the pancreas. This hormone elevates blood sugar level by prompting glycogen breakdown in the liver.

Epinephrine is a powerful blood sugar stimulant, but it is secreted by the adrenal medulla. Its role is also to stimulate a breakdown of glycogen in the liver and therefore elevate glucose in the bloodstream.

Hormones

Thyroxine, which is manufactured by the follicular cells of the thyroid, plays a role in carbohydrate metabolism and protein metabolism. Patients with hypothyroidism may see their basal metabolic rate fall from 30% to 50%. Thyroxine affects protein metabolism by increasing the rate of metabolism in all cells.

Glucocorticoids, such as cortisol, raise blood glucose levels by stimulating gluconeogenesis. These hormones counteract the effects of insulin by reducing glucose use in the body and increasing the rate at which protein is turned into glucose.

ACTH is secreted from the pituitary gland, and works to reduce the effects of glucose by stimulating the adrenal cortex to grow and release glucocorticoids. This hormone is part of the neuroendocrine response and is stimulated by stress, allowing the body to mobilize resources, such as amino acids stored in the muscle, to be used as energy.

Digestion

The basic steps of digestion:
- Mouth: Food is chewed here and mixed with salvatory secretions that help prepare food for swallowing.
- The esophagus passes the food to the stomach. The food in the stomach is then diluted with fluids and mixed with enzymes.
- The food is then pushed through the pyloric value and into the small intestine (where food is completed digested and absorbed).
- Food that is not digested passes through the ileocecal valve to the large intestine (colon).
- The large intestines also allow for temporary storage of waste products.

There are 4 hormones that regulate the digestive tract:
- **Gastrin,** which originates in the pyloric region, stimulates the flow of stomach enzymes and acid. Gastrin is produced in greater response to the stimuli of coffee, alcohol, spices, and protein
- **Gastric inhibitory peptide** reduces stomach motility and also inhibits the secretion of stomach acid and enzymes. Fats and proteins stimulate the secretion of this hormone, which originates in the duodenum and jejunum.
- **Cholecystokinin,** also referred to as CCK, originates in the duodenum and jejunum, and is released especially in response to the presence of fat and protein in the duodenum. This hormone causes the gallbladder to contract, releasing bile into the duodenum. CCK also causes the release of enzyme-rich pancreatic juices and bicarbonate-rich pancreatic juices.
- **Secretin** functions by stimulating the secretion of thin bicarbonate-rich pancreatic juice, offering a buffering effect, and it also reduces stomach motility. Secretin is stimulated by the acidic substance chyme entering the stomach. This hormone originates in the duodenum and the jejunum.

Peristalsis
Peristalsis is a series of coordinated muscular movements that propels food from the esophagus to the anus. A circular group of muscles constricts and relaxes behind and in front of the ingested food, allowing it to move down the GI tract. A second group of muscles that runs lengthwise along the GI tract then contracts, which makes the GI tract shorter. This coordinated squeezing and shortening moves the food through the esophagus in 2 main waves to the stomach, where the peristalsis action functions in a mixing and grinding fashion as frequently as 3 times a minute. The small intestine has rapid peristalsis movements, which function more to mix the chyme rather than to move the food along. The colon features less frequent movements, employing occasional large waves that coordinate contraction along the length of the colon to help produce bowel movements.

Intestinal tract
The valves, or sphincters, located throughout the intestinal tract include:
- The **upper and lower esophageal sphincters** control the flow of food through the esophagus. The lower esophageal sphincter plays an important role in preventing heartburn, as it stops food from flowing from the stomach back into the esophagus.
- The **pyloric sphincter**, located at the base of the stomach, allows the acidic contents of the stomach to enter the small intestine a few milliliters at a time.
- The **sphincter of Oddi**, located at the end of the gallbladder, relaxes in response to the hormone Cholecystokinin, allowing bile to enter the duodenum.

- The **ileocecal valve**, located at the end of the small intestine, prevents the bacteria-laden contents of the large intestine from entering the small intestine.
- At the end of the rectum are 2 **anal** sphincters, which are under voluntary control and allow for the release of fecal waste.

Small intestine

Absorption: Passive absorption requires no carrier molecules or energy in order for the nutrient to pass through the wall of the intestine. The substance must be present in a higher concentration in the lumen of the small intestine than in the absorptive cells for this to take place.

Active absorption uses energy to pump the nutrient, such as amino acids, into the intestine's villi. This process requires the use of ATP as the driving energy force. Facilitated absorption uses a carrier molecule to transport the nutrients from the lumen of the intestine into the absorptive cells, but no energy is needed. Phagocytosis means the absorptive cell actually surrounds and engulfs the nutrient. Breast milk antibodies ingested by infants are absorbed this way.

Villi: The villi in the small intestine are drained by the bloodstream and the lymphatic system. Blood laden with nutrients collects in capillary beds inside the intestine's villi. This blood leaves the intestine via the portal vein, which flows directly to the liver. This allows the liver to process and filter any ingested substances before they enter the general circulation. The lymphatic vessels assist in draining the villi by removing any particles too large to pass into the capillaries. Large proteins and fat byproducts are 2 examples of nutrients that travel through this system. The particles then travel to the thoracic duct, which connects to the bloodstream near the neck.

Large intestine

While the small intestine is the major site for nutrient absorption, the large intestine functions to prepare the last undigested remnants to be excreted as feces. The ingested foodstuffs that eventually reach the colon consist mostly of water, some minerals, and some plant fibers and starches. Only a very small percentage of carbohydrate, protein, and fat remain. The colon does function to absorb some water, although nearly 90% has already been absorbed by the small intestine. The colon absorbs vitamin K, sodium, and potassium along the first half. By the time the stool reaches the descending colon, peristaltic waves push the mass toward the rectum, and the urge to eliminate stimulates the anal sphincters to relax.

Carbohydrate digestion

Mouth: The process begins in the mouth when the salivary enzyme amylase is released. Amylase breaks down the starch into small polysaccharides and maltose.

Stomach: Once the bolus (swallowed food) reaches the stomach, the stomach acid inactivates salivary enzymes, halting starch digestion. The stomach contains no enzymes to digest carbohydrates. Fiber lingers in the stomach and delays gastric emptying.

Small Intestine: Most of the carbohydrate digestion occurs here. The pancreas produces pancreatic amylase through the pancreatic duct into the small intestine. Starch --→ pancreatic amylase --→ small polysaccharides and disaccharides. The final steps take place on the surface of the small intestinal cells.

Maltase
Maltose ----------→ glucose + glucose

Sucrase
Sucrose ----------→ fructose + glucose

Lactase
Lactose ---------→ galactose + glucose

Intestinal cells then absorb these monosaccharides.

Protein catabolism

Amino acid to energy pathway:
- Step 1: Deamination is the reaction that removes the amino group (NH_2) from the amino acid.
- Step 2: The amino group is then converted to NH_3 (ammonia). Most ammonia can be converted to urea and excreted; some ammonia is converted to purines and then to uric acid; other ammonia is used to make new amino acids.
- Step 3: the non-N form ketoacid can enter the tricarboxylic acid (TCA) cycle.

Fat digestion

- Mouth: the salivary glands secrete a lipase enzyme and hard fats begin to melt as they reach body temperature.
- Stomach: little fat digestion takes place. Lipase initiates lipid digestion by hydrolyzing triglycerides to diglycerides and fatty acids.
- Small Intestine: fat in the intestine triggers the release of the hormone cholecystokin (CCK), which then signals the gallbladder to send bile. Bile is an emulsifier.

Bile
Fat ----------→ emulsified fat

Pancreatic lipase is secreted from the pancreas and breaks down the emulsified fat (triglycerides) into monoglycerides, glycerol, and fatty acids. Glycerol is absorbed into the blood.

Polysaccharides

Cellulose is a plant fiber that forms the structure of cell walls. The same properties that give structure to plants also contribute to the tough, fibrous texture of fruits and vegetables. This undesirable quality can be lessened in the cooking process. Humans do not possess the ability to break cellulose down, thus the function of this polysaccharide is to add bulk in the diet.

Dextrins are produced during the breakdown of starch. They have many uses in the food industry, for example, the maltodextrin derived from cornstarch is commonly added to many products. Dextrins are easily digested and inexpensive.

Glycogen is an animal starch with many branches in its structure. More branching in a starch molecule means more sites for enzymes to work on. This makes glycogen very easy to break down, and therefore makes it a good way to store carbohydrates in the body.

Krebs cycle

The Krebs cycle is also called the TCA cycle. It handles glucose, protein, and fat. Acetyl-CoA is made from pyruvic acid (irreversible reaction), oxidation of fatty acids and amino acids.
- Step 1: making citric acid
- Step 2: releasing CO_2 and water
- Step 3: alpha-ketoglutaric acid (needs thiamin) to form oxaloacetic acid. Oxaloacetic acid is the major carbohydrate fuel that keeps the cycle going.
- Step 4: oxaloacetic acid reacts with acetyl-CoA and starts the cycle again.
- 38 ATP are yielded

Citric acid cycle

The citric acid or Krebs cycle involves a sequence by which carbon atoms are converted into ATP, which is used for energy, and carbon dioxide, which is exhaled by the lungs. The cycle begins with the reaction of a 2-carbon acetate molecule with the 4-carbon compound oxaloacetate. The resulting 6-carbon compound citrate is then turned back into a 4-carbon oxaloacetate molecule, thus completing the cycle. The significance of this cycle is that in the process, substances are produced that can be converted in the electron transport chain for energy-yielding ATP and water. The overall result is that the energy present in the chemical bonds of glucose is turned into a form of energy the body can use, which is ATP.

Ketogenesis

Ketone bodies are products of acetyl-CoA metabolism that are normally present in small amounts and can be burned for energy. However, large numbers of ketone bodies may build up when too many fatty acids enter the bloodstream, overwhelming the liver's ability to metabolize acetyl-CoA into carbon dioxide. This can occur in diabetes, when there is not enough insulin produced to allow for normal fat metabolism. This can also be a problem when carbohydrate intake is insufficient, as in some weight-loss plans.

Cells pick up ketones for energy and remove enough carbon atoms to turn them into acetyl-CoA, which is then pushed through the citric acid cycle. The resulting acetone byproduct leaves the body through the lungs, resulting in a distinctive, sweet-smelling breath. If the number of ketone bodies in the bloodstream rises too high, the excess spills into the urine, taking sodium and potassium with it. This can lead to ion imbalances in the body.

Nitrogen balance

Nitrogen balance is the amount of nitrogen consumed compared with the amount of nitrogen excreted in a certain time period. It is based on the fact that about 16% of the mass of protein is nitrogen.

Nitrogen balance (NB): NB is calculated to determine infidivudal protein requirements:
NB = Nitrogen Intake − Nitrogen Output
Nitrogen intake is estimated from protein intake where grams of nitrogen equal grams of intact protein/6.25 or grams of crystalline amino acids/6. Nitrogen output is assessed as 24-hour total urinary nitrogen + 2 g of nitrogen to account for normal losses via feces, skin, etc. One gram of nitrogen should be added to nitrogen output for each 500 mL of diarrhea, fistula, or gastric output

(any collectable body fluid can be analyzed for total nitrogen content if extra-urinary losses are in question). To accurately assess NB, a steady metabolic state needs to be achieved.

At least 3 days of steady nutrient intake are desirable prior to obtaining the total urinary nitrogen (TUN). Ideally, 3 consecutive 24-hour urine collections are analyzed and averaged for a best estimate of nitrogen output. Careful and complete urine collection and intake records are imperative.

Zero balance – N in = N out → a healthy adult who consumes adequate protein.
Positive (+) balance – N in > N out → indicates growth: infant, pregnancy, teenager, or healing.
Negative (-) balance – N in < N out → inadequate protein intake.

Formula:
$$\frac{\text{Protein intake (grams)}}{6.25} - (\text{urinary urea nitrogen} + 4)$$

For every 6.25 g of dietary protein consumed, 1 g of N is excreted.
Nitrogen balance is invalid with renal patients, and patients with burns, vomiting, diarrhea, and fistulas.

Absorption of nutrients

Absorption of nutrients into intestinal cells occurs by one of the following methods.
- Simple diffusion: some nutrients, such as water and small lipids, are absorbed by small diffusion. They cross into intestinal cells freely. Net movement is from higher to lower concentration.
- Passive diffusion: Some nutrients, such as water-soluble vitamins, are absorbed by passive diffusion. These nutrients need a specific carrier to transport them from one side to the other. This is also called facilitated diffusion. Movement is from higher to lower concentration.
- Active transport: Most nutrients are absorbed this way, such as glucose and amino acids. These nutrients move against the gradient (lower to higher concentration), requiring energy from ATP.

Calcium
Calcium is best absorbed in the acidic environment of the duodenum. Vitamin D plays an important role in calcium absorption by stimulating production of calcium binding protein. Calcium is also absorbed through passive diffusion throughout the intestine. Calcium is absorbed only in water-soluble form and usually 70% to 80% remains unabsorbed and is excreted in waste.

Iron
The transfer of iron is dependent on a protein carrier synthesized in the liver called transferrin. This protein makes iron available to the cells responsible for heme synthesis. Dietary iron occurs in heme form, found in hemoglobin and myoglobin, and nonheme form, present in plant sources. Gastric acidity increases the availability and absorption of iron from foods. Ascorbic acid increases absorption by forming a compound with iron that is more soluble in the alkaline environment of the small intestine. Lack of gastric acidity or consumption of alkaline products such as antacids decreases iron absorption.

Vitamins A, D, and B$_{12}$

Vitamin A is released from proteins in the stomach. Natural vitamin A in the form of retinyl esters are broken down in the small intestine to form retinol, which is transported in the lymphatic system and then to the liver, where most storage takes place. When vitamin A is needed in the body, it binds with retinol-binding protein and travels from the liver through circulation. Vitamin D is absorbed from the intestine with the aid of bile. Vitamin D is bound to a protein for transport and stored in the liver, skin, bones, and brain. Thiamin is easily absorbed in the first part of the small intestine by active transport, and absorption is inhibited by folate deficiency and alcohol intake. The absorption of riboflavin occurs in the small intestine and is enhanced by the presence of food in the GI tract. The bonds of vitamin B$_{12}$ are broken down in the acidic environment of the stomach. However, it is poorly absorbed from the intestine without the presence of the intrinsic factor enzyme.

Nutritional status

Physical and psychosocial factors

With age, the senses of taste, sight, and smell diminish, which adversely affects food intake. Medications commonly taken by elderly people can change the taste of food or give food a metallic taste.

Impaired function of the gastrointestinal tract can affect nutritional status in several ways. Tooth decay or ill-fitting dentures may interfere with mastication, forcing individuals to give up foods they previously enjoyed. Diminished salivary function due to normal aging or medications also interferes with mastication and swallowing. The large intestine exhibits decreased motility, leading to constipation, which can inhibit appetite. Dementia or depression found in some elderly people may contribute to poor nutritional status, especially if the person lives in isolation. The inability to shop for or prepare food can be one of the leading reasons elderly individuals enter a nursing home. Many senior citizens also struggle with financial difficulties when they stop working. Although two-thirds of these individuals may qualify for the Food Stamp Program, less than half use it.

Nutritional requirements

Exercise

Water functions in the body to transport nutrients and waste products to and from cells, and allows the body to maintain temperature control. The water lost during exercise comes from increased respiration and sweating. Fluid lost from sweat comes from the blood volume, so dehydration can impair cardiovascular functioning. Fluids should be consumed in adequate amounts to maintain pre-exercise weight.

The first source of energy for exercising muscles is glycogen stored in the muscle. When that is exhausted, the liver maintains the glucose supply via gluconeogenesis and glycogenolysis. The liver can maintain blood glucose for extended periods this way, but depletion can occur after long distance events. After heavy training, it can take up to 24 hours to renew glycogen stores. For an athlete, protein is more important in terms of functioning as an energy source than for building muscle. The amount of protein needed to build new muscle is met by the average diet, and the Recommended Daily Allowance (RDA) for protein for athletes is the same as for the general population.

Childhood

Children need extra energy and nutrients in relation to their size because they are growing and developing bones, muscle, and blood. Children also have higher basal metabolic rates, which increases their need for calories even at rest. Children triple their birth weight in the first year of life, and increase their length by 50%. Growth slows until adolescence, when the child will gain 20% of his or her adult height and 50% of his or her adult weight.

Protein intake should range from 1.2 g/kg in early childhood to 1 g/kg in late childhood. Protein deficiency in children is rarely a problem in the United States because of the abundance of protein-rich foods. Iron deficiency anemia is common in preschool-aged children because the rapid rate of growth may not be supported by enough iron-rich foods in the diet. Calcium is essential for mineralization and maintenance of growing bones. Vitamin D is necessary for proper calcium absorption, and may be found in fortified milk.

Pregnancy

Vitamin D is essential in skeletal formation in the fetus and for the metabolism of calcium. Calcium metabolism increases during pregnancy, so the recommended dietary allowance (RDA) for vitamin D doubles from 5 to 10 mcg/day. This increase may be satisfied by regular sunlight exposure, increasing one's consumption of vitamin D milk, or via supplementation.

Folate plays an important role in the synthesis of nucleic acids, and is therefore necessary to DNA formation. Beginning one's pregnancy with an adequate store of folic acid is important in reducing certain birth defects, such as spinal malformations. The RDA for folate increases from 180 mcg for adult females to 400 mcg, which ideally should begin before conception.

Red blood cell formation increases dramatically during pregnancy, so the RDA for iron doubles from 15 to 30 mg/day. Although it remains important to seek out iron-rich foods such as red meat or spinach, supplementation is usually necessary to provide adequate amounts to prevent problems such as premature delivery and low birth weight.

Important terms

Biological Value (BV): measures protein quality. It is the amount of protein nitrogen that is reattained from growth and maintenance of the body.

Chylomicrons: type of lipoprotein that transports lipids from the intestinal cells into the body. Triglycerides, cholesterol, and phospholipids are assembled into chylomicrons. Dietary fat enters the blood as a chylomicron.

Deamination: reaction that removes the nitrogen from the amino acid.

Gelatinization: Achieved by dispersing a starch in boiling water. At the appropriate temperature, weaker hydrogen bonds between molecules break and the granule swells as it takes up water, causing an overall increase in viscosity.

HDL (high-density lipoprotein): the smallest of all the lipoproteins and composed primarily of protein.

LDL (low-density lipoprotein): derived from VLDL as cells remove triglycerides from them. It is composed mostly of cholesterol.

Lipoprotein: clusters of lipids associated with proteins that are used to transport lipids in the lymph and blood.

Net protein utilization (NPU): a measure of protein quality. It is the amount of protein nitrogen retained from the diet. BV measures retention of absorbed nitrogen, but NPU just measures retention of food nitrogen.

Pasting: This refers to changes that occur in gelled starch. These include loss of amylose and implosion of the granule.

Syneresis: The loss of water from a gel. It is also an important mechanism in the production of curds in cheese manufacture.

Transamination: the transfer of an amino acid from one amino acid to a ketoacid, producing a new nonessential amino acid and a new ketoacid.

VLDL (very low-density lipoprotein): a type of lipoprotein, but smaller than chylomicrons and carrying half the triglycerides.

Education and Communication

Nutritional education plans

Design and development
The development of a solid educational plan begins with an analysis of the existing information. The material should be matched to the objectives the instructor wants to achieve, and the information should be organized in a logical fashion that complements the retention of the material. A detailed lesson plan should include a summary of each section, the time set aside for each lesson, and the formative and summative assessment tools that will be used. Learning should have everyday applications in order to bring the subject matter to life. Quality visual aids such as posters or PowerPoint presentations make the presentation more engaging. In some cases, short video presentations may be appropriate to supplement the instructor's lessons.

Conducting an educational needs assessment

In order to develop appropriate educational interventions, it is necessary to assess the needs and readiness to learn of the intended audience or population. One should assess how motivated the target audience is to learn. Highly motivated individuals may be very interested in the topic and will attend counseling sessions whether they are mandatory or not, those with low motivation will feel the education is not useful to him or her. Educational level should be assessed to plan the most effective teaching style. An audience with a high level of education can understand complex messages, those with a low level of education need simple messages and benefit from repetition. Level of sophistication may tie in with education. Highly sophisticated people may already consider themselves self-styled experts in the field; those with little sophistication include children or those never exposed to nutrition messages before. Socioeconomic status should also be considered. Upper income adults tend to be more interested in health foods. Poor individuals are focused on coping with immediate problems.

Teaching framework

Listen
Explain
Acknowledge
Recomend
Negotiate

The LEARN framework is a 5-step plan that can improve the communication between a clinician and a patient so that the implementation of the treatment plan will go smoothly. The first step is to use active listening skills and attend to the patient's concerns with empathy. Putting oneself in the shoes of the patient can facilitate understanding. The second step is to explain one's perception of the problem, or to justify one's opinions about the situation to the patient. Using "I" statements instead of "you" statements will avoid putting the patient on the defense. The third step is to acknowledge and discuss differences. This should be done with empathy, for example, "I can understand why you are anxious about this change, but this is why it is so important to your health." The fourth step is to recommend the appropriate treatment. The last step is to negotiate treatment, or reach a middle ground where the patient agrees to participate at a level satisfactory to both patient and clinician.

Methods of instruction

Large groups
Large group instruction is appropriate when a clear, unambiguous message needs to be relayed to a large group of people without the need for much discussion. Examples include conferences, where professionals are usually speaking to their peers, and lectures, where groups of students are taking in a great deal of subject matter in an abbreviated period.

<u>Small groups</u>
Small group discussion is beneficial when a group of several people have similar backgrounds. In this setting, the lecture is interspersed with frequent discussion, which allows the participants to learn from and support one another.

<u>Self-paced</u>
Self-paced instruction is usually computer-based, such as a web-based module that a health care professional completes for continuing education credits. This form of learning is better for the highly motivated and educated learner.

<u>Question-and-answer</u>
Question-answer techniques place a high value on student participation. Examples include role play, which stimulate thought about real-life implications of the materials.

Group discussion leader

Providing good leadership when conducting a group counseling session can help propel the group towards its goals smoothly. Groups are by nature inclusive, so the leader should promote group harmony and make everyone feel accepted.

Skillful leaders do not monopolize the interactions; rather, they make suggestions or offer ideas to facilitate discussion, and then wait patiently for the group to converse. However, if the conversation wanders off topic or exchanges become heated, the leader should step in to resume control. The leader may involve non-participants in a tactful way, without putting them on the spot. Sometimes it may be necessary to wrest control away from an overly dominating member. Praise should be offered equally, so that no one feels silenced because one member is favored over another. It is helpful to have an agenda planned in advance; organization keeps the control with the leader and thus reduces the opportunity for conflict.

Communication

Good nutritional instruction requires excellent communication and critical thinking skills. Establishing rapport with the client allows him or her to share anxieties about lifestyle changes, and lets the instructor know where to focus his or her support. Even small changes in lifestyle can seem overwhelming to the client, so offering as many alternatives as possible to give control back to the client can help to reduce fears. Empathizing with the client can help build rapport by allowing the client to feel understood.

The educational message should be clear but not rigid. Including the client in the learning process also empowers the client and can enhance retention of knowledge. Good listening skills include paraphrasing the client's message or asking for clarification to reduce ambiguity. Soliciting feedback from the client can help the instructor tailor the message and teaching method as the learning continues.

<u>Communication channels</u>
Organizational communication utilizes different channels to carry messages both vertically and horizontally within an organization. In order to have purposeful, meaningful communication in one's office, it is helpful to be aware of how these channels function to pass information from the sender to the receiver. Downward communication happens when a supervisor sends an email or a

memo to his or her employees, or leads a staff meeting. This kind of communication is usually more formal in tone. Establishing good upward communication is the role of the supervisor, who may want to use comment boxes or an open-door policy to encourage employees to share information. Horizontal communication occurs between departments, such as the information sharing that takes place between nursing and dietary services in a nursing home. Diagonal communication takes place between departments that have a different placement in the organizational hierarchy. Informal communication often occurs as gossip or "water-cooler" talk, and can serve both an information-sharing function and a socializing function.

Characteristics of effective communication

Effective communication is evidenced by mutual understanding, body language, and follow-through on information discussed. Some characteristics of effective communication include the following:
- Good eye contact. Eye contact shared by both parties conveys interest and understanding between the individuals. Looking down or away from the presenter may indicate that a topic is not well understood, is an uncomfortable subject, or needs further discussion.
- Effective oral communication. When communicating orally, it is imperative that all parties understand one another. Slow, clear speech greatly improves understanding and comprehension of material discussed. Additionally, hearing devices and/or translators should be used when necessary.
- Open dialogue. Even when presenting nutritional information to another, an open dialogue is important. Questions asked to and from both individuals helps drive critical points and clarify weakly communicated topics.
- Quiet, undisturbed environment. Communication in any counseling setting is most effective in a quiet environment with little distraction.

Gender differences in communication

Men
Emphasize status
Nonverbals (less eye contact)
Use "I"
Ritual opposition
Offer advice or solutions
Direct style of giving orders

Women
Downplay their status
Nonverbals (more direct eye contact)
Focus on social connections ("we")
Ritual apology
Offer social support
Indirect style of giving orders

Focused recitation

Focused recitation uses class discussion to arrive at a solution or answer to a problem under the guidance of the instructor. The solution has been preordained, but the creative process of brainstorming and working together gives the students ownership of the problem and improves the retention of knowledge.

Guided practice involves allowing the students to try a new skill under the tutelage of the instructor before returning home to try the skill alone. An example is a healthy cooking class where the dietitian guides the students as they prepare low-fat, high-flavor dishes.

Role-playing helps the student become more comfortable with an upcoming lifestyle change by pretending to adopt the behavior with a classmate acting in a supporting role.

For example, a child preparing to go on dialysis may act out the process with a peer, which can reduce anxiety about the procedure. The teacher provides feedback and uses the dialogue to further the discussion.

Kinds of learning

Perhaps the most important aspect of the situation is the kind of learning that is to be facilitated. Knowing about the kinds of learning helps us to do a better job of teaching them. The most basic distinction is Benjamin Bloom's 3 domains:
- Cognitive learning (thoughts), such as teaching someone to add fractions.
- Affective learning (feelings, values), such as teaching someone to not want to smoke.
- Physical or motor learning (actions), such as teaching someone to touch type.

Levels of cognitive learning
The major levels of cognitive learning can be classified as memorizing, understanding, and applying:
- Memorization. This is rote learning. It entails learners encoding facts or information in the form of an association between a stimulus and a response, such as a name, date, event, place, or symbol.
- Understanding. This is meaningful learning. It entails learners relating a new idea to relevant prior knowledge, such as understanding what a revolutionary war is.
- Application. This is learning to generalize to new situations, or transfer learning. It entails learners identifying critical commonalities across situations, such as predicting the effects of price increases.

Bloom's taxonomy

Bloom's taxonomy argues that there are multiple learning styles, and this can be helpful to recognize before preparing educational nutritional programs. The cognitive domain can be understood in terms of the acquisition of knowledge. This type of learning would include recalling facts, such as being able to explain the different levels in the food pyramid. Comprehension is also a part of cognitive learning, and getting someone to describe the healthy fats in his or her own words can show comprehension. The affective domain encompasses one's attitudes and emotions about the subject material. The willingness to listen respectfully and respond to questions asked by the discussion leader is an example of affective learning. The formation of values regarding the learning material also falls in the affective realm, such as when the individual changes his or her schedule to make time to prepare healthy meals. Psychomotor learning can be thought of in terms of skills gained. The ability to check one's blood glucose is an accomplishment of psychomotor learning.

Portion size food models

When educating a client in regards to portion size, it is helpful to provide everyday comparisons, or models, for portion size. This allows a client to more adequately "eyeball" the correct portion size. Some common comparison models are as follows:

Meat, 1 oz. = Matchbox
Meat, poultry, 3 oz. (typical serving size) = Deck of cards or palm of hand
Cheese, 1 oz = 4 dice
Potato, medium = Computer mouse
Peanut butter, 2 Tbsp = Ping pong or golf ball
Pasta, ice cream, 1/2 cup = Tennis ball or a cupped hand
Bagel = Hockey puck
Fruits/Vegetables = Baseball
Pancake/Waffle = CD
Fish, 3 oz. = Checkbook

Nutritional education resources

There are many resources available to individuals wishing to change their eating habits. Resources are available in the community and virtually. Some of those resources include:

Virtual Resources
- Choosemyplate.gov
- American Heart Association website
- American Cancer Society website
- American Diabetes Association website
- American Dietetics Association website
- USDA website

Community Resources
- Home healthcare agencies
- Local nursing associations
- Local dietary associations
- Meals on Wheels
- Senior Services/Centers

Structure of dietary counseling

It is important that dietary counseling/education be methodically prepared and presented. In order to do so, the client's health and dietary needs are first assessed by the dietary manager and the patient's care team. After the assessment, a plan with future dietary changes and goals must be developed and followed. In order for the plan to be implemented, the developed plan must be realistic in its expectations. Finally, ongoing evaluations must be performed in order to ensure that the needs found by the assessment are, in fact, being addressed by the developed plan and implemented by the patient and care team. An evaluation of the plan may be used to revise dietary goals and plan expectations.

Effectiveness of written materials

Written materials are essential elements of patient education as they serve as a source of reference outside of dietary counseling sessions. Patients with impaired memory, who experience difficulty concentrating, and/or are suffering from fatigue may rely on written materials to guide their nutritional choices. The most effective written materials are printed in an easy to read font, that is both stylistically simplistic and of adequate size.

Capitalization and punctuation should be properly utilized. Additionally, the materials should be kept as simple as possible, minimizing the use of complex sentences, large words, vocabulary consisting of medical and/or scientific jargon, and inclusion of excessive information. Spacing between lines and paragraphs should be such that the information may be easily read. Graphics and/or diagrams may be used to help explain topics, though excessive use of pictures may detract from the message being conveyed.

Active listening techniques and questioning techniques

Active listening techniques include seeking understanding through asking for clarification of the message, paraphrasing to make sure you have understood the message, encouraging dialogue through empathic remarks, and refraining from interrupting and making judgmental remarks.

Examples of questioning techniques are using open-ended questions that call for more than a "yes" or "no" answer, using follow-up questions to obtain additional information, and avoiding leading questions that put the respondent under pressure to respond in a certain way.

Illegal interview questions

Where were you born?
Where are your parents from?
What's your heritage?
What religion are you?
Are you married?
Is this your maiden or married name?
With whom do you live?
How many kids do you have?
Do you plan to have children?
How old are you?
What year were you born?
When did you graduate from high school?
Which religious holidays will you be taking off from work?
Do you attend church regularly?
Have you ever been arrested?
Have you ever spent a night in jail?
Do you have any disabilities?
What's your medical history?
How does your condition affect your abilities?

Best practices

Successful recruiting can be done from in-house candidates, or can be done outside of the organization. In-house recruiting has the advantages of selecting someone who has shown that he or she fits into the culture of the organization, and retaining skilled employees who might otherwise look for opportunities elsewhere. External recruiting can be done with the aid of advertising, placement services, or college career services.

Employee interviews can be structured or unstructured. Structured interviews are conducted from a predetermined list of questions used for each applicant. Advantages include consistency in information gathering among applicants.

Disadvantages include insufficient information gathered from ill-prepared questions. Unstructured interviews use open-ended, unplanned questions and conversations to elicit information. Inexperienced interviewers need to be aware of the possibility of including questions that are not permissible in the interview process, such as those relating to age or marital status.

Proven counseling techniques

Various counseling techniques may be used to convey nutritional information, implement a healthy program, and set goals for future progress. Some of the following techniques may be helpful:
- Assess whether the patient is ready and motivated to make behavior changes and modification. If so, proceed with nutritional counseling. If not, it is imperative that the counselor impresses upon the client the need for change. If the individual is not willing to make changes, further counseling will be for naught.
- Help the client set realistic goals. If the client feels empowered, s/he is more apt to reach his/her goals. Setting goals for the client may undermine the counseling and his/her motivation to change.
- Ask the patient if s/he feels comfortable involving a support system. If so, bring these individuals into counseling to help "check" and motivate the patient when s/he needs it.
- Stress the importance of keeping an accurate journal, to include information about food, biological markers (including blood glucose measurements, if necessary), and emotions about food and/or goals.

Tactics to customize a nutritional counseling

It is crucial that nutritional counseling be tailored to the individual, as each person has specific and unique needs. Even among individuals prescribed the same diets, it is imperative that each person receives specialized and individual counseling. Elements of counseling should include information about the patient's nutritional needs and restrictions, which should be personalized based upon the individual's taste preferences, regional recipes, and religious and/or cultural observances. Additionally, learning materials, including visual aids, videos, food portion models, and other similar tools should also be tailored to the individual being counseled. An individual with impaired vision, for example, should be provided large print reading materials and/or audio notes. Finally, take into account any adaptive equipment that an individual may use during mealtime. The adaptive equipment may influence the individual's willingness and ability to eat certain items. Patients may also need to be taught how to effectively utilize adaptive equipment.

Research

Descriptive research

Descriptive research involves gathering new data to generate hypotheses regarding causal relationships. Descriptive research is useful when one seeks to study current descriptions of things and explore possible reasons that describe things as they are now. This kind of research cannot establish a causal relationship between variables. The only way to get evidence about cause-and-effect relationships is through some form of experimentation. Descriptive research designs are useful in establishing goals, and as such may examine the question, "Where should we be?" Another emphasis may be on developing methods, which examines the question, "What is best to do?" Qualitative methods may be used in descriptive research, in which observations are described in non-numerical terms. An example includes the case study, which is an intensive inquiry about a single event or population. Surveys are a commonly used quantitative method, which use questionnaires or interviews to reveal descriptive characteristics of a population.

Analytical research

Analytical research allows the study of the effects of variables for the purpose of establishing a cause-and-effect relationship. Clinical trials are a frequently used analytical research method in the field of medicine. Randomization is a basic requirement for any sound experimental design, and this involves assigning subjects at random so that they have an equal likelihood of belonging to the experimental group or the control group. This ensures that sources of variation will be controlled so that no one individual difference, such as gender or intelligence, will influence the conditions of the experiment more than another. The experimental group receives the new program or treatment being studied. The control group may receive the standard treatment, or they may receive a placebo, which is an inactive substance.

Experiments

An experiment is a set of actions and observations, performed to verify or falsify a hypothesis or research a causal relationship between phenomena. Experiments have 2 parts:
- *Control group* - group under normal conditions (nothing unusual done to it).
- *Experimental group* - the test group in which variables are changed.

Only one condition in an experiment is changed at a time; the conditions that affect the outcome are called variables. Factors in experiments that do not change are called constants.

Variables
Research questions must involve at least two variables. Researchers then try to show a relationship between one variable and another. A variable is a symbol to which numbers may be assigned. The two major variable types are dependent and independent. The dependent variable can be thought of as the consequence or output in the hypothesis. In the hypothesis, "Obese children have higher levels of anxiety than non-obese children," the dependent variable is anxiety. An independent variable is the input that predicts outcomes in the hypothesis statement. In the hypothesis, "Native American mothers will wean their children from the bottle earlier than will Mexican American mothers," the independent variable is the ethnic background of the mother. Nominal variables can fit into a category without order, such as the variables Native American and Mexican American fit

into the category of race. Ordinal scale variables are ordered, such as a ranking that ranges from highly dissatisfied to highly satisfied.

Independent Variable: The independent variable is a manipulated variable in an experiment or study whose presence or degree determines the change in the dependent variable.

Dependent Variable: The dependent variable is the observed variable in an experiment or study whose changes are determined by the presence or degree of one or more independent variables.

Control Variable: This is the inputs and outputs that a control system manipulates and measures to keep proper control.

Decision errors
The decision errors associated with the null hypothesis:
- Type I error: Rejecting the null hypothesis when it is actually true.
- Type II error: Failing to reject the null when it is false.

Quasi-experiments

Quasi-experiments: The word "quasi" means as if or almost, so a quasi-experiment means almost a true experiment. There are many varieties of quasi-experimental research designs, and there is generally little loss of status or prestige in doing a quasi-experiment instead of a true experiment, although you occasionally run into someone who is biased against quasi-experiments. Some common characteristics of quasi-experiments include the following:
- Matching instead of randomization is used.
- Time series analysis is involved
- The unit of analysis is often something different than people

Of course, any type of research can study anything, for example, people, medicine, crime statistics. However, quasi-experiments are well suited for "fuzzy" or contextual concepts such as sociological quality of life, morale, climate, and nutrition. This kind of research is sometimes called contextual analysis.

Constructing a problem statement

Problems are stated in clear, unequivocal language, and are usually phrased as questions. Most problem statements contain at least two variables, with the exception of simple descriptive studies. Studies that contain only one variable, such as "How many African-American women breastfeed their babies?" do not gather much new information or extend the field of study. Problems must be testable, so that more than one answer is possible. Asking, "How can dietitians get patients with diabetes to adhere to their diet?" has limitless answers, and is not testable. Problems should not contain value-laden statements. Asking if something "should" be done is a cue that the problem contains a value judgment. Finally, the problem must follow standard grammatical rules and be free of error. Asking, "Do college students eat fewer vegetables?" is missing the part of the sentence that explains, "Fewer than whom?"

Constructing a hypothesis

A hypothesis provides the expected answer to the question posed by the researcher's question. A hypothesis is not just an educated guess, it is a rationalized prediction that may be based on the results of previous research, or it may have a theoretical basis that lends credence to an expectation of what will happen. Hypotheses should predict a relationship between the variables in the problem statement. They should not be so far-fetched as to be at odds with all previous research or theories. Like problem statements, hypotheses must be testable. Stating "Diets in wealthy families differ from diets in poor families" is too vague to be tested.

A null hypothesis states that there is no relationship between the variables. A directional hypothesis will use the phrases "more than" or "less than." A non-directional hypothesis predicts that there will be a relationship between variables without using quantifying language.

Types of studies

Randomized controlled studies

A randomized controlled study is one in which: There are 2 groups, 1 treatment group and 1 control group. The treatment group receives the treatment under investigation, and the control group receives either no treatment or some standard default treatment. Patients are randomly assigned to all groups.

Assigning patients at random reduces the risk of bias and increases the probability that differences between the groups can be attributed to the treatment. Having a control group allows us to compare the treatment with alternative choices. For instance, the statement that a particular medication cures 40% of cases tells us very little unless we also know how many cases get better on their own. With certain research questions, randomized controlled studies cannot be done for ethical reasons. For instance, it would be unethical to attempt to measure the effect of smoking on health by asking a group to smoke 2 packs a day and another group to abstain, since the smoking group would be subject to unnecessary harm. Randomized controlled trials are the standard method of answering questions about the effectiveness of different therapies.

Double-blind studies

A double-blind study is one in which neither the patient nor the physician knows whether the patient is receiving the treatment of interest or the control treatment. For example, studies of treatments that consist essentially of taking pills are very easy to do double–blind. The patient takes one of two pills of identical size, shape, and color, and neither the patient nor the physician needs to know which is which.

A double-blind study is the most rigorous clinical research design because, in addition to the randomization of subjects that reduces the risk of bias, it can eliminate the placebo effect, which is a further challenge to the validity of a study.

Cohort studies

A cohort study is a study in which patients who presently have a certain condition and/or receive a particular treatment are followed over time and compared with another group who are not affected by the condition under investigation. For instance, since a randomized controlled study to test the effect of smoking on health would be unethical, a reasonable alternative would be a study that identifies 2 groups, a group of people who smoke and a group of people who do not, and follows them forward through time to see what health problems they develop. Cohort studies are not as reliable as randomized controlled studies, since the 2 groups may differ in ways other than in the variable under study. For example, if the subjects who smoke tend to have less money than the nonsmokers, and thus have less access to health care, that would exaggerate the difference between the 2 groups. The main problem with cohort studies, however, is that they can end up taking a very long time, since the researchers have to wait for the conditions of interest to develop.

Case-control studies
Case-control studies are studies in which patients who already have a certain condition are compared with people who do not. For example of a case-control study would be a study in which lung cancer patients are asked how much they smoked in the past and the answers are compared with a sample of the general population. Case-control studies are less reliable than either randomized controlled trials or cohort studies. Just because there is a statistical relationship between two conditions does not mean that one condition actually caused the other. For instance, lung cancer rates are higher for people without a college education (who tend to smoke more), but that does not mean that someone can reduce his or her cancer risk just by getting a college education. There are 2 main advantages of case-control studies. First, they can be done quickly. By asking patients about their past history, researchers can quickly discover effects that otherwise would take many years to show themselves. Second, researchers do not need special methods, control groups, etc. They just take the people who show up at their institution with a particular condition and ask them a few questions.

Cross-sectional studies
Cross-sectional studies measure the prevalence of a disease or condition in a population during one point in time. Such studies may examine etiology, for example the relationship between alcohol consumption and the development of liver disease.

Sampling

Sampling allows researchers to draw conclusions about events without having to gather data on every possible event. In the context of sampling, a population is all of the events, and the sample contains the carefully selected events that the researcher will study. The goal of effective sampling is to choose events that will accurately represent the population. The size of the sample depends on the scope of the study and how much sampling error the researcher is willing to accept.

Random sampling is conducted so that any one event in the population has an equal chance of being included in the study. Random sampling is not done in a haphazard way; great care must be taken to ensure that all events have an equal chance of being selected. Random sampling is not always possible; for example, a researcher cannot decide to randomly assign some subjects to a group of people who have cystic fibrosis and other subjects to a group that does not have cystic fibrosis.

Test validity

A test is valid when it measures what it is supposed to. How valid a test is depends on its purpose, for example, a ruler may be a valid measuring device for length, but is not very valid for measuring volume. If a test is reliable, it yields consistent results. A test can be both reliable and valid, one or the other, or neither. Reliability is a prerequisite for measurement validity.

Types of validity
- Face validity: Does it appear to measure what it is supposed to measure? There would be low face validity when the researcher is disguising intentions.
- Content Validity: Is the full content of a concept's definition included in the measure? It includes a broad sample of what is being tested, emphasizes important material, and

requires appropriate skills. A conceptual definition can be thought of as the "space" that contains ideas and concepts.

- <u>Criterion Validity</u>: Is the measure consistent with what we already know and what we expect?
- <u>Construct Validity</u>: Shows that the measure relates to a variety of other measures as specified in a theory.

Internal validity: Internal validity means the researcher can conclude that the variable being studied is causing the observed effects. If a researcher cannot remove all of the potential sources of invalidity, then he or she should add equivocal statements to their conclusions, such as, "if…" or, "maybe…" Some sources of problems to internal validity include assigning subjects to experimental or control groups at will, subjects dropping out of the study before completion, or changes in the use of interviewers for who administer tests in different ways.

External validity: External validity means that the experimental results can be generalized to other populations. Researchers usually comment on the degree to which their findings are limited, and call for further study to expand on the application of test results to other groups. External validity can be compromised when subjects become sensitized to variables after taking a pre-test, or when groups are sampled in a way that does not make them representative of a larger population.

Test reliability

A sound study is expected to have measures that are reliable. A consistent measure produces the same results time and time again. Reliability can be numerically expressed as a coefficient that ranges from 0 (no reliability) to 1 (perfect reliability). A good measure should have a reliability coefficient of 0.8 or greater. There are several ways to assess the reliability of a test. Test-retest reliability involves running the same test multiple times, resulting in consistent scores. Parallel-forms technique involves administering different forms of the same test from a common group of measures, and determining the consistency between the two forms. Split-half reliability can be checked by dividing a test in two, administering the test, and checking the separate scores for consistency. Intercoder reliability examines the way different researchers will categorize the same behavior or response, given a check sheet.

Test sensitivity and specificity

Sensitivity and specificity are measures that assess the validity of diagnostic and screening tests. These measures reflect how well the test is detecting the disease and classifying individuals into disease and non-disease groups. Sensitivity (Se) describes how well the test detects disease in all who truly have disease, or the percent of diseased individuals who have positive test results. Specificity (Sp), on the other hand, describes how well the test is detecting non-diseased individuals as truly not having the disease, or the percent of non-diseased individuals who have negative test results.

Research reports

Research reports begin with an abstract, which is a summary of the study. The abstract may include a background, or rationale for conducting the study; the methods used to gather and analyze the data; the results of the study; and the conclusion. A general introduction follows where the researcher may share objectives, operationalize the definitions used, and provide a brief overview of the research that has preceded the current study. This may expand into a more extensive review of the literature that inspired the current study.

The methodology section will share the hypothesis of the researcher, what procedures were used to gather data, and what statistical analyses were used. Results are shared, along with any charts or diagrams that help to illustrate the findings. The discussion might share the researcher's ideas about why the study did or did not show what the author thought it would. The conclusion section sums up the results, and usually invites others in the field to expand on the study or replicate its results.

Pie charts

Pie charts illustrate the relationship or proportions of parts to the whole. A pie chart always contains one data series.

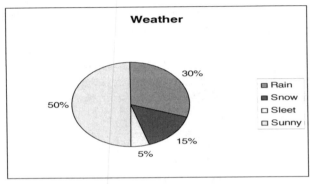

This pie chart is illustrating the precipitation in a given area for the entire year. It is sunny 50% of the year, it rains 30% of the year, it snows 15% of the year, and there is sleet 5% of the year.

Statistics

Descriptive statistics use numbers to characterize information. Examples include measures of central tendency, such as mean or median, and distributions, such as the standard normal curve. Inferential statistics use tools that allow the researcher to draw conclusions about populations from which the samples do not belong. Examples include analysis of variance and probability

Chi-square
Chi-square is a non-parametric test of statistical significance for bivariate tabular analysis (also known as crossbreaks). Any appropriately performed test of statistical significance lets you know the degree of confidence you can have in accepting or rejecting an hypothesis. Typically, the hypothesis tested with chi-square is whether or not 2 different samples (of people, texts, etc.) are different enough in some characteristic or aspect of their behavior that we can generalize from our samples that the populations from which our samples are drawn are also different in the behavior or characteristic.

A non-parametric test, such as chi-square, is a rough estimate of confidence; it accepts weaker, less accurate data as input than parametric tests (like t-tests and analysis of variance, for example) and therefore has less status in the pantheon of statistical tests. Nonetheless, its limitations are also its strengths; because chi-square is more "forgiving" in the data it will accept, it can be used in a wide variety of research contexts.

Spearman's rho:
Spearman's rho is a measure of the linear relationship between 2 variables.

ANOVA
Analysis of variance (ANOVA) performs comparisons like the t-test, but for an arbitrary number of factors. Each factor can have an arbitrary number of levels. Furthermore each factor combination can have any number of replicates. ANOVA works on a single dependent variable. The factors must be discrete. The ANOVA can be thought of in a practical sense as an extension of the t-test to an arbitrary number of factors and levels. It can also be thought of as a linear regression model whose independent variables are restricted to a discrete set.

T-test
The t-test compares means from two populations to each other to see if their difference is statistically significant. There are several applications and formulas for administering the t-test, depending on what the researcher is trying to ascertain. In the one sample t-test, a researcher may explore the reasons that a new sample mean is different from the known population mean if the population's standard deviation is not available for study. If the null hypothesis is rejected based on the results of this test, one might conclude that the new sample did not come from the original population. If one wishes to compare two independent, unrelated samples, a t-test for independent samples may be used. This formula allows the researcher to combine standard deviations from any two samples without taking an average, which would imply an order that does not exist.

Correlation coefficient (r)
Correlation is a measure of the degree to which variables have a relationship with one another, as shown with various mathematical formulas. Correlations are assigned values from -1.00 to 1.00. The closer the number is to -1 or 1, the stronger the relationship between the variables. The numbers can tell a researcher that either a direct relationship or an inverse relationship exists to some degree. A direct relationship means that as one variable increases or decreases, the correlating variable increases or decreases accordingly. Direct relationships are expressed as positive coefficients. An inverse relationship exists if an increase in one variable is accompanied by a decrease in the other variable, and vice versa. Inverse relationships are expressed as negative coefficients. It is important to remember that the negative sign does not mean an absence of correlation; a correlation of -0.92 is very strong.

The value of r is such that $-1 < r < +1$. The + and – signs are used for positive linear correlations and negative linear correlations, respectively.
- Positive correlation: If x and y have a strong positive linear correlation, r is close to +1. An r value of exactly +1 indicates a perfect positive fit. Positive values indicate a relationship between x and y variables such that as values for x increases, values for y also increase.
- Negative correlation: If x and y have a strong negative linear correlation, r is close to -1. An r value of exactly -1 indicates a perfect negative fit. Negative values indicate a relationship between x and y such that as values for x increase, values for y decrease.
- No correlation: If there is no linear correlation or a weak linear correlation, r is close to 0. A value near zero means that there is a random, nonlinear relationship between the 2 variables.

P value
The probability value (P value) of a statistical hypothesis test is the probability of getting a value of the test statistic as extreme as or more extreme than that observed by chance alone, if the null

hypothesis H_0, is true. It is the probability of wrongly rejecting the null hypothesis if it is in fact true. It is equal to the significance level of the test for which we would only just reject the null hypothesis. The P value is compared with the actual significance level of our test and, if it is smaller, the result is significant. That is, if the null hypothesis were to be rejected at the 5% significance level, this would be reported as " $P < 0.05$."

Small P values suggest that the null hypothesis is unlikely to be true. The smaller it is, the more convincing is the rejection of the null hypothesis. It indicates the strength of evidence for say, rejecting the null hypothesis H_0, rather than simply concluding "reject H0" or "do not reject H_0."

Standard deviation

Standard deviation is a measure of how much the scores vary from the mean. In the sample, the standard deviation is 3.76, indicating that the average difference between the scores and mean is around 4 points. The higher the standard deviation, the more different the scores are from one another and from the mean. Approximately 68% of the data points or observations will fall within 1 SD of the mean. Approximately 95% of the data points or observations will fall within 2 SD of the mean.

The standard deviation makes it possible for researchers to use the standard normal curve to identify unusual patterns that exist in their data distribution. The standard normal curve is the ideal data distribution one would achieve if perfect random sampling occurred. The curve visually explains the way that most data clusters around the average, and as one moves away from the average, fewer and fewer data can be found. The tails, or outlying pieces of data on the curve, never reach zero, but hypothetically go on forever. In this idealistic data distribution, the mean, median, and mode are all located at the peak in the center of the curve. At each point on the curve where the slope changes, or deviates, a line is dropped to the base to indicate a change. Each change in slope is called a standard deviation. Approximately two-thirds of the data will be contained in the first standard deviations above and below the mean.

Skewed distributions

A distribution is skewed if one of its tails is longer than the other. The first distribution shown has a positive skew. This means that it has a long tail in the positive direction. Distributions with positive skews are more common than distributions with negative skews. One example is the distribution of income. Most people make less than $40,000 a year, but some make quite a bit more with a small number making many millions of dollars per year. The positive tail therefore extends out quite a long way whereas the negative tail stops at zero.

Distribution forms: In the mathematically perfect standard normal curve, the mean, median, and mode are the same. In most real distribution forms, the data can take on several different patterns or "skews." When the distribution is skewed left, or negatively skewed, the tail of the curve extends to the left and the data hump is located on the right. If the skew is positive, or skewed to the right, the tail of the curve extends to the right and the data hump is on the left. In either type of skew, the mean is located closest to the tail, the mode is located closest to the data hump, and the median is in between. A bimodal curve will have two data humps, and the mean and median will be located between the humps.

Hawthorne effect

The Hawthorne effect is a phenomenon in group-based observational research. It is an effect on an outcome variable caused by the fact that the participants of the study know they are participating in the study.

The theory speculates that a process is improved by the psychological stimulus of those being singled out and made to feel important. In other words, if participants know they are a part of an experiment that can lead to improved efforts of the people involved, this creates a distortion of research results caused by the response of participants to the special attention they receive from researchers.

Important terms

Alternative Hypothesis (H_1): This is set up to deal with any other possibility besides that stated in the null hypothesis and thus the null and alternative hypotheses are mutually exclusive and exhaustive.

CARF - Commission on Accreditation of Rehabilitation Facilities

Experimenter bias: Expectations of an outcome may inadvertently influence participant or cause the experimenter to view data in a different way.

Focus group - a small group selected from a wider population and sampled, as by open discussion, for its members' opinions about or emotional response to a particular subject or area, used especially in market research or political analysis.

HCFA – Health Care Financing Agency

Morbidity rate - Can refer either to the incidence rate or to the prevalence rate of a disease.

Mortality rate - the number of people dying from a particular disease during a given time interval.

Null Hypothesis (H_0): This is the hypothesis that is tested and states that differences between a sample and the population (or another sample) is 0. Any observed difference is simply the result of sampling error.

OSHA - Occupational Safety and Health Administration

Parallel-forms: Two tests of different forms that supposedly test the same material will give the same results.

Placebo effect: Improvement due to expectation rather than the treatment itself; can occur when participants receive a treatment that they consider likely to be beneficial.

Selection bias: The sample is not representative of the population demographically.

Split-half reliability: If the items are divided in half (e.g., odd vs. even questions), the 2 halves give the same results.

Statistical regression: Tendency to regress towards mean makes scores higher or lower. If a measure is not extremely reliable, there will be some variation between repeated measures. The chances are that the measurements will move towards a mean instead of towards extremes.

Test-retest: A measure at 2 different times with no treatment in between will yield the same results.

Management Copncepts

This section is covered in detail under Domain III, Topic A – Functions of Management.

Nutrition Care for Individuals and Groups

Screening and Assessment

Nutritional screening

Nutritional screening determines the need for a nutritional assessment. The purpose is to see which patients are malnourished and who are at risk for malnutrition. The nutritional screen can be completed by any health care provider (e.g., diet tech, nurse, physician). Once it is completed, those patients who are at nutritional risk are referred to the registered dietitian. The Nutrition Screening Initiative (NSI) is a project developed to focus on and improve the quality of nutritional care available to elderly people. It includes social service, mental health, nutrition support, education, oral heath, and counseling.

Nutritional assessment

Nutritional assessment is a comprehensive approach that defines nutritional status using the following: medical, social, nutrition, and medication histories; physical examinations; anthropometric measurements and laboratory data. The purpose is to define nutritional status, determine what risk a patient is at (low, moderate, high), monitor changes in status, and determine if nutrition interventions need to be administered. A nutritional assessment precedes the care plan and intervention. From admit, you should allow 24 to 48 hours for assessment, then 3 to 5 days for the registered dietician (RD) to see patients for follow-up. The RD must talk to the patient; they cannot get everything from the chart.

Obtaining dietary information
- Diet history – a review of a person's usual patterns of food selection variables that determine food intake. May include previous diet changes, use of supplements, and food intolerances.
- Food record – also called food diary. It is a written record of the exact amounts of foods and liquids consumed during a specific period of time, usually between 3 to 7 days. It often includes time, place, and what was happening while eating.
- 24-hour recall – a method of estimating daily intake by asking a person to mentally recall what he/she has been eating in the last 24 hours.
- Food frequency lists – Data that are collected to determine how often a specific food or foods were consumed. This is often used in a community setting.

Body measurements
- Triceps skinfold is an anthropometric measurement that can be used to estimate an individual's body fat. A device called a caliper is used to pinch the skin and underlying fatty tissue without disturbing the muscle layer.
- Waist-to-hip ratio is indicative of the distribution of abdominal fat deposits. A WHR of greater than 1 in men or 0.8 in women indicates that the individual is at a higher risk for cardiovascular disease and diabetes.

- Arm muscle is an important measurement used in children to assess whether the child has an adequate skeletal muscle mass. If a growing child is not receiving enough carbohydrates in the diet, protein that would otherwise be used to build muscle mass is burned as energy.
- Body mass index is a formula that can be used to screen for the presence of excess adipose tissue that may cause weight-related problems. The formula is weight (kg) / [height (m)]^2.

Tricep skinfold: Triceps skinfold (TSF) measures body fat reserves and calorie reserves. Calipers measure the thickness of the triceps at mid-portion of the non-dominant arm. Three measurements are taken, and then averaged. Standard results: male 12.5 mm; female 16.5 mm. Invalidate if: Total body edema or when upper body is edematous, or when individual is > 150 % IBW. Hydration is also a source of error.

Waist to hip ratio: Waist to hip ratio (WHR) is the ratio of the waist measurement to the hip measurement. It is used for assessing fat distribution in a person. It allows us to determine if a patient has android obesity or gynoid obesity. WHR for men > 1 or > 0.8 for women is an indicator for android obesity. This means that the person is at an increased risk for obesity-related diseases such as heart disease or diabetes.

Midarm muscle circumference: Measures skeletal muscle mass (somatic protein). Three MAC are taken, and then averaged. Standard results: men: 25.3 cm; female: 23.2 cm. Obesity = >90th percentile. Nutritional Risk = < 40th percentile.

Midarm muscle circumference (MAMC) (cm) = midarm circumference (MAC) (cm) – TSF (mm)

Invalidated if: Total body edema or when body is edematous, or when individual is > 150 % IBW.

Body mass index: Weight is often evaluated by looking at it in relation to height, using the body mass index (BMI). To calculate BMI:
- Multiply your weight (in pounds) by 705.
- Multiply your height (in inches) by itself, that is, square it.
- Divide the result of step 1 by the result of step 2.

Here's an example of a woman who is 5'9" and weighs 160 pounds. First, multiply 160 by 705 to get 112,800. Then, multiply her height, which is 69 inches, by itself to get 4,761. Dividing 112,800 by 4,761 gives a BMI of 25.5. According to the National Institutes of Health (NIH), this BMI level indicates that the woman is just a bit above normal weight.

Interpreting results:
- < 18.5 = underweight
- 18.5 to 24.9 = normal
- 25 to 29.9 = overweight
- > 30 = obese
- > 40 morbid obesity

Limitations to BMI: Overestimates body fat in muscular people. Underestimates body fat in some underweight people because they have lost lean muscle mass. BMI of 24 to 29 is still a healthy weight for most elderly people.

Biochemical measurements

- Albumin is the most prevalent protein in the plasma. Normal values should range between 3.5 and 5 g/dL. Anything below normal values may be a sign of liver cirrhosis, diabetic kidney disease, or anorexia.
- Transferrin is the protein responsible for carrying iron through the body's blood to allow for heme synthesis. The amount of iron available that can be bound by plasma can be used to estimate this value.
- Hemoglobin is present in red blood cells in normal amounts ranging from 11 to 17 gm/dL. Hemoglobin by itself is not an adequate measure of iron deficiency, because it is only affected later in the disease process and values can vary widely in healthy individuals.
- Blood urea nitrogen is present in the body as a waste byproduct of protein breakdown. Normal values range from 10 to 20 mg/dL, and can be affected by protein intake. Dialysis lowers BUN amounts in renal patients.

Estimating height

- Arm Span measurement: Measure the distance between the tip of one middle finger to the tip of the other middle finger OR measure the distance between the tip of the middle finger to mid-sternum on the dominant hand and times that number by 2. This method is an acceptable alternative, but it must be charted as estimated weight.
- Knee height stature: Measure from the bottom of the heel to the anterior surface of the thigh at the knee. The knee should be at 90 degree angle.
- Adult recumbent height: Start from head and inch down to heel.
- Children younger than 24 months: Measure the child lying down. If they can't stand alone by over 24 months, then you can measure lying down up to 36 months. Growth chart is used for recumbent length up to 36 months.

Criteria set

A criteria set is a series of statements developed by a body of professionals that guide the practitioners in their pursuit of the provision of quality care. Professional organizations such as the American Dietetic Association or the Dietary Managers Association may develop their own statements that describe the structures, processes, and outcomes the organization feels a professional should adhere to in order to provide high quality products or services. The structures discussed in criteria sets may include a description of the quality standards found in the workplace environment, policies, accounting methods, or employee-related factors. The processes described in criteria sets may describe best practices or benchmarking procedures the profession uses to accomplish clinical activities such as delivery of care, or the chronology of events, such as the steps necessary to conducting a successful catering event. Outcomes are described in criteria sets as measurable success or failure resulting from the process, such as improvement in health status.

Weight measurements

- <u>ABW</u> – actual body weight. This is what should be taken at admit.
- <u>UBW</u> – usual body weight; what a person weighs at normal circumstances, not when sick.
- % UBW = actual weight / usual weight x 100.
  - 85% to 95% = mildly malnourished.
  - 75% to 84% = moderately malnourished.
  - < 74% = severely malnourished.
- <u>% Weight loss</u> = (usual wt – actual wt) / usual wt x 100.

- IBW – ideal body weight, found by using the Hamwi formula:
  - ➤ 106 + 6 x (inches over 5 ft) = IBW for men.
  - ➤ 100 + 5 x (inches over 5 ft) = IBW for women.
- %IBW = ABW / IBW x 100.

Anthropometrics in children

Recumbent length
Reflects long-term nutritional adequacy. Infants and children younger than 2 or 3 years of age. Plot on a growth chart.

Weight
Reflects recent short-term nutritional adequacy. It is a more sensitive measure. Children who are between the 10th and 90th percentile on the growth chart are considered normal weight. Those children who are < 10th or > 90th percentile are at risk. The curve might change with neglect, abuse, or illness.

Head Circumference
Indicator for nonnutritional abnormalities. Used for children younger than 3 years of age.

Laboratory tests

Prealbumin
Prealbumin is more sensitive than albumin. It is the best visceral protein to analyze. It quickly responds to decreased energy intake. It is sensitive to protein and calories, so it is a good indicator of how medical nutrition therapy is working. It is not an indicator of low protein intake in chronic renal failure on dialysis because protein is being pulled out through the dialysis process. A decrease in value is seen in inflammation, surgical trauma, stress, and cirrhosis. Normal Value = 19 to 43 mg/dL

Serum albumin
Serum albumin (visceral protein) is the indicator for chronic malnutrition because of the slow turnover. It indicates protein status over the past 3 months. It is a poor indicator of protein depletion. It is a strong indicator of morbidity and mortality in hospital patients. It responds well to protein depletion. An increase in serum protein values is seen with growth hormones or steroids. Normal Value = 3.5 to 5 g/dL

Tests for anemia
Hemoglobin (Hgb): Iron containing oxygen carrying protein in the blood.
Increased with dehydration. Decreased with anemia, cancer antigen (CA), renal, cirrhosis, and chronic infection. Normal Values: Males, 14 to 17 g/dL; females, 12 to 15 g/dL; pregnancy, $\geq$ 11 g/dL.

Hematocrit (Hct): The percentage of packed cells in the volume of whole blood. Increased with hydration, diabetic ketoacidosis (DKA), trauma, surgery and burns. Decreased with anemia, CA, renal, chronic infection. Normal values: males, 40% to 54%; females, 36% to 47%.

Mean corpuscular hemoglobin (MCH): A measurement of the average weight of hemoglobin in red blood cells. Increased with macrocytic anemia. Decreased with microcytic anemia. Normal: 26 to 34.

Mean corpuscular volume (MCV): A measurement of individual cell size. Increased with macrocytic anemia. Decreased with microcytic anemia.

Glucose

Glucose is an energy source that is formed from the digestion of carbohydrates and conversion of glycogen by the liver. Normal range is 70 to 110 mg/dL fasting. Increased with diabetes, acute stress, severe infection, surgery, burns, chronic steroid use. Decreased with hypoglycemia, malnutrition, liver damage, postgastrectomy, and bacteria sepsis. Normal range for diabetes mellitus = 80 to 120 mg/dL fasting.

Lymphocyte assessments

Lymphocytes assess immune competence and are expressed as a percentage. White blood cells are expressed in thousands (a white blood cell count (WBC) of 17 is actually 17,000)). Total lymphocyte count (TLC) = lymphocytes x WBC. Normal range for TLC is 3,000 to 5,000. TLC can be affected by infection, steroid therapy, CA, chemo, radiation, or surgery.

Example: WBC = 17 and lymphocyte = 10%
TLC = 17,000 x 0.10 = 1,700

Conditions that increase TLC:
Leukemia, infectious disease of bacteria origin, leukocytes.

Conditions that decrease TLC:
Anesthetics, aging, CA, chronic obstructive pulmonary disease (COPD), corticosteroids, stress, chemo, radiation, surgery.

Renal function assessments

Blood urea nitrogen (BUN)
Related to protein intake. Indicator of renal disease. Normal value = 10 to 20 mg/dL. Increased with renal failure, chronic heart failure, dehydration, a high protein diet, and protein catabolism.

Creatinine
Related to muscle mass. Measures somatic protein. Indicator for renal disease. Normal value = 0.6 to 1.4 mg/dL. Increased with renal failure, muscle loss, surgery, trauma, chronic heart failure, and diabetes. Both are elevated in renal disease. Increased BUN and normal creatinine = dehydration.

Laboratory tests affecting hydration

Normal values
Na^+: 135 to 147 mEq/L
K^+: 3.5 to 5 mEq/L
BUN: 10 to 20 mg/dL

Dehydration
Elevated BUN
Decreased K^+

Overhydration
Decreased Na+ and BUN

Patient counseling

Interviewing

In the context of patient counseling, the interview is a chance to obtain complete information from the patient about his or her eating habits, and it can reveal other social, cultural, environmental, or socioeconomical issues that will affect the patient's willingness or ability to take part in the counseling. The first step is to collect factual data, such as age, weight, and height, giving the client time to become comfortable with the interview process. Open-ended questions are important, as this gives the patient the opportunity to expand upon his or her answer and provide information the interviewer might not otherwise have received.

Instead of, "Are you watching your fat grams?" say, "Describe your typical breakfast/lunch/dinner." If the client pauses frequently, avoid leading them to an answer in order to move the interview along. Summarize what you heard and note at the end of the interview to give the client a chance to correct any errors, and tell him or her how you will use the information that was gathered.

Nonverbal communication: Kinesics refers to the movement of any body part that is done in a communicative way. For example, affective displays add emotion to what is being said. This can vary widely across cultures. A member of one culture may shake his or her fist in anger, while an equally angry person from another culture may sit with their arms folded across their chest. Regulators are kinesic nonverbal communication methods that keep the flow of conversation moving. Sometimes the interviewer may mistake nodding of the head for understanding, when the person is just politely agreeing with what is said.

Paralinguistics refers to anything that can differ about one's speech except the words themselves. Features such as volume, rate, and pitch can reveal anxiety, fear, or irritation.

Proxemics: The term proxemics was introduced by anthropologist Edward T. Hall in 1963 to describe the measurable distances between people as they interacted. Hall pointed out that social distance between people is reliably correlated with physical distance, and described 4 distances:
- Intimate distance for embracing, touching, or whispering (15 to 45 cm, 6 to 18 in).
- Personal distance for interactions among good friends (45 to 120 cm, 1.5 to 4 ft).
- Social distance for interactions among acquaintances (1.2 to 3.5 m, 4 to 12 ft).
- Public distance used for public speaking (over 3.5 m, 12 ft).

Principle: Nonmaleficence ("do no harm"). The dietitian has a duty to refrain from harming the patient.

This principle expresses the concept that professionals have a duty to protect the patient from harm. Under this principle, the dietitian's primary obligations include keeping knowledge and skills current, knowing one's own limitations and when to refer to a specialist or other professional, and knowing when and under what circumstances delegation of patient care to auxiliaries is appropriate.

Nutrition assessment of a particular population

The rationale for the Nutritional Assessment of Populations is to gain an understanding of the biological, cultural, and environmental factors that contribute or take away from the nutritional status of communities determined to be at risk. The program also seeks to assess how well existing programs are serving the health needs of the community and how problem areas identified in the assessment process can be addressed so that health is enhanced.

Research relies on a variety of epidemiologic and anthropologic methods applied to areas that are deemed to be socially or economically depressed. The tools that serve as sources of information include assessment of growth and physical activity of the population; the existence and utilization of social services such as WIC, school foodservice programs, and free health clinics; analysis of socioeconomic factors coming from data on public housing usage or census data; and demographics, morbidity, and mortality rates.

Food security

Food security is a term coined by the Food and Agriculture Organization of the United Nations to assess the level of access to food. It does not assess the nutritional status of individuals; rather, it describes a state in which people have adequate access to food in order that they may lead healthy lives. Furthermore, the access should be through socially approved channels of acquisition, such that individuals do not have to resort to scavenging or stealing.

Insecurity: When taking a census of households affected by hunger, food-insecure individuals are those considered to have inconsistent or limited access to the food that would allow them to lead healthy, active lives. People may be considered to be food insecure with hunger or food insecure without hunger. The difference is concerned with the quality and quantity of food consumed: those with hunger experience a decrease in these measures.

Community Food Security Initiative: The Community Food Security Initiative (CFSI) is the USDA's response to the problem of food insecurity in the United States. The goal of this program is to reduce hunger by 50% by the year 2015 by utilizing grassroots efforts and local government agencies to improve nutrition, increase the efficacy of local food programs, and help low-income families help themselves. Local organizations may be awarded federal grants to assist in this endeavor. An example may be a small community lacking a grocery store: grants and partnerships may help farmers in the community market their produce directly to the community. Food recovery programs may redistribute to the community foods from institutions or restaurants that might otherwise be discarded. Social service agencies that focus on helping under- or unemployed individuals are also targeted to help families rise above the poverty line and achieve self-sufficiency.

Nutrition Screening Initiative

The Nutrition Screening Initiative (NSI) helps elderly individuals in the United States at risk for compromised nutritional status by identifying those at risk because of their financial, social, or functional status. It also considers one's access to food. The "DETERMINE" acronym can be used to describe the list of factors health care providers or social service agencies look at when determining risk:
D- Disease
E- Eating Poorly
T- Tooth loss or mouth pain
E- Economic hardship

R- Reduced social contact
M- Multiple medications
I- Involuntary weight loss or gain
N- Needs assistance in self care
E- Elder years older than 80

The benefits of the screening tool include ease of use and ability to identify patients in need of more comprehensive screening. Limitations include the tool's dependency on patient's ability or willingness to cooperate.

National Health and Nutrition Examination Survey

The National Health and Nutrition Examination Survey (NHANES) is a program of studies under the guidance of the CDC's National Center for Health Statistics. The program, which began in the 1960s, uses a combination of interviews and physical examinations to assess the health and nutritional status of adults and children in the United States.

The survey examines about 5,000 people each year, the survey process is continuous, and the focus of the survey changes each year to look at different populations and emerging issues in health and nutrition. The interview process includes demographic, socioeconomic, and nutritional intake questions. The exam includes a variety of physiological and laboratory tests administered by trained medical personnel, such as hemoglobin or cholesterol levels. The medical conditions that are studied may include anemia, diabetes, renal disease, obesity, and others. Survey results are used to further epidemiological and health science research, and findings are used to develop responsive public health policy and increase the nation's health knowledge.

Third National Health and Nutrition Examination Survey: The Third National Health and Nutrition Examination Survey (NHANES III), 1988–1994, contains data for 33,994 persons 2 months of age and older who participated in the survey. This survey looked at the effects of nutrition on aging. There was no upper age limit in this survey and the survey included a large number of individuals older than 65 years of age.

USDA's Healthy Eating Index

The Healthy Eating Index is the USDA's tool designed to assess how well Americans are eating based on the federal government's dietary guidelines. Points ranging from zero to 20 are assigned to each dietary component according to how compliant the individual has been with following the recommendation. For example, when assessing the whole grain category, with the standard for maximum score being consumption of 1.5 oz or more per 1,000 kcal consumed, zero points are assigned to "no whole grains," and 5 points are assigned for meeting the standard. Compliance in all areas earns a score of 100. The Healthy Eating Index tool can be useful in monitoring nutrition and conducting research and consumer education.

Nutrition surveillance systems

The CDC has 2 major programs in place to monitor the health and nutritional status of low-income women, infants, and children. The Pediatric Nutrition Surveillance System (PedNSS) uses data from the Women, Infants, and Children program (WIC), the Early and Periodic Screening, Diagnosis, and Treatment (EPSDT) Program, and the Title V Maternal and Child Health Program. Data are analyzed to discover trends in birth weight, anemia, breastfeeding, stature, and other nutrition-related indicators. The goal of the program is to use this surveillance data to implement and evaluate existing health programs and formulate public policy.

The Pregnancy Nutrition Surveillance System (PNSS) looks at maternal health and nutritional status of low-income women, but is more concerned with maternal nutrition as it relates to the outcome of the infant. Data on maternal weight gain, prenatal vitamin intake, and pregnancy-related complications such as diabetes are evaluated in the context of birth outcomes such as preterm delivery and low birth weight. Results are used to guide public health policy.

Special needs populations

Migrants: The lifestyle of migrants provides several challenges for nutritional assessment and intervention. The families move from season to season, making continuity of care difficult. The public health systems they utilize do not communicate across communities, so medical records and other health documents need to be transported with the patient. Language and cultural barriers can interfere with nutrition education and counseling. Nutrition education may focus on issues specific to the group, such as prenatal care and diabetes services.

Homeless: Individuals experiencing homelessness frequently have mental health issues that interfere with their ability to seek social services available to them. Emergency food programs may not provide balanced nutrition, and many programs are ill-equipped to meet the needs of infants and children. Homeless families who qualify for WIC may not have the transportation to reach the provider. For homeless individuals who do not routinely use shelters, storage and proper preparation of food is an issue.

Prevalence

Prevalence is the measure of a condition in a population at a given point in time (referred to as point prevalence). Prevalence can also be measured over a period of time (e.g., a year). This second type of prevalence is called period prevalence; it is a combination of point prevalence and incidence. Prevalence data provide an indication of the extent of a condition and may have implications to the provision of services needed in a community.

Formula:

$$\frac{\text{\# existing cases *}}{\text{population at risk *}}$$

*During a specified time period.

Incident Cases

An incident case can be determined based on the first occurrence in the data of a condition (e.g., first diagnosis) or of an event representing the condition. True incidence is often difficult to get since access to earlier data that might contain an indication of the condition may not be available.

Formula:

$$\frac{\text{\# new cases *}}{\text{population at risk *}}$$

*During a specified time period.

Native American and Alaskan native populations

As Native Americans and Alaskan natives have traded traditional foods such as deer meat and buffalo for foods high in calories and saturated fat such as hamburger and fast foods, the population has seen an obesity epidemic. Accompanying obesity-related diseases such as diabetes, heart disease, and hypertension have risen accordingly. Limited food availability on reservations can also contribute to intake patterns. Processed meats and sugar-sweetened drinks are popular mainstays in many reservation markets, while fresh produce is often limited. Baby bottle tooth decay is another nutritional problem that affects a large number of both Native Americans and Alaskan Natives. Prolonged bottle use is common and sugar-sweetened drinks are offered throughout the day. Although fluoridated water is available, drinking water may be obtained from rainwater or wells, with drinking water saved for other household use. Native Americans and Alaskan natives have higher rates of alcohol abuse, which contributes to the malabsorption of several nutrients, as well as liver disease.

Diagnosis

Nutrition care plan

The nutrition care plan (NCP) is designed to meet changing nutritional needs. The process may be initiated by the referral of a doctor who discovers a patient experiencing or at risk for nutrition-related problems. The methods used in this type of care require the use of critical thinking and problem-solving skills. The process is made up of assessment of nutritional status, diagnosis of nutritional needs or problems, implementation of interventions necessary to meet care objectives, and monitoring and evaluation of the nutritional care. The rationale of the NCP is to give dietitians a common structure and method to promote better decision making and to obtain data that may be evaluated quantitatively and qualitatively. The process also serves to validate the care provided by dietitians and allows for continual improvement in the nutrition care cycle.

The care plan should specify the objectives, the areas of content, and a tentative time frame. It consists of 5 steps:
1. Assess the nutritional status of the individual by using the ABCD's (anthropometrics, biochemical data, clinical, and dietary).
2. Organize (analyze the data to identify nutritional needs or problems.
3. Plan and prioritize the objectives to meet the nutritional needs of the individual.
4. Implement the plan.
5. Evaluate the effectiveness of the plan.

Critical thinking skills
Dietitians should think about verbal or nonverbal cues the patient provides so that they can tailor their interview appropriately. When thinking about which data to collect and which tools to use, the information gathered should be accurate, appropriate to the patient, and interpreted using only those tools and methods pertinent to the situation. Types of data collected should be relevant to the situation and may cover such broad concerns as health, nutritional, functional, and behavioral status.

Documentation
Documentation should be organized and should exclude information that does not help to identify nutrition-related problems or concerns. The screening and assessment should also help the dietitian identify when consultation with other health care providers is needed. The NCP process does not end with the initial screening but is an ongoing process that may require repeated assessments until a reason for discharge or discontinuation of therapy is reached.

SOAP note: SOAP is a method for charting legal documents of nutrition care provided. It is a comprehensive assessment regarding nutritional support or nutrition education for patients/family, written communication regarding nutritional goals of therapy, and documentation for reimbursement.
- S = Subjective. Information provided by the patient, family, or caretaker on diet history, current dietary intake and habits, previous diet education.
- O = Objective. Factual information such as age and gender, height, weight, admitting diagnosis and significant medical history, tests results, diet order, medications, calculation of nutrient needs.

- A = Assessment. Interpretation of current weight status, statement of perceived nutritional status, assessment of lab data and diet order, expected compliance, and anticipated problems.
- P = Plan. Goals, recommendations, referrals.

Diet order: Diet prescribed by the physician. It needs to be written very specifically. The diet manual is a book compiled by dietitians that describes the foods allowed and restricted on specific diets. It outlines the rationale and indications for use of each diet, and provides sample menus.

Nutrition diagnosis

When charting a patient's nutrition diagnosis the dietitian should describe the problem in standardized language that includes the problem, etiology, signs, and symptoms (PESS).
- In order to write the problem, a dietitian must use an approved diagnostic label. This is a statement that includes an adjective to capture how the patient deviates from the desired state of health. Examples include "altered mental status," "impaired bowel function," "chronic renal failure," or "at risk of liver cirrhosis."
- The next step is to define the etiology, or the cause/contributing risk factors that contribute to the problem. The appropriate way to chart this is to use the language "related to." Contributing factors in etiology may be physical, situational, cultural, developmental, or anything found to be an underlying cause of the problem.
- The last step is to chart the signs and symptoms present in the patient. This may include findings from lab tests, anthropometric measures, or descriptions given by the patient.

Nutrition diagnostic labeling

Clinical domain
When conducting a nutrition diagnosis, the dietitian may identify nutritional problems in the patient that relate to the medical problem the patient is experiencing; this is not to be confused with a medical diagnosis. The clinical domain encompasses 3 classes: functional balance, biochemical balance, and weight balance:
- Functional balance problems can be physical or mechanical and interfere with one's ability to achieve normal nutritional status, for example, inability to chew.
- Biochemical balance represents a loss of the ability to metabolize foods normally, because of medicine, surgery, or a disease process. An example would be the malabsorption of short bowel syndrome.
- Weight balance describes involuntary weight changes that deviate from the patient's normal or desired body weight. This includes excessive weight loss or gain.

Intake domain
The intake domain of nutrition diagnosis includes problems related to the ingestion of energy, vitamins, minerals, and fluids, whether the patient receives nutrition orally, enterally, or parenterally. This domain encompasses 5 classes of concern:
- Calorie energy balance is used to describe observed or potential changes in energy expenditure, due to diagnoses such as anorexia, dialysis, trauma, or other conditions that can place one in catabolic or anabolic state.
- Oral or nutrition support intake is described as adequate or excessive compared with the goal.

- Fluid intake balance is also described as adequate or excessive compared to the goal. This can be significant in many disease processes of the kidney, where fluid intake is strictly regulated.
- Bioactive substance charting gives the dietitian an opportunity to chart miscellaneous substances ingested by the patient, such as vitamin supplements or alcohol.
- Nutrient balance expands on the patient's use of vitamin or mineral supplements by examining the practice of ingesting large amounts of single nutrients, as is sometimes done with vitamin C.

Behavioral-environmental domain

The behavioral-environmental domain describes problems or findings that relate to a patient's knowledge, attitudes, beliefs, environment, food safety, or access to food. Knowledge and beliefs may encompass cultural practices that are harmful to one's nutritional status, such as the Native American's practice of feeding sugar-sweetened beverages in bottles to young children, leading to dental decay.

Examples of concerns in the class of physical activity balance and function might include an elderly person no longer able to prepare food, or a sedentary person whose inactivity places him or her at risk for obesity.

Food safety and access encompasses problems related to the ability to obtain the foods needed to maintain good nutrition and the ability to store and prepare food safely. A homeless person unable to refrigerate foods would be described in this category.

Diagnostic related groupings

The DRG is a classification of more than 500 illness categories into which a patient is placed when he or she is hospitalized. The illnesses are further categorized by organ system, and this grouping plays a large factor in determining how hospitals will be reimbursed for the services they render. The system assumes that patients with similar disorders will have a similar disease process, and will therefore require similar treatments and services. It is significant to note that hospitals receive the same amount of reimbursement per DRG, regardless of how many days the patient was hospitalized or how many/what kinds of services were rendered. Critics argue that health care providers may not be able to perform as many services as they deem necessary; or conversely, that they will be pressured to perform unnecessary but profitable services. Quality control is overseen by the Peer Review Organization, which uses explicit criteria to assess the appropriateness of services provided.

Nutrient requirements

Dietary Reference Intakes
Dietary Reference Intakes (DRIs) are reference values used to estimate nutrient intakes to be used for planning and assessing diets for healthy people. The DRI is a type of umbrella term that includes EARs, RDAs, AIs, and ULs.

Estimated Average Requirement
An Estimated Average Requirement (EAR) is the level of a nutrient estimated to meet the requirement of half the healthy people in a life stage and gender group. Of course, at this intake level, 50% of the group would not meet its nutrient needs. The EAR is used to evaluate the adequacy of nutrient intake in groups and to develop RDAs.

Nutrient's RDA

A nutrient's RDA is the average daily intake that is sufficient to meet the nutrition requirement of nearly all (97% to 98%) individuals in a life stage and gender group. The RDA is based on the EAR plus an added amount.

Adequate Intake

Adequate Intake (AI) is used instead of the RDA if sufficient scientific evidence is not available to calculate an EAR. The AI is based on estimates of average nutrient intake in 1 or more groups of healthy people.

Tolerable Upper Intake Level

The Tolerable Upper Intake Level (UL) is the highest level of daily nutrient intake that is likely to pose no risk of adverse health effects to almost all people in the general population. The higher the intake of a nutrient at levels above the UL, the greater the risk of adverse side effects. Even though there may not be enough evidence to establish a UL for every nutrient, an excessive intake of that nutrient may still cause negative side effects.

Dumping syndrome

Dumping syndrome is when food is dumped into the small intestine directly from the esophagus. It usually occurs following a gastrectomy using the Billroth I or Billroth II procedures. Dumping syndrome is a group of symptoms that occur after eating. Symptoms include increased heart rate, nausea, diarrhea, flushing, sweating, and weakness. It is more likely to occur with simple sugars.
- Billroth I: partial removal of the stomach and reattachment to the duodenum.
- Billroth II: partial removal of the stomach, but duodenum is passed and reattached to the jejunum.

Nutrition recommendations: Many small meals (6), restricted simple carbohydrates, high protein, moderate fat, have fluids before or after meal, B_{12} injections (anemia can occur). Medium chain triglycerides may be helpful if steatorrhea is present.

Peptic ulcer disease

An ulcer is a circumscribed loss of tissue on the surface of the mucosa or the skin. It can extend through the mucosa, submucosa, and sometimes to the muscle. Peptic ulcer occurs in any area that is exposed to pepsin and acid. It can be with either gastric (stomach), esophageal, duodenal, or jejunal. Only 15% of peptic ulcers occur in the stomach. Duodenal ulcers are the most common at 85%. One of the most common causes of peptic ulcers is *H. pylori* infection. These spiral-shaped bacteria inhabit the GI tract around the pyloric valve.

Nutrition recommendations: Small, frequent, well-balanced meals as tolerated. High protein, vitamin C for healing. Limit gastric stimulants if not tolerated. Avoid pepper, chili powder, alcohol, excess caffeine, and late-night snacks. Primary goal is tissue healing and maintenance of healthy tissue.

Sprue

Nontropical

Celiac disease is an example of a nontropical sprue. It is also called gluten-induced enteropathy. It is caused by a reaction to gliadin, the alcohol-soluble component of gluten, which affects the jejunum and ileum (not the stomach). The damage to the intestines leads to malabsorption of almost all nutrients, including fat-soluble vitamins.

Nutrition recommendations: Gluten-restricted diet: no wheat, rye, oats, barley, bran, graham, or malt. Substitute corn, potato, rice, soybean, tapioca, and arrowroot.

Tropical

Tropical sprue is a chronic GI disease of unknown etiology that causes diarrhea and malabsorption. Malabsorption can lead to B_{12} deficiency and folate deficiency because of decreased HCL and intrinsic factor. A big difference between the 2 types of sprues is that a tropical sprue can also affect the stomach.

Nutrition recommendations: High calorie, high protein, B_{12}, and folate supplements.

Nontropical sprue, or celiac sprue, occurs when gliadin, a component of gluten, damages the villi of the small intestine. The resulting damage can affect the absorption of all nutrients. Atrophy and flattening of the villi reduce the amount of surface area available for nutrient absorption, especially in the proximal bowel. Cells in the villi also lack the enzymes needed for digestion and the carriers needed to transport nutrients in the bloodstream. Symptoms can be severe in extensive disease because of the wide-ranging effects of the nutrient losses, and can include anemia because of iron deficiency, hemorrhage due to vitamin K losses, muscle cramps and tetany due to calcium depletion, and osteoporosis due to impaired vitamin D absorption. Freedom from symptoms may be achieved following a gliadin-free diet, making wheat, rye, barley, and oats off limits.

Tropical sprue is also a disorder that damages intestinal villi, but is much less severe than celiac sprue. Control of the disease is achieved following administration of tetracycline and folate therapy.

Lactose intolerance

Lactose intolerance is due to lactase deficiency and is the most common carbohydrate intolerance. Lactase is the enzyme that digests lactose (sugar in milk) into glucose and galactose. When this does not happen, the lactase stays intact and remains in the gut, allowing water to be drawn into the intestines. This leads to distention, cramps, and diarrhea. Bacteria can then ferment the undigested lactose, causing carbon dioxide and hydrogen gas to be released. A lactose tolerance test is used to detect the deficiency. A person takes an oral dose of lactose (1 qt or 50 g) after a fast. If the person is intolerant to lactose, the blood glucose from the lactose increases less than 25 mg/dL above fasting. If they are tolerant to lactose, the blood glucose will rise above 25 mg/dL.

Nutrition recommendations: Lactose-free diet. Calcium and riboflavin supplements because of the lack of animal products. Yogurt and cheese may be tolerated, but only in small amounts

Vitamin deficiency

Neutrophil hypersegmentation
One of the earliest clinical signs of both folate and vitamin B_{12} deficiency is hypersegmentation of neutrophils. Deficiency should be suspected when greater than 5% of cells have 5 or more lobes or when any 6-lobed cells are seen within a random sample of 100 cells. Hypersegmentation may also occur in uremia, myeloproliferative disorders, myelofibrosis, and as a congenital lesion in 1% of the population.

Short Gut Syndrome
Patients with an absence of the terminal ileum should be evaluated for fat-soluble vitamin and fat malabsorption by measurement of either serum beta-carotene concentration and/or 72-hour quantitative fecal fat. Patients with resected ileum are at risk for vitamin B_{12} malabsorption requiring intramuscular or aerosol supplementation and periodic serum vitamin B_{12} monitoring.

Vitamin B_{12} deficiency
Plasma vitamin B_{12} is the available test for evaluating vitamin B_{12} stores. Plasma vitamin B_{12} will be elevated in myeloproliferative disorders and hepatic tissue damage. A low plasma vitamin B_{12} is almost always indicative of deficiency. Vitamin B_{12} deficiency can result from either dietary deficiency or impaired absorption. Pernicious anemia, inadequate secretion of intrinsic factor, achlorhydria, a history of gastric or ileal resections, or diseases associated with malabsorption (e.g., Crohn disease) may cause impaired vitamin B_{12} absorption. The Schilling test can be used to distinguish insufficient secretion of intrinsic factor from malabsorption syndromes. In this test, radioactive B_{12} is taken orally, and its urinary excretion is measured over 24 hours. A flushing dose of unlabeled B_{12} is given with the labeled B_{12} to saturate liver storage and enhance labeled B_{12} excretion. Normally, greater than 7% of the labeled B_{12} is recovered in the urine. If absorption is low, it is necessary to repeat the test with administration of intrinsic factor.

One of the earliest clinical signs of both folate and vitamin B12 deficiency is hypersegmentation of neutrophils.

Deficiency should be suspected when greater than 5% of cells have 5 or more lobes or when any 6-lobed cells are seen within a random sample of 100 cells. Hypersegmentation may also occur in uremia, myeloproliferative disorders, myelofibrosis, and as a congenital lesion in 1% of the population.

Iron deficiency

To confirm iron deficiency as a cause of microcytic anemia, it is recommended to first evaluate the zinc protoporphyrin/heme ratio (ZPP/H). ZPP/H is an inexpensive screening test for iron deficiency. Zinc protoporphyrin is produced during heme synthesis in the developing erythron when iron availability is limited, thus iron deficiency is characterized by an increase in the ZPP/H. Confirmation of iron deficiency following an elevated ZPP/H (greater than 80 mcmol/mol) requires determination of serum ferritin. Ferritin concentration of less than 20 ng/mL is considered iron deficient. Both ZPP/H and serum ferritin can be elevated by chronic inflammation. Under conditions of chronic inflammation, a serum ferritin less than 70 ng/mL may be considered iron deficient. ZPP/H can also be elevated in lead toxicity and protoporphyria (a rare congenital disease). Serum iron, total iron binding capacity (TIBC), and % transferrin saturation may also be used in the diagnosis of iron deficiency; however, these tests are less predictive of iron stores. Percent saturation is very useful in evaluation of iron overload.

Marasmus syndrome

Calorie deficiency
Criteria:
1. Wt < 80% of desirable body weight (DBW) or wt loss > 10% in last 6 mo.
2. Serum albumin > 3 g/dL (relatively preserved visceral proteins).
   ↳ *blood PR*

Characterized by gradual loss of fat and muscle tissue, lethargy, and weakness. Nitrogen losses decrease to 2 to 4 g/d as fat and ketone utilization increases.

Kwashiorkor syndrome

"Nutritional" edema with dyspigmentation of skin and hair.
Criteria:
1. Wt > 90% of DBW.
2. Serum albumin <3 g/dL.

Characterized by edema, fatty liver, muscle catabolism, weakness, neurologic changes, and dyspigmentation. Found almost exclusively in the tropics and associated with famine, infection, and markers of inflammation. Not simply due to deficient protein intake. (Sometimes inappropriately used to describe hypoalbuminemia postoperatively or with catabolic illness.)

Protein-calorie malnutrition

Protein-calorie (energy) malnutrition (PEM), moderate to severe.
Criteria:
1. Wt < 80% of DBW or > 10% wt loss in last 6 mo (edema may mask wt loss).
2. Serum albumin often < 3 g/dL.

The moderate to severe forms of PEM typically are associated with exposure to stress and may include edema, hypercatabolism, poor wound healing, and increased risk for infection. In stressed metabolism, hormonal and cytokine signals promote acute phase protein synthesis but net proteolysis, altered immune responses, accelerated gluconeogenesis, and lipolysis. Urinary nitrogen losses are often > 15 to 20 g/d. Elevated resting energy expenditure (hypermetabolism) may also be present.

Pregnancy

Weight gain
A proper diet and adequate weight gain during pregnancy are essential for good health of the mother and optimum development of her baby. If a mother doesn't gain enough weight, her baby may be born small. On the other hand, if weight gain is excessive, the baby may grow too large. This could complicate the birth process and increase the risk of problems during pregnancy. Pregnant patients should gain 5 lbs in the first trimester, and approximately 1 lb/wk in the second and third trimesters. The appropriate weight gain during a pregnancy depends on several factors, including mother's pre-pregnant weight and age. A woman who is of average weight is encouraged to gain somewhere between 25 and 30 pounds during pregnancy. Underweight women need to gain a bit more weight, and high weight women a bit less. No one should ever try to lose weight during pregnancy. Maternal weight loss results in excess blood ketone levels. Ketones are toxic to fetuses.

High Risk Conditions

- Diabetic mothers: Severity of affects on the infant is affected by severity of disease. Hypoglycemia can occur in infants after birth within 1.5 to 4 hours. Drug exposed-narcotics readily cross the placenta, caused by maternal infection (especially viral during early gestation).
- T-Toxoplasmosis, O-other (hepatitis, parvovirus,...), R-Rubella, C-Cytomegalovirus, H-Herpes simplex virus
- Mothers who smoke: Significant birth weight deficit and lower Apgar score. Developmental delays, passive smoking at home increases sudden infant death syndrome (SIDS), respiratory infections, and deficits in learning.
- *Fetal alcohol syndrome (FAS):* Fetal alcohol effects show cognitive, behavioral, and psychosocial problems without facial dysmorphia and growth retardation. This is a leading cause of intellectual disability. Early diagnosis and treatment are beneficial.

Lactation

Human lactation has 4 phases that differ in the composition and volume of milk produced: colostral, transitional, mature, and involutional. Colostrum is secreted for the first 3 to 5 days after delivery, transitional milk until the end of the second week, mature milk during full lactation, and involutional milk at the end of lactation.

Notably, colostrum is rich in secretory immunoglobulin A (IgA), lactoferrin, vitamin A, and sodium compared with mature milk but has relatively low concentrations of fat, lactose, and vitamin B_1. Involutional milk is characterized by low lactose content and high concentrations of protein, fat, and sodium. Because milk volume is low during the colostral phase, rising slowly during the first week to the higher levels of established lactation, the daily intake of most milk components by breastfed babies increases after birth, reaching a peak after several weeks. The exception is secretory IgA and, hence, total protein intake, which is maximal in the first week. Mature breastmilk composition also changes during the course of lactation, although not as markedly as in the early weeks. Many nutrients show a gradual decrease in concentration of around 10% to 30% during the first year of lactation, often reaching a low plateau thereafter. Some components show little change, including lactose and sodium, whereas a few, notably lysozyme, increase.

Burn management

3 Phases of Burn Management:

The Emergent Phase, Resuscitative
Lasts from onset to 5 or more days but usually lasts 24 to 48 hours; begins with fluid loss and edema formation and continues until fluid motorization and diuresis begins. Basal metabolic rate (BMR) increases 50% to 100%

Arrhythmias, hypovolemic shock, which may lead to irreversible shock. Circulation to limbs can be impaired by circumferential burns and then the edema formation. Escharotomies (incisions through eschar) done to restore circulation to compromised extremities.

Acute Phase
Begins with mobilization of extracellular fluid and subsequent diuresis. Is concluded when the burned area is completely covered or when wounds are healed.

Rehabilitative

May take weeks or months. Patient is no longer grossly edematous because of fluid mobilization, full and partial thickness burns more evident, bowel sounds return, patient more aware of pain and condition. Needs high levels of protein, vitamin K and C, and zinc

The pathological condition of T3/T4

Both are stimulated by TSH release from the pituitary gland:
- T4 control basal metabolic rate.
- T4 becomes T3 (active form) within cells.
- T3 radioimmunoassay: Check T3 levels.
- Hyperthyroidism: T3 increased, T4 normal (in many cases).

Medications that increase levels of T4
Methadone, Oral contraceptives, Estrogen, Cloffibrate.

Medications that decrease levels of T4
Lithium, Propranolol, Interferon alpha, Anabolic steroids, Methiamazole.

Hypothyroidism

Hypothyroidism is poor production of thyroid hormone.
- Primary -- Thyroid cannot meet the demands of the pituitary gland.
- Secondary-- No stimulation of the thyroid by the pituitary gland.

Causes:
Surgical thyroid removal, irradiation, congenital defects, Hashimoto thyroiditis (key).

Symptoms:
Constipation, weight gain, weakness, fatigue, hoarse vocal sounds, joint pain, depression, muscle weakness, poor speech, color changes.

Tests:
Decreased BP and HR, Chest x-ray, Elevated liver enzymes, prolactin, and cholesterol, decreased T4 levels and serum sodium levels, presence of anemia, low temperature, poor reflexes.

Treatment:
Increase thyroid hormone levels, levothyroxine, weight reduction plan, decreased BMR.

Nephrotic syndrome

The nephrotic syndrome is defined by:
Proteinuria: greater than 3 g per 24 h in adults
0.05 g/kg per 24 h in children.
Hypoalbuminemia, with albumin concentration less than 30 g/L edema, which is periorbital and in the upper limbs
This triad is commonly accompanied by hyperlipidemia.

Points worth consideration are:
In severe cases of nephrotic syndrome, the proteinuria may be less than 3 g per 24 h: in these cases, the levels of plasma proteins are low.
With increasing age patients are more vulnerable to severe proteinuria and hypoalbuminemia. The level of hypoalbuminemia at which edema develops varies between individuals and with age. Other measures of renal function, such as urea and creatinine, are usually normal.
Renal failure may develop.

Although the nephrotic syndrome has long thought to be due to protein loss resulting in a low albumin and low plasma oncotic pressure, patients may have a normal or increased plasma volume.

Diverticulitis

Abnormal pouch formation that becomes inflamed in the intestinal wall.

Symptoms: Fever, Diarrhea, Nausea, Vomiting, Constipation
Tests: Barium enema, WBC count, Colonoscopy, CT Scan
Sigmoidoscopy
Clear liquids diet progressing to high fiber.
Note: low-fiber diets can cause constipation.

Gestational diabetes

Gestational diabetes (GDM) is defined as glucose intolerance of variable degree with onset or first recognition during the present pregnancy. It can be screened by drawing a 1-hour glucose level following a 50 g glucose load, but is definitively diagnosed only by an abnormal 3-hour oral glucose tolerance test (OGTT) following a 100 g glucose load. The growth and maturation of the fetus are closely associated with the delivery of maternal nutrients, particularly glucose. This is most crucial in the third trimester and is directly related to the duration and degree of maternal glucose elevation.

The (American Diabetes Association (ADA) recommends that all pregnant women, who have not been identified with glucose intolerance earlier in pregnancy, be screened with a 50 g 1-hour glucose challenge test (GCT) between 24 and 28 weeks of pregnancy.

Cystic Fibrosis

CF is an inherited disease caused by an abnormal protein that does not allow the normal passage of chloride (which, along with sodium, makes up salt) into and out of certain cells, including those that line the lungs and pancreas. As a result, these cells produce thick, sticky mucus and other secretions. The mucus clogs the lungs, causing breathing problems. The thickened digestive fluids made by the pancreas are prevented from reaching the small intestine, where they are needed to digest food. Individuals with CF tend to cough and wheeze frequently.

They may develop repeated lung infections, such as pneumonia. Many of these infections are caused by a bacterium called Pseudomonas aeruginosa, which rarely causes problems in healthy people. Many, but not all, children and adults with CF have digestive problems due to blockage of digestive chemicals from the pancreas. Affected children often have a big appetite, but gain weight or grow slowly.

CF is a condition of malabsorption and pancreatic enzyme deficiency. Treatment includes a high-calorie, high-protein, and unlimited fat diet.

Pancreatitis

Pancreatitis may occur when gallstones are blocking the pancreatic duct. The common bile duct and the pancreatic duct join at the ampulla of Vater. At the ampulla of Vater, both of these structures empty into the small bowel. Thus, if stones in the bile duct block the pancreatic duct, gallstone pancreatitis may result. The endocrine function reflects the secretion of hormones, primarily insulin, into the bloodstream. The exocrine function is to aid in digestion. The pancreas secretes a combination of pancreatic enzymes and bicarbonate that are mixed with bile in order to digest food. When the pancreas becomes inflamed, it is called pancreatitis. The enzymes that usually aid in digestion begin to digest the pancreas. Thus, as its own enzymes digest the pancreas, more enzymes are released into the pancreas. This continues to inflame the pancreas and causes complications of pancreatitis. Acute pancreatitis may be related to alcohol, gallstones, medications, or surgery.

No food should be given throughout the upper GI in acute cases. Chronic pancreatitis occurs after there have been repeated injuries to the pancreas. It is perplexing that approximately one-third of all causes of acute pancreatitis are due to unknown causes. Limit fatty foods and alcohol in chronic conditions.

HIV and AIDS

H - Human: because this virus can only infect human beings. I - Immunodeficiency: because the effect of the virus is to create a deficiency, a failure to work properly, within the body's immune system. V - Virus: because this organism is a virus, which means one of its characteristics is that it is incapable of reproducing by itself.

Some people newly infected with HIV will experience some "flu-like" symptoms. These symptoms, which usually last no more than a few days, might include fevers, chills, night sweats and rashes (not cold-like symptoms). Other people either do not experience "acute infection," or have symptoms so mild that they may not notice them. When immune system damage is more severe, people may experience opportunistic infections (called opportunistic because they are caused by organisms that cannot induce disease in people with normal immune systems, but take the "opportunity" to flourish in people with HIV). Zidovudine (AZT) is a common drug used for HIV. HIV-infected mothers should not breastfeed. Patients with HIV should be on a high protein, high calorie plan.

Addison disease

Addison disease is an endocrine or hormonal disorder that occurs in all age groups and afflicts men and women equally. The disease is characterized by weight loss, muscle weakness, fatigue, low blood pressure, and sometimes darkening of the skin in both exposed and nonexposed parts of the body. Addison disease occurs when the adrenal glands do not produce enough of the hormone cortisol and, in some cases, the hormone aldosterone. The disease is also called adrenal insufficiency, or hypercortisolism. Cortisol's most important job is to help the body respond to stress. Among its other vital tasks, cortisol helps maintain blood pressure and cardiovascular function, helps slow the immune system's inflammatory response, helps balance the effects of insulin in breaking down sugar for energy, and helps regulate the metabolism of proteins, carbohydrates, and fats.

Aldosterone helps maintain blood pressure and water and salt balance in the body by helping the kidney retain sodium and excrete potassium. When aldosterone production falls too low, the kidneys are not able to regulate salt and water balance, causing blood volume and blood pressure to drop. Diet should be high salt and protein with frequent feedings.

Phenylketonuria

In phenylketonuria (PKU), phenylalanine is not broken down into tyrosine because of an enzyme deficiency. This results in build up of phenylalanine and other metabolites, which can lead to severe intellectual disability if not treated by diet therapy. Most newborns are screened at birth using the Guthrie blood test, and those with a positive result should be screened again by checking for elevated phenylalanine levels in the blood and urine to confirm the diagnosis. Low phenylalanine formula and evaporated milk products should provide 90% of the protein needs of infants and toddlers.

Classical PKU is an autosomal recessive disorder, caused by mutations in both alleles of the gene for phenylalanine hydroxylase (PAH), found on chromosome 12. In the body, phenylalanine hydroxylase converts the amino acid phenylalanine to tyrosine, another amino acid. Mutations in both copies of the gene for PAH means that the enzyme is inactive or is less efficient, and the concentration of phenylalanine in the body can build up to toxic levels. In some cases, mutations in PAH will result in a phenotypically mild form of PKU called hyperphenylalanemia. The diet should limit the amount of subtrate or (PHE) and patients should avoid aspartame.

Phenylalanine-containing foods may be slowly offered as long as the blood phenylalanine content is checked frequently and remains below 10 mg/dL. Energy intake should be carefully regulated, especially in times of increased need such as illness. If tissue catabolism occurs because of insufficient energy intake, the protein breakdown will cause phenylalanine levels to rise in the blood.

Rheumatoid arthritis

Rheumatoid Arthritis: inflammatory autoimmune disease that affects various tissues and joints.

Symptoms
Fever, fatigue, joint pain and swelling, range of motion (ROM) decreased, hand/feet deformities, numbness, skin color changes

Tests
Rheumatoid factor tests, C-reactive protein, Synovial fluid exam, X-rays of involved joints, Erythrocyte sedimentation rate (ESR) increased.

Treatment
Physical therapy, moist heat, anti-inflammatory drugs, Corticosteroids, anti-malarial drugs, COX-2 inhibitors, Splinting. Not treated with supplements. Normal balanced diet.

Cerebral palsy

Cerebrum injury causing multiple nerve function deficits.

Types
Spastic cerebral palsy (CP) 50%, Dyskinetic CP 20%, Mixed CP, Ataxic CP.

Symptoms
Poor respiration status, intellectual disability, spasticity, speech and language deficits, delayed motor and sensory development, seizures, joint contractions.

Tests
Sensory and motor skill testing, check for spasticity, CT scan/MRI, EEG.

Treatment
PT/OT/ST, surgery, seizure medications, spasticity-reducing medication. Spastic CP should have diet high in fiber and fluid, but low calorie. Dyskinetic or athetoid CP should have high protein, and calorie diets.

GERD

Gastroesophageal reflux disease (GERD); Reflux esophagitis.

Pathology
Decreased tone with smoking, alcohol, fatty meals. Reflux worse with obesity, pregnancy, impaired gastric emptying, prone positioning and peristaltic dysfunction.

Clinical
Heartburn typical, cough or hoarseness (irritation larynx) less common. Often asymptomatic, dissociation between symptoms and degree of reflux, prolonged exposure (especially nocturnal) -> mucosal damage. Damage can include ulceration, erosion, and Barrett metaplasia (intestinal metaplasia)

Histology
Squamous epith replaced by columnar cell glandular mucosa.

Diagnosis
pH monitoring.

Treatment
Decrease acid, alter diet, raise head of bed, surgery.

Achalasia

Achalasia is a motor disorder of the esophagus characterized by complete loss of peristalsis. The exact cause of achalasia is unknown; several theories exist regarding loss of nerve endings or loss or hormones. The symptoms are somewhat similar to GERD, thus patients may be treated for reflux before the diagnosis of achalasia is made. Maybe be characterized by patients putting their arms above their heads to get food to go down, heartburn, regurgitation, and chest pain. Most patients will experience weight loss, and some may present with complications such as inhalation of debris from their esophagus. The diagnosis of achalasia may be suspected by barium x-ray or by endoscopy.

Barium studies will show a dilated esophagus down to a "bird beak" at the level of the lower esophageal sphincter (LES). Upper endoscopy is performed to exclude cancer as a cause of blockage. The primary diagnosis, however, is based on the lack of peristalsis documented on manometry. Manometry may also show a failure of the LES to relax with swallowing. Since there is currently no treatment for the loss of peristalsis, treatment focuses on removing the resistance of the LES.

Anorexia

People with anorexia starve themselves, avoid high-calorie foods, and exercise constantly. Anorexia may also cause hair and nails to grow brittle. Skin may dry out, become yellow, and develop a covering of soft hair called lanugo. Mild anemia, swollen joints, reduced muscle mass, and light-headedness also commonly occur as a consequence of this eating disorder. Severe cases of anorexia can lead to brittle bones that break easily as a result of calcium loss.

Bulimia

Bulimia is characterized by episodes of binge eating followed by inappropriate methods of weight control (purging). Inappropriate methods of weight control include vomiting, fasting, enemas, excessive use of laxatives and diuretics, or compulsive exercising. A binge is an episode where an individual eats a much larger amount of food than most people would in a similar situation. It is usually a response to depression, stress, or self-esteem issues.

Signs/Symptoms:
Eating uncontrollably, purging, strict dieting, fasting, vigorous exercise, vomiting, or abusing laxatives or diuretics in an attempt to lose weight, vomiting blood, using the bathroom frequently after meals, preoccupation with body weight, depression or mood swings, feeling out of control, swollen glands in neck and face, heartburn, bloating, indigestion, constipation, irregular periods, dental problems, sore throat, weakness, exhaustion, bloodshot eyes.

Food Allergies

Usually, the gastrointestinal system and the immune system provide a barrier to proteins that have the ability to interact with the immune system and cause an allergic response. Foreign substances, or antigens, are cleared from the body by the immune system's macrophages, T lymphocytes, and B lymphocytes. The B lymphocytes play an important role in food allergies. These cells produce antibodies specific to antigens encountered in the body. Five types of antibodies are recognized: IgG, IgM, IgD, IgA, and IgE. When IgE antibodies bind with the allergen in special cells in the intestine, skin, and respiratory tract, chemicals are released that begin what is recognized as an allergic reaction. Histamine, bradykinin, and serotonin can cause abdominal pain, coughing, or itching in mild reactions; anaphylaxis, shock, and death can occur in severe cases. The symptoms can begin within seconds of ingesting the offending food or up to 2 hours later. Common culprits include eggs, fish, wheat, soy, peanuts, and milk.

There is no catchall test used to diagnose food allergies, so several tests are usually done to pinpoint the offender. A diet history is taken to determine the symptoms, a list of foods that were ingested around symptom development, duration between consumption and symptom development, and family history of allergies. A 2-week food and symptom diary provided by the patient is helpful.

The skin prick test is a reliable immunologic test that cannot be used alone, but can help narrow down suspicious foods to use in a food challenge. A welt larger than 3 mm from a skin test is useful for children older than 3 years of age; younger children may not have positive skin test reactions to allergens.

A double-blind food challenge can help to identify multiple food allergies. The food is administered in capsule form, along with a placebo, and neither the patient nor the health care professional knows which capsule has been offered until the end of the test.

Hirschsprung disease

Hirschsprung disease (congenital megacolon). People with Hirschsprung disease lack the nerve cells that enable intestinal muscles to move stool through the large intestine (colon). Stool becomes trapped in the colon, filling the colon and causing it to expand to larger than normal. Hirschsprung disease is also called megacolon. It is a congenital disease, which means a person is born with it. The disease may also be hereditary, which means a parent can pass it to a child.

Hirschsprung disease affects mainly infants and children. Although symptoms usually begin within a few days after birth, some people do not develop them until childhood or even adulthood. In infants, the primary symptom is not passing meconium, an infant's first bowel movement, within the first 24 to 48 hours of life. Other symptoms include constipation, abdominal swelling, and vomiting.

Symptoms in older children include passing small watery stools, diarrhea, and a lack of appetite. Physicians diagnose Hirschsprung disease through rectal manometry, a lower gastrointestinal series, and rectal biopsy. Colostomy is the most effective treatment for Hirschsprung disease.

Pancreatitis

The pancreas has cells that fall into the endocrine or exocrine category of functioning. The endocrine pancreas produces insulin, and the exocrine pancreas manufactures enzymes that help to digest carbohydrates, fats, and proteins in the intestine. Pancreatitis is an inflammation of the pancreas characterized by accumulation of pus in the intracellular space, fat necrosis, and edema. Pancreatitis can be acute or chronic, mild or severe enough to cause total loss of function. Symptoms can range from mild stomach discomfort to severe abdominal pain, shock, or even death. Diagnostic tests that may assess pancreatic function include checking for increased serum amylase levels, secretin stimulation test, 72-hour stool fat test, and glucose tolerance test.

The exact cause is unknown but a leading contributing factor is alcoholism. The flow of pancreatic juice can be blocked, causing digestive juices to begin digesting the pancreas itself. Enzymes can also leak from the pancreas and begin to digest surrounding tissues.

Nutritional management for pancreatitis
The painful symptoms of pancreatitis flare up when pancreatic enzymes and bile are stimulated by the ingestion of food. When an individual is suffering from acute, severe pancreatitis, all oral nutrition should cease and hydration should be given intravenously. Forty-eight hours after the absence of severe symptoms clear liquids may be introduced slowly as tolerated. If the patient is

unable to tolerate even a prescribed liquid diet containing a small amount of fat, glucose, and amino acids, parenteral nutrition is needed. In moderate attacks, several small meals a day with a very low fat content may be offered. Chronic pancreatitis is characterized by failure of inflammation to subside or recurrent attacks. Large meals, high-fat foods, and alcohol should be avoided. Over a period of several years, the function of the pancreas may deteriorate to the point that enzyme replacement is necessary. The enzyme Pancrease can be given after meals to decrease the presence of fat in the stools.

Cystic fibrosis

Cystic fibrosis is an inherited disease that involves a malfunction of the exocrine glands. This results in the production of thick, mucous-like secretions that obstruct the airway, pancreatic ducts, and ducts in other organs. Thick plugs block the pancreas from releasing digestive enzymes into the small intestine. This results in a cascade of negative effects, beginning with the malabsorption of all of the major nutrients. The excess mucous functions to further interfere with absorption. Damage to the pancreas over time can lead to diabetes. Patients may have poor oral intake due to shortness of breath and coughing, pain, weight loss accompanying infections, and impaired sense of smell.

Enzyme replacement therapy is offered to control nutrient malabsorption. Calorie requirements are 120% to 150% of the RDA. High-calorie snacks and larger portions at mealtimes should be offered. Fat malabsorption may require supplementation of fat-soluble vitamins. Sodium intake should be liberal to compensate for excess amounts lost in sweat.

Atherosclerosis

A large body of research supports the link between serum cholesterol levels and the incidence of cardiovascular disease. Cholesterol is absorbed in the small intestine and transferred to the liver, where lipoprotein lipase (LDL) removes the triglycerides for use by cells.

LDL is the also the main transport vehicle for cholesterol and triglyceride in the circulation. High-density lipoproteins (HDL) contain less cholesterol than LDL. LDL helps to transport cholesterol into the arterial walls. HDL seems to offer a protective effect, suggesting that HDL removes cholesterol from the arterial walls, or perhaps takes cholesterol away from the liver before LDL can deposit it in arterial plaques. So while cholesterol associated with LDL and HDL transport is often classified as bad or good, it is actually the mechanism of the protein rather than the cholesterol itself that has positive or negative effects on the circulatory system. Lipoprotein ratios considered to be at risk include LDL above 130 mg/dL and HDL below 35 mg/dL, or total cholesterol above 200 mg/dL.

LDL > 130   HDL < 35   Total > 200

Dietary modifications

The dietary recommendations for atherosclerotic disease focus on the effects of fatty acid intake and cholesterol on serum cholesterol, especially the less desirable LDL. A desired outcome is to reduce total cholesterol to less than 200 mg/dL and LDL cholesterol to less than 130 mg/dL. This can be achieved in part by monitoring serum cholesterol; following a low-fat, low-cholesterol diet; and prescribing medication as needed. A patient who adheres to the recommendation of less than 30% of kcal from fat and less than 10% of kcal from saturated fatty acids may see an average reduction in cholesterol of at least 30 mg/dL. If saturated fats are reduced to less than 7% of kcal, cholesterol may be lowered an additional 15 mg/dL. Depending on the individual's need for weight loss, the servings can be adjusted to meet kcal needs of 1,200 to 2,500. Low-fat sweets and snacks are included to make the adjustment to a permanent lifestyle change easier.

Hypertension

Hypertension is defined as a systolic blood pressure of 140 or greater and a diastolic blood pressure of 90 or greater. Blood pressure levels are managed in the body by a variety of mechanisms, including the volume of fluid in the vascular system, the contractions of the heart pushing the blood through the blood vessels, and the strength of the muscular walls of the arterioles. Several organs work in coordination to maintain normal blood pressure levels, including the kidney, heart, and nervous system.

If the kidney is unable to excrete excess sodium, the elevated sodium and water levels in the blood cause an increased plasma volume. The increase in sodium in cells may also cause a rise in calcium in the vessel musculature, increasing rigidity and raising pressure. Obese persons have a higher risk for hypertension, perhaps due to the increased insulin levels triggering the kidneys to increase sodium reabsorption.

Management

The standard pharmacological approach for the management of hypertension is the administration of diuretics and antihypertensive drugs. Diuretics can lower the volume of fluid in the circulation and decrease sodium in the body. However, potassium loss can be an unwanted effect of treatment with thiazide diuretics, increasing the possibility of hypokalemia. Additional potassium should be given unless potassium-sparing drugs are used. Conservative treatment for mild cases of hypertension includes using weight loss, low-sodium diet, alcohol reduction, and aerobic exercise. Even moderate weight loss can reduce the activity of the sympathetic nervous system, which plays a big role in blood pressure management. Reducing sodium intake to less than 1500mg/day or less can help the individuals who are truly salt sensitive; in others it may help the medications work more effectively. Limit intake of high-fat foods. Try baking or broiling rather than frying. Limit alcohol. Overconsumption contributes to weakening of the heart muscle and to hypertension. Follow the DASH diet. The DASH diet was designed to prevent high blood pressure, but it's also low in fat. The DASH diet is based on a 2,000 calories/day meal plan and is a salt-restrictive plan.

Dietary Interventions for Hypertension

Limit salt. Most medical experts recommend salt-sensitive persons limit salt to 2,000 mg/day. Watch out for "hidden" salt, found in butter flavorings, seasonings, tomato sauces, condiments, and canned foods. Patients should check with their health care practitioner before using a salt substitute.

Limit intake of high-fat foods. Try baking or broiling rather than frying.

Limit alcohol. Overconsumption contributes to weakening of the heart muscle and to hypertension.

Follow the DASH diet. The DASH diet was designed to prevent high blood pressure, but it's also low in fat. The DASH diet is based on a 2,000 calories/day meal plan and is a salt-restrictive plan.

Congestive heart failure

Congestive heart failure is the result of a long process of deterioration in which the heart loses its ability to function normally. The organ may be able to function in the early stages of disease by enlarging and increasing pulse rate. When normal blood circulation can no longer be maintained, patients experience shortness of breath, chest pain, and changes in blood pressure, causing increased resorption of sodium and edema in the legs. Decreased blood flow to the brain can also cause altered mental status, headache, and anxiety.

Edema can disguise the disease in assessment by making typical anthropometric measures inaccurate. Dietary history and mid-upper arm circumference are appropriate tools. CHF patients experience decreased circulation to the kidneys, which allows sodium and fluid to accumulate in tissues. A low-sodium diet and diuretics are needed to prevent further heart damage and to relieve edema. Use of diuretics can deplete potassium. Potassium supplementation may prevent digitalis toxicity.

Cholesterol management

The Adult Treatment Panel (ATP) III is the National Cholesterol Education Program's clinical guidelines for cholesterol testing and management. The program periodically updates its ATP reports based on advances in cholesterol research, and the third report focuses on prevention of coronary heart disease in people with multiple risk factors.

This report informs health practitioners that elevated LDL cholesterol levels are the main contributing cause to heart disease. The first step in prevention is determining the individual's risk, with a complete lipoprotein profile for all adults older than 20 years of age being recommended. LDL cholesterol levels below 100 are optimal. Smokers, hypertensive people, diabetics, and those with a family history of CHD have the highest risk and should strive for optimal levels. The program recommends reducing saturated fat and cholesterol intake, exercise, and weight control. The therapeutic lifestyle diet (TLC) calls for increased fiber intake (10 to 25 g/day), lowered saturated fat intake (less than 7% calories), and lowered cholesterol intake (less than 200 mg/day). Moderate physical activity and maintaining normal body weight are also advocated.

Kidney disease

As necessary, the kidney functions to maintain a balance of fluids, electrolytes, and organic solutes by continuously filtering the blood and secreting or reabsorbing substances. The end result of this filtering process is the generation of approximately 1.5 liters of urine each day. The functioning unit of the kidney is the nephron, which consists of a glomerulus connected to a series of tubules. The tubules can further be described by segments as the proximal convoluted tubule, the loop of Henle, the distal tubule, and the collecting duct. The glomerulus is a mass of capillaries surrounded by a membrane, and it functions to produce large amounts of ultrafiltrate similar in composition to blood. The tubules reabsorb the majority of the components of ultrafiltrate, producing the final urine product. The kidney has other functions apart from urine production, including blood pressure regulation, erythropoietin production, and maintaining calcium-phosphorus balance.

Hormones related to kidney function

Vasopressin: Vasopressin is produced in the pituitary gland but one of its primary mechanisms of action involves the kidney. The hormone is released when plasma volume is reduced, meaning that the body is moving into a state of dehydration. Vasopressin acts as an antidiuretic, signaling the kidneys to concentrate the urine and therefore conserve water.

Renin: Renin is a hormone that plays a major role in blood pressure regulation. Decreased blood volume stimulates the glomerulus cells in the kidney to release renin, which then forms the substance angiotensin in the plasma. Angiotensin triggers sodium reabsorption by acting as a vasoconstrictor and by stimulating the adrenal gland to secrete aldosterone, thus returning blood pressure to normal.

Erythropoietin: Erythropoietin is a hormone released by the kidney that plays a critical part in the formation of red blood cells in the bone marrow. A deficiency of this hormone can cause severe anemia in those suffering from renal disease.

Nephrotic syndrome

Nephrotic syndrome describes a group of diseases that have loss of the glomerular barrier to protein in common. This leads to large albumin protein losses in the urine, the consequences of which include edema, high cholesterol, abnormal bone metabolism, and abnormally thick blood. Some diseases that commonly account for this syndrome include diabetes and lupus. The goal of dietary management is to replace the proteins lost from the plasma through the urine. Protein intake should be high enough to reduce edema and increase the albumin level in the plasma. Protein should range from 0.8 to 1 g/kg per day, with the majority coming from sources with a high biologic value to ensure optimal use. Edema usually indicates a state of sodium overload in the body. However, because of the hypoalbuminemia in these patients, the volume of blood is actually reduced. Therefore, edema cannot be totally controlled and sodium restriction should be modest.

The nephrotic syndrome is defined by:
- Proteinuria: greater than 3 g per 24 h in adults, 0.05 g/kg per 24 h in children.
- Hypoalbuminemia, with albumin concentration less than 30 g/L edema, which is periorbital and in the upper limbs.
- This triad is commonly accompanied by hyperlipidemia.

Nephrolithiasis

Nephrolithiasis, or kidney stones, can form when the concentration of calcium salts, uric acid, cystine, or other salts reach a high enough concentration to cause crystallization. The problem tends to recur, so patients may benefit from a metabolic assessment to help identify the underlying problem. The most common stones are calcium oxalate stones, usually occurring in middle-aged men. Causes may include hyperparathyroidism, hypercalciuria, and hyperoxaluria. The over-absorption of oxalate is commonly seen in Crohn disease, celiac sprue, and excessive supplementation of vitamin C. A low-oxalate diet combined with calcium supplements, which bind the oxalate, provides relief. Patients with stones resulting from hypercalciuria may have problems with increased absorption of calcium, impaired renal absorption of calcium, or excessive resorption of calcium from the bones. Treatment in these patients includes 1.5 to 2 liters of fluid a day and thiazide diuretics to decrease urinary calcium. Patients with uric acid stones can be managed with an alkaline diet to raise urine pH, and adequate fluid intake.

Chronic renal failure

Once three-quarters of kidney function is lost, eventual renal failure is inevitable, resulting in end-stage renal disease (ESRD). Most ESRD patients lost their kidney function because of diabetes, glomerulonephritis, or hypertension. As the kidney becomes unable to excrete urine, maintain fluid balance, or secrete hormones, uremia results. This is a condition of nitrogen waste accumulation marked by nausea and vomiting, weakness, muscle cramps, a BUN above 100, and a creatinine over 12.

Treatment of ERSD involves kidney transplant or dialysis. Dialysis methods include peritoneal dialysis or the more common hemodialysis. The goals of nutritional care include maintaining adequate energy and nutrient status, controlling edema and electrolyte imbalance, and preventing kidney-related bone disease.

Sodium in the diet should be adjusted to urinary sodium and fluid excretion, usually 3 g/day. Dialysis drains body protein, so intake should be adjusted upwards from 1.2 to 1.5 g/kg of body weight, depending on dialysis type. Calcium intake should be high and phosphorus intake low to avoid worsening the hyperparathyroidism, phosphate retention, and hypocalcemia of renal failure.

Acute renal failure

Acute renal failure (ARF) is characterized by the sudden loss of previously healthy kidneys to process urine. The symptoms can include a decrease in or cessation of urine production, edema, altered mental status, nausea or vomiting, metallic taste in mouth, hypertension, tremors, or seizures. Many conditions can cause acute kidney damage, including burns, trauma, infection, urinary tract obstruction, or clotting of the blood vessels in the kidney.

Limit fluid intake according to the amount of urine the patient can produce. If no urine is being produced or hyperkalemia occurs, dialysis may be necessary. In patients with chronic renal failure, the goal is to minimize toxicity or prevent further degradation of renal status; in ARF, extra nutrition is required to aid in wound healing and support the immune system. Protein needs can range from 1.2 to 1.5 g/kg body weight for catabolic patients. The hyperkalemia and hyperphosphatemia associated with ARF should be addressed by providing 8 to 15 mg/kg of phosphorus, and 2 to 3 g of potassium, depending on serum levels and whether dialysis is necessary.

Descending and Ascending Aspects of the Loop of Henle

Because the descending limb is highly permeable to water, water moves by osmosis here. It moves out of the tubule and into the medullary interstitial fluid for reabsorption. The descending limb epithelial cells just do not have the protein channels on them.

In the ascending limb, the sodium-potassium pump is working like mad to keep shoving sodium out into the medullary interstitial fluid. This is a large part of the reason that the medullary interstitial fluid has its solute concentration gradient to begin with. As the positive ions leave the ascending limb cells, the negative ions tend to follow, and chloride ions also leave in the ascending limb. Note that the ascending limb is not permeable to water, which is unusual. Most cells allow some water to slip through at any time. These cells are specialized to prevent it. Even their tight junctions to one another are excessively tight so that water will not slip by between the cells.

Diabetes

Diabetes is a disorder in which the body has a reduced ability to metabolize carbohydrates and fats, which are then present in abnormal concentrations in the blood. The impaired metabolism results from a lack of insulin, or the reduced efficacy of the insulin that is present.

Type I

Literally this means the overproduction of a sweet urine. Type I (Insulin-Dependent Diabetes Mellitus [IDDM]). (Formerly called childhood-onset diabetes because typically it surfaces early in life, before the age of 30). In these individuals, the beta cells of the islets of Langerhans have suffered damage, usually due to autoimmunity, childhood disease, exposure to toxins, or congenital damage. As a result, the pancreas produces inadequate amounts of insulin, sometimes none.

Because of this, the individual is unable to maintain normal plasma glucose concentration, and is unable to uptake and use glucose in metabolism. Treatment is by means of insulin administration, either by injection or orally, depending on the individual.

Complications include → *low bld sugar*
- Hypoglycemia from overdose of insulin. This results in weakness, sometimes fainting, and, in the extreme, coma, all reversible with administration of glucose. *< 70*
- Ketoacidosis from fat metabolism when insulin is under-administered. This complication can be life threatening.
- Hyperglycemia when insulin administration is imprecise. Hyperglycemia damages cells and tissues. Insulin therapy should be incorporated with normal eating plans. Important to monitor blood glucose. *7126*

high bld sugar ↙

Type II

Type II diabetes, or noninsulin-dependent diabetes, is more common in individuals older than the age of 40. Symptoms may come on slowly, and a family history of the disease is common. Weight loss can induce remission of the disease, but sometimes insulin is needed in addition to nutritional therapy for maximum control. This type is caused by insulin-resistant receptors on the target cells. Insulin resistance can be the result of:
- Abnormal insulin. This might result from mutation to the beta cells.
- Insulin antagonists. This can be the result of adaptation to hypersecretion of insulin.
- Receptor defect. This can be:
  - The result of an inherited mutation.
  - Due to abnormal or deficient receptor proteins. This is the result of adaptation to hypersecretion of insulin.

Glucose tolerance test

The glucose tolerance test (GTT) consists of drinking 100 g of glucose solution and measuring the blood glucose values every hour to get a curve. The values obtained tell a lot about the body's sugar metabolism. The following results are typical and are interpreted briefly. A 2-hour GTT is used to diagnose diabetes, but a 6-hour test might also diagnose diabetes plus hypoglycemia, because symptoms of hypoglycemia occur after the 5th hour. Twenty-five percent of the normal population will also show a blood glucose content of less than 50 mg/dL (2.8 mmol/l) but do not show any other symptoms of hypoglycemia. Therefore, to diagnose a person as hypoglycemic, not only are the blood glucose values important but also the person must experience the symptoms of hypoglycemia in the course of the test.

Fasting Blood Glucose
- 70 to 99 mg/dL (3.9 to 5.5 mmol/L) Normal glucose tolerance.
- 100 to 125 mg/dL (5.6 to 6.9 mmol/L) Impaired fasting glucose (pre-diabetes).
- 126 mg/dL (7 mmol/L) and above on more than 1 testing occasion: Diabetes.

Medications

Several types of oral medications are available for people with type II diabetes to help these patients maintain normal blood glucose levels.
- One class of drugs, known as insulin secretagogues, stimulates the pancreas to make more insulin. Sulfonylureas and meglitinides are examples of secretagogues.
- Biguanides, such as glucophage, cause the liver to produce less glucose, which enhances the action of whatever insulin is being produced.

- **Thiazolidinediones**, such as Actos and Avandia, make the body's tissues more sensitive to the action of insulin.
- **Alpha glucosidase inhibitors**, such as Acarbose and Precose, slow down the absorption of the carbohydrates patients ingest by acting as an enzyme inhibitor.

Insulin is only available in injection form. There are 6 different types of insulin. Each act at different speeds, so they are taken in different intervals to allow the insulin to coincide with the meal or other surges of glucose patients may experience.

Insulin
The major function of insulin is to counter the concerted action of a number of hyperglycemia-generating hormones and to maintain low blood glucose levels. In addition to its role in regulating glucose metabolism, insulin stimulates lipogenesis, diminishes lipolysis, and increases amino acid transport into cells. Insulin also modulates transcription, altering the cell content of numerous mRNAs. It stimulates growth, DNA synthesis, and cell replication, effects that it holds in common with the insulin-like growth factors (IGFs) and relaxin. Insulin is synthesized as a preprohormone in the b cells of the islets of Langerhans. Its signal peptide is removed in the cisternae of the endoplasmic reticulum and it is packaged into secretory vesicles in the Golgi, folded to its native structure, and locked in this conformation by the formation of 2 disulfide bonds. Specific protease activity cleaves the center third of the molecule, which dissociates as C peptide, leaving the amino terminal B peptide disulfide bonded to the carboxy terminal A peptide. Insulin secretion from b cells is principally regulated by plasma glucose levels.

Types of insulin
Very Fast acting - The fastest acting insulins are called lispro (Humalog) and insulin aspart (Novolog). Should be injected under the skin within 15 minutes before eating. Remember to eat within 15 minutes after a shot. These insulins start working in 5 to 15 minutes and lower blood sugar most in 45 to 90 minutes. It finishes working in 3 to 4 hours. With regular insulin you have to wait 30 to 45 minutes before eating. Many people like using lispro because it's easier to coordinate eating with this type of insulin.

Fast acting - The fast-acting insulin is called regular insulin. It lowers blood sugar most in 2 to 5 hours and finishes its work in 5 to 8 hours.

Intermediate acting - NPH (N) or Lente (L) insulin starts working in 1 to 3 hours, lowers blood sugar most in 6 to 12 hours, and finishes working in 20 to 24 hours.

Degenerative disorders
Much of the morbidity and mortality associated with a diagnosis of diabetes is a result of the increase in renal disease, vascular disease, ophthalmologic disease, and infections. Coronary heart disease, stroke, and peripheral vascular disease are more common in diabetics and constitute a major cause of mortality in patients. Diabetics suffer from reduced circulation to the extremities, especially the legs and feet, putting them at risk for complications due to poor wound healing and the possibility of gangrene and eventual amputation.

Microvascular disease occurs in tissues where the extracellular levels of glucose are high, causing osmotic accumulation of water and subsequent swelling. The lens of the eye is particularly susceptible, leading to glaucoma or cataracts. After two decades of managing diabetes, patients are at increased risk for renal disease as nitrogenous wastes accumulate in the blood and the kidneys eventually fail.

Diabetic ketoacidosis

Ketoacidosis can occur when the patient fails to take his or her prescribed insulin, or when the hormones glucagon, cortisol, or epinephrine increase in response to stress or illness. These hormones act against the effects of insulin, causing hyperglycemia and losses of sodium and water, causing dehydration and further hyperglycemia. The citric acid cycle is unable to handle the fatty acids in the body, resulting in the accumulation of ketone bodies that dangerously lower the body's pH. If not checked, coma and eventually death can occur. If patients show signs of drowsiness, nausea, fruity breath, dizziness, or extreme weakness, treatment should be administered immediately. Treatment consists of intravenous insulin, rehydration, and electrolyte support. In severe cases, hydration takes precedence over blood glucose control, and patients may receive saline solution with or without potassium and phosphate.

Hypoglycemia

Hypoglycemia is defined as a blood glucose level of 70 mg/dL or less, and can be caused by an imbalance of too much of insulin in the presence of too little blood glucose. Symptoms may include sweating, trembling, irritability, hunger, faintness, or headache. Hypoglycemia can be brought on by excessive exercise, waiting too long to eat, not eating the prescribed amount of food, or taking too much insulin. Patients should monitor their blood glucose levels to avoid overcorrecting with carbohydrates, resulting in hyperglycemia. Patients may respond by ingesting 15 g of a rapidly absorbed form of carbohydrate such as fruit juice or sugar, waiting 15 minutes, testing blood glucose, and then ingesting more carbohydrates if glucose levels are still below 70 mg/dL. This is often referred to as the 15/15 rule.

Reactive hypoglycemia: Postprandial or reactive hypoglycemia occurs when blood glucose levels drop below 40 mg/dL within 2 to 5 hours after the ingestion of a meal. Individuals may have this response when they have an excessive insulin response to the presence of glucose in the bloodstream, or patients may develop this as a result of having dumping syndrome. The insulin response is delayed to 90 minutes or more after a meal, as opposed to the normal 30 to 60 minutes after a meal. The liver has already started taking up glucose by this time, resulting in an abnormal drop in glucose levels. Symptoms include trembling, weakness, hunger, headache, or confusion. Dietary management is similar to the diabetic plan, with 5 to 6 small meals rich in complex carbohydrates allowing for slow, even release of glucose into the bloodstream.

Diet recommendations

Protein needs of the diabetic patient should be calculated in a similar way to the protein needs of the general population, varying from 0.8 g/kg for adults to somewhere between 1 and 2.2 g/kg for infants and children. This results in protein providing between 15% and 20% of total energy intake. Some research suggests that keeping the protein intake on the lower end of the spectrum, between 12% and 15% of total energy intake, can delay kidney disease.

To help guard against the vascular disease common in diabetics, fat should make up less than 30% of total energy intake, and cholesterol intake should stay under 300 mg/day. Saturated fats should account for less than 10% of lipids in the diet.

The recommended amount of carbohydrate in the diet can vary depending on the patient's blood glucose response, but usually ranges from 55% to 60%. Research suggests that providing approximately 10% of energy in the form of monounsaturated fats instead of carbohydrates results in a more favorable lipid profile for diabetics.

Glycemic index: A glycemic index has been developed for many foods to evaluate the effect of those foods on blood glucose levels. Many factors affect the rate of carbohydrate absorption and metabolism, including how the food was prepared, the amount of fiber, what other nutrients were ingested during the meal, and how the food was processed. For example, in processing, the high-gluten flour found in pasta is absorbed more slowly than the regular flour found in bread. The glycemic index looks at the rise in blood glucose after it is ingested, and compares it with the rise in blood glucose after a standard food is consumed, usually bread or glucose, which has a value of 100. The glycemic index has limited utility in the nutritional management of diabetics because of the many different features that contribute to the complexity of a meal and affect the index.

Glycemic load: The glycemic load (GL) is a relatively new way to assess the impact of carbohydrate consumption that takes the glycemic index into account, but gives a fuller picture than does glycemic index alone. A GI value tells only how rapidly a particular carbohydrate turns into sugar. It doesn't tell how much of that carbohydrate is in a serving of a particular food. Knowledge of both is necessary to understand a food's effect on blood sugar.

That is where glycemic load comes in. The carbohydrate in watermelon, for example, has a high GI. But there isn't a lot of it, so watermelon's glycemic load is relatively low. A GL of 20 or more is high, a GL of 11 to 19 inclusive is medium, and a GL of 10 or less is low.

Pregnancy with diabetes

Diabetes places additional stress on the body of the pregnant mother, and patients who previously controlled their glucose levels with diet alone may be required to take insulin. The goal is to meet the nutritional needs of the fetus, avoid large fluctuations of blood glucose during the day, and provide appropriate nutrition so that the mother's stores do not become exhausted. Babies born to diabetic women are larger, because the elevated glucose levels cross the placenta and result in overfeeding of the fetus. This results in increased insulin levels in the fetus, which can cause the newborn to become hypoglycemic after birth.

In healthy women with normal pregnancies, the increased hormones secreted by the placenta stimulate the mother's body to produce more insulin. If the mother's body does not respond by secreting more insulin, gestational diabetes can result. All pregnant women should be screened using fasting glucose at 24 weeks gestation, and dietary management is usually effective.

Hyperthyroidism

Hyperthyroidism results from the release of excessive T3 and T4 hormones, and these hormones have important roles in regulating metabolism. These hormones increase the body's metabolism and heart rate, and patients may experience trembling, irritability, weight loss, and weakness. Treatment options include antithyroid medication, radioactive iodine, and surgical removal of the thyroid. Dietary management includes an increase in caloric intake to counter undesired weight loss.

Hypothyroidism

Hypothyroidism happens when the thyroid does not produce enough T3 or T4 hormone. This may be caused by a disease process that damages the cells of the thyroid, such as Hashimoto thyroiditis, or can result from medical treatments that damage the thyroid. Symptoms include weight gain, weakness, fatigue, hair loss, and intolerance to cold. The treatment includes thyroid replacement therapy, coupled with a weight-reduction diet if necessary.

Gastrointestinal ulcer

Gastric ulcers are caused by factors leading to impairment of the mucosal barrier, allowing stomach acid to enter the gastric tissue where erosion and eventual ulceration can occur. One cause of this process can be a malfunction of the pyloric sphincter, which allows the alkaline contents of the duodenum to back up into the stomach, where the base content of the fluid acts to lower the mucosal defense. Taking NSAID drugs and infection with the *H. pylori* bacteria also increases the risk of ulcer development.

↳ non-steroid anti-inflam drugs = asprin, ibuprofen, advil, motrin, naproxen, aleve

Drugs commonly used to treat gastric ulcers include antacids, which neutralize gastric acids; cimetidine, which inhibits acid secretion; and sucralfate, which coats and protects the ulcer site.

Nutritional care focuses on patient comfort, neutralization of stomach acids, and maintenance of healthy gastric mucosa. Most foods can be allowed as tolerated. Alcohol in high amounts is damaging to the mucosa. Pepper and spicy foods may stimulate acid secretion and can irritate the stomach lining.

Diverticular diseases

Diverticulosis is a disease of the large intestine in which pouches collect in the wall of the colon. These pouches may develop as a result of high intracolonic pressure due to a low-fiber diet or the reduction of strength of the muscle wall in the colon. The incidence of the disease is increased in elderly populations. Diverticulitis occurs when fecal matter accumulates in the herniations of patients with diverticulosis. This can lead to infection, inflammation, ulceration, and even rupture of the colon wall.

It was once believed that adherence to a low-fiber diet eased the symptoms of diverticular diseases. It is now understood that high-fiber diets increase the movement of waste through the colon and decrease intracolonic pressure, relieving symptoms. For those patients experiencing a flare-up of diverticulitis, a low-residue diet can be followed, with gradual introduction of high-fiber foods as tolerated.

Crohn disease

Crohn disease is a disorder of unknown etiology that is characterized pathologically by involvement of all bowel wall layers in a chronic inflammatory process with noncaseating granulomas. Can lead to megaloblastic anemia if there is a B_{12} deficit. The granulomatous inflammation most frequently affects the terminal ileum but it may affect any part of the gastrointestinal tract and frequently affected areas are in discontinuity. There is a tendency to form fistulae. Probable presence of anorexia, weight loss, and diarrhea. If acute, treat with parenteral nutrition or a low-fiber diet.

Ulcerative colitis

Chronic inflammation of the rectum and large intestine.

Symptoms
Weight loss, Jaundice, Bloody Diarrhea, Negative nitrogen balance, abdominal pain, Fever, Joint pain, GI bleeding, Anorexia, Electrolyte disturbance.

Tests
Barium enema, ESR, C-reactive protein (CRP), Colonoscopy.

Treatment
Corticosteroids, Mesalamine, Surgery, Ostomy, Azathioprine, Sulfasalazine-antidiarrheal. If acute, treat with elemental diet. Needs high-protein, high-calorie, low-fat diet.

Lactase-deficiency

Lactase is the enzyme responsible for digesting the sugar lactose found in milk. When lactose is not broken down into glucose and galactose, it acts osmotically to draw water into the intestines, stimulating rapid peristalsis and resulting in watery diarrhea. The diarrhea can result in excessive loss of fluids and loss of electrolytes. Bacterial action metabolizes some of the lactose in the colon, causing lactic acid, carbon dioxide, and hydrogen gas to form. This causes pain, gas, and bloating. The condition is common among African Americans, Asians, and South Americans.

A lactose tolerance test may be administered to symptomatic individuals. If blood glucose does not elevate and symptoms occur upon oral administration of lactose, a diagnosis may be made. The omission or reduction of dairy foods may alleviate symptoms. Cheese and yogurt are sometimes tolerated because of low lactose content. Milk products with added lactase are available, or the enzyme may be taken with milk products.

Diarrhea

Infants and children
Diarrhea is an abnormality of excretion that occurs when stools are frequent and high in liquid content. It is also characterized by an excessive loss of electrolytes, especially sodium and potassium, which can lead to dangerous complications in children. Diarrhea can be the result of the rapid passing of small intestinal contents, preventing the action of digestive enzymes and disallowing for the absorptive action of fluid and nutrients. Diarrhea can also result from changes in the intestinal mucosa. Diarrhea is a symptom of a disease process rather than a disease in itself, so treatment should aim to manage the underlying disorder. Acute diarrhea can become serious quickly in infants and young children, as their small body mass increases their susceptibility to dehydration and electrolyte imbalances.

Aggressive replacement of fluids and electrolytes should be given in the form of an oral rehydration solution. The glucose electrolyte solution recommended by the World Health Organization is composed of specified amounts of glucose, sodium, potassium, chloride, and bicarbonate in a water solution.

Chronic nonspecific infantile diarrhea: There is no significant malabsorption with this. This happens mainly in the United States. Diet: Give 40% calories as fat and balance with limited fluids.

Adults
Allow bowel to rest. Replace lost fluids and electrolytes by increasing the oral intake of fluids, those high in sodium and potassium such as broths are best. When diarrhea stops, start feeding with low-fiber foods, followed by protein. Fat doesn't have to be limited. Avoid lactose at first.

Steatorrhea

Most diseases of malabsorption cause steatorrhea, a condition characterized by the presence of undigested fat in the stool. Regular stools contain 2 to 5 g of fat; however, the stools of patients with steatorrhea may contain up to 60 g of fat. Diagnosis can be made by keeping a food diary and analyzing the fat content of stools over a 72-hour period, focusing on the ratio of ingested fat to stool fat.

Treatment should be tailored according to the underlying condition. Disease processes associated with malabsorption include inadequate digestion, bile salt deficiency, mucosal cell damage, inflammatory disorders, and malfunctions of the intestine's lymphatic system.

Weight loss in patients due to fat loss may be countered with increased energy intake in the diet from carbohydrates and protein. Reduced absorption of vitamins and minerals due to the lack of fat as a transport mechanism can be problematic. Supplementation of calcium, iron, zinc, magnesium, and fat-soluble vitamins may be required.

Short bowel syndrome

The small or large intestine may need to be surgically resected for a variety of reasons. Removal of more than two-thirds of the small intestine is sometimes necessary in the treatment of cancer, Crohn disease, radiation damage, or bowel obstruction, resulting in problems collectively referred to as short bowel syndrome.

Symptoms include severe malnutrition and metabolic problems leading to weight loss, diarrhea, muscle wasting, dehydration, and electrolyte imbalances. The severity of the syndrome depends on how much and which sections of bowel are removed. Loss of the ileum is not tolerated as well as loss of the jejunum because of ileum's role in absorbing vitamin B_{12}. Other problems accompanying this syndrome can include excessive gastric acid due to loss of the buffering effects of the small intestine; increase in peristalsis due to loss of small intestine hormones that regulate bowel activity; formation of kidney stones due to excess oxalate absorption; and gallstone formation due to decrease in bile production.

Nutritional care
Following resection, the remaining bowel has the ability to adapt to make up for loss of function. If adequate nutrition is provided for several months following surgery the bowel will gradually increase its absorptive surface area by forming larger villi and deeper crypts of Lieberkühn. In the first several weeks after surgery, nutrition needs to be provided directly into the circulatory system of the patient. Gradually the patient may begin to receive nutritional support delivered into the stomach, duodenum, or jejunum. An easily digested liquid diet may be prescribed at first, avoiding sucrose and lactose.

Vitamin supplementation with the fat-soluble vitamins is usually necessary, and vitamin B_{12} status may need to be assessed depending on the area of resection. Supplementation with calcium, iron, and zinc may also be necessary. Several months after surgery oral intake may begin as tolerated. Setbacks are common and small meals are better tolerated than 3 main meals.

Liver cirrhosis

Cirrhosis is the final stage of liver damage that occurs when normal liver tissue is gradually destroyed and replaced by scar tissue. This condition is found in 15% or more of heavy drinkers, but other causes may include poisoning, hepatitis, cystic fibrosis, or biliary obstruction.

When normal tissue in the liver is replaced with connective or scar tissue, the liver becomes segmented with fibrous bands. Abnormal nodules form that limit blood circulation, and the damage is irreversible. Obstruction of the portal vein can cause pressure that stimulates a new circulatory system to form that bypasses the damaged liver tissue. A consequence of this is the accumulation of fluid in the peritoneal cavity and enlargement of the veins providing the additional circulation. The pressure on these additional veins causes them to be thin-walled and places an individual at high risk of hemorrhage from venous rupture. Altered mental status can also occur because of toxins being carried across an abnormally porous blood-brain barrier.

Symptoms
People with cirrhosis often experience loss of appetite, nausea, vomiting, and weight loss, giving them an emaciated appearance. Diet alone does not contribute to the development of this liver disease. People who are well nourished, for example, but drink large amounts of alcohol are also susceptible to alcoholic disease.

Diet recommendations
Adults with cirrhosis require a balanced diet rich in protein, providing 2,000 to 3,000 calories a day, to allow the liver cells to regenerate. However, too much protein will result in an increased amount of ammonia in the blood; too little protein can reduce healing of the liver. Patient should also have low fiber if varices are noted.

Malnutrition in alcoholics with liver disease
In the case of light drinkers, alcohol can function as an additional energy source, providing 7 kcal/g, although no protein, fat, vitamins, or minerals are provided. In heavy drinkers, consumption of alcohol may take the place of food altogether. When alcohol is metabolized in the liver, triglycerides are formed that are deposited in the liver.

Pyruvate metabolism is disrupted, and if glycogen stores are not being replenished, the alcoholic may become hypoglycemic. Alcohol consumption causes inflammation of the stomach, pancreas, and intestine, which decreases the ability of these organs to absorb vitamin C, vitamin B_{12}, thiamin, and folic acid. Alcohol-related thiamin deficiency is a common cause of dementia. When alcohol is metabolized to acetaldehyde, hepatic toxicity occurs, impairing the liver's ability to help the body use vitamins A, D, B_6, and folic acid. The problem in vitamin B impairment is furthered by the alcoholic's need for increased levels of the vitamin in the metabolism of alcohol.

Functions of the liver
The liver is the most important organ in the body involved in the metabolism of food. Most ingested foods are digested and then transported to the liver where they are stored, synthesized into something else, or transported to other parts of the body. The liver plays a role in energy production and maintenance by acting as a storage facility for glycogen, which can be made into glucose when needed. When carbohydrate intake is insufficient to meet glucose needs, the liver can make protein into glucose. The liver makes cholesterol and turns it into bile salts or lipoproteins as needed. Fatty acids are oxidized into acetyl-CoA, which can be used in the citric acid cycle for energy. Protein metabolism in the liver takes place when amino acids are broken down and

- 98 -

ammonia is detoxified by turning it into urea. The liver retrieves iron from discarded red blood cells and stores the reserve. All fat-soluble vitamins are stored in the liver.

Esophageal varices

Esophageal varices are dilated blood vessels within the wall of the esophagus and caused by portal hypertension. Patients with cirrhosis develop portal hypertension. When portal hypertension occurs, blood flow through the liver is diminished. Thus, blood flow increases through the microscopic blood vessels within the esophageal wall. As this blood flow increases, the blood vessels begin to dilate. This dilation can be profound. The original diameter of the blood vessels is measured in millimeters while the final, fully established esophageal varix may be 0.5 to 1 cm or larger in diameter. Blood cannot enter the liver with esophageal varices. These blood vessels then continue to dilate until they become large enough to rupture. When esophageal varices rupture, patients become acutely ill.

Liver failure

Liver failure is defined as the function of the liver being reduced to 30% or less. The liver will no longer be able to absorb or metabolize fat properly, and the liver may become fatty. Fat should be reduced to 25% of caloric intake, and medium-chain triglycerides may be substituted for the more difficult-to-digest long-chain fats. If medium-chain fats are used exclusively, supplementation with linoleic acid will avoid the development of an essential fatty acid deficiency. Fat in the stools is present in many cirrhotic patients because of lack of bile salts, pancreatic insufficiency, or portal vein blockage. This indicates the need for supplementation of the fat-soluble vitamins A, D, and E. In patients with advanced cirrhosis, injections of vitamins A, D, and K may be necessary. Folate, thiamin, and vitamin B_{12} deficiencies should also be addressed with supplementation. Because of liver impairment, nutrient toxicities occur at low levels of supplementation so close monitoring is essential.

Protein metabolism is greatly altered in advanced liver disease, and the ratio of aromatic amino acids to branched-chain amino acids (BCAA) becomes unbalanced, putting patients at risk for hepatic encephalopathy. However, this is complicated by the body's need for adequate protein to nourish the patient and provide building blocks for liver repair. Blood ammonia may be reduced by supplementing with neomycin, an antibiotic that destroys the flora in the gut that produces ammonia. Lactulose is also given, which removes intestinal contents by osmotically inducing diarrhea to help remove nitrogen. When these methods are unsuccessful, supplementing protein intake with BCAA may help to improve encephalopathy.

Ascites, or accumulation of fluid in the peritoneal cavity, can be managed by restricting sodium to 500 to 2,000 mg/day, depending on the severity of the problem. Diuretics may also be given, and monitoring should include daily weight and abdominal examinations. As ascites dry up, normal fluid and sodium intake should resume.

Gallbladder disease

After bile is secreted by the liver, the gallbladder concentrates and stores the bile. The mucosa of the gallbladder absorbs water and electrolytes from the bile, leaving a concentrated product containing high levels of bile salts and cholesterol. Bile helps in the absorption of fats, vitamins A, D, E, and K, as well as calcium and iron. When food is ingested, the sphincter of Oddi relaxes, releasing bile into the duodenum through the common bile duct. The bile duct is joined with the liver and pancreatic ducts, so diseases involving the gallbladder often involve these other organs as well.

The most common diseases of the gallbladder include gallstones (cholelithiasis) and inflammation (cholecystitis). Gallstones result from stones slipping into the common bile duct, causing cramps and pain. Inflammation can occur when gallstones block the duct opening, causing bile to back up into the gallbladder. The organ then becomes red, swollen, or possibly infected.

Nutritional management for gallbladder disease
Surgery is usually the best treatment modality for gallbladder disease. The gallbladder is removed, and bile is stored in the common duct connecting the liver and small intestine. The duct expands to accommodate its new role, and bile moves directly from the liver to the small intestine. After surgery, enteral feedings may be offered until normal bowel sounds return, usually within the first few days. A low-fat diet may be followed for the first month after surgery, and then normal dietary intake may gradually resume as inflammation subsides.

Some patients are not surgical candidates, and must be treated conservatively with diet changes. For acute attacks of cholecystitis, the gallbladder should be rested by following a low-fat diet, as fat can painfully stimulate the sphincter of Oddi. For chronic disease, a diet providing 25% of kcal from fat may be followed, with supplementation of fat-soluble vitamins necessary in some individuals.

Gout

Gout is a disease in which abnormal metabolism of purines result in excessive levels of uric acid in the blood. This results in the formation of sodium urate crystals, which accumulate in joints and cartilage. Over time, the excessive crystals can increase one's risk of kidney stones or cause damage in the joints, leading to arthritis. Obesity is a risk factor for developing gout, which is usually diagnosed after age 35. Both excessive eating and fasting resulting in ketosis can trigger attacks.

Low-purine diets are not effective in treating gout, as uric acid formation can occur within the body in the absence of purines. However, a low-purine diet may be useful in acute attacks to reduce their severity. A gradual reduction in weight to ideal levels is recommended. A diet low in fat and moderate in protein from sources low in purines such as dairy and bread is recommended. Liberal intake of water is encouraged to dilute the uric acid in the urine.

Metabolic disorders

Galactosemia
Galactosemia is a metabolic disorder that describes 2 different syndromes that make the body unable to convert galactose into glucose. This causes the accumulation of galactose and/or galactose-1 phosphate in body tissues or intercellular fluid. Galactosemia occurs when one of two enzyme activities that ultimately allow lactose to be broken down into glucose is not functioning. If the galactose-1-phosphate uridyl transferase enzyme is dysfunctional at birth, infants may present with vomiting, diarrhea, susceptibility to infections, and failure to thrive. If not diagnosed and treated promptly, death can occur. Nutritional management includes lifelong galactose elimination from the diet. This includes avoiding all dairy products, dates, bell peppers, organ meats, and papaya.

Urea cycle defects
Urea cycle defects, including ornithine transcarbamylase (OTC) deficiency, citrullinemia, and argininosuccinic aciduria result in accumulations of ammonia in the blood that can cause vomiting, seizures, and death. The goal of therapy is to prevent excessive ammonia in the blood and

accompanying neurological deficits. Acute attacks may require the elimination of all dietary protein, while long-term management restricts protein from 1 to 2 g/day.

Goiters

If the thyroid gland does not produce enough T3 or T4 hormone, the pituitary gland may release additional thyroid-stimulating hormone to try to up the thyroid's production. This causes an enlargement of the thyroid gland, or compensatory goiter.

Endemic goiter is common in regions where iodine is absent from the diet. Iodine is stored in the thyroid where it is used to make T3 and T4 hormones. Iodine content is variable in foods; common sources include seafood, eggs, and milk. In areas where goiter is common, preparation of foods with iodized salt should be emphasized in order to reach the RDA of 150 micrograms/day.

Goitrogens, substances in foods that block the absorption or use of iodine in the body, can also contribute to goiter. Goitrogen-rich foods include turnips, peanuts, and soybeans.

Osteoporosis

Bone loss is a normal part of aging, and is defined by loss of density and mass. If bone density decreases to the point that the skeleton is susceptible to fractures under normal stresses, osteoporosis is diagnosed. Type I osteoporosis is found in postmenopausal women within two decades of the onset of menopause and involves the spongy material of the long bones. Type II disease affects both sexes and usually occurs after age 70, involving both the spongy and hard layers of bone.

Many factors can contribute to the development of osteoporosis, including age, race, gender, body type, medications, and other lifestyle factors. Being female, white or Asian, and slight of build increases the risk. Engaging in weight bearing exercise stimulates bone formation, while leading a sedentary lifestyle encourages bone loss. Many medications exacerbate bone loss, by preventing calcium absorption (steroids) or causing calcium loss from bones. Smoking and alcohol use contribute to osteoporosis by damaging the bone-forming osteoblast cells.

Prevention and treatment
Hormone replacement therapy is the standard of care for preventing type I osteoporosis in postmenopausal women. It has the greatest efficacy for preventing bone loss when taken in the first decade after menopause. However, it cannot help to rebuild bone in those patients who have already suffered a significant loss in density. Weight bearing exercise is an effective treatment of both types of osteoporosis. The pull of muscles on the bones stimulates the activity of osteoblasts to form new bone.

Dietary calcium is the most important from birth through the teen years, when peak bone mass is reached. Although calcium may not help build new bone in osteoporosis patients, adequate calcium may help to prevent further losses. Vitamin D intake is important in housebound individuals who are not exposed to enough sunlight to manufacture this hormone.

Epilepsy

Epilepsy is a neurological disorder in which the cerebral neurons release excessive, disordered electrical discharges, causing a condition of chronic seizures. The anticonvulsant drugs phenobarbital, phenytoin, and primidone increase the metabolism of vitamin D and therefore decrease the absorption of calcium in the intestine. Patients on these drugs are at an increased risk of osteomalacia and rickets, so vitamin D supplementation is necessary. Phenobarbital is absorbed poorly with meals, so the medication should be taken between meals.

A ketogenic diet is recommended as a last resort in some patients with moderate to severe seizures that cannot be adequately controlled by medication. The mechanism of action is thought to be an inhibitory effect of ketone bodies on neurotransmitters. The efficacy of the diet wears off after a few years. Nearly all of the energy needs in this diet are supplied by fat, and vitamin supplementation is required. The diet is unpalatable and side effects can include nausea and irritability, making compliance low.

Anemia

Megaloblastic anemias

Megaloblastic anemias are usually caused by a folic acid or vitamin B_{12} deficiency, but can also be caused by certain medications or cancers.

- Folate deficiencies severe enough to cause anemia may be found in pregnancy, tropical sprue, or infants born to deficient mothers. If serum folate levels are less than 3 ng/ml, erythrocyte protein cannot be manufactured in the body and large, immature red blood cells result. Treatment includes supplementation with 1 mg of folate daily for 2 weeks. After that, 50 to 100 micrograms/day of folate should be consumed to maintain functional status.
- Vitamin B_{12} deficiency can cause pernicious anemia, which affects not only red blood cell formation but also the GI tract and the nervous system. The deficiency is often related to a lack of intrinsic factor, a protein necessary in the absorption of vitamin B_{12}. Treatment therefore bypasses oral supplementation and requires injections of 50 to 100 micrograms/day of B_{12} until adequate levels are achieved.

Microcytic anemias

Microcytic anemia, characterized by small red blood cells and low levels of circulating hemoglobin, is the last stage of a long period of iron deficiency. The main causes of iron deficiency anemia are heavy blood loss, inadequate iron intake or absorption, or increased iron needs due to pregnancy, infancy, or adolescence. First, the storage forms of iron in the form of ferritin and hemosiderin are depleted. Second, the amount of iron supplied to the bone marrow is not sufficient to produce healthy blood cells. Those that are produced are small and low in hemoglobin. This eventually results in anemia.

Treatment should focus on restoring iron stores, not just alleviating the anemia. Supplementation of 50 to 200 mg of elemental iron is recommended, depending on severity of anemia. Children may receive 6 mg/kg body weight. Foods high in iron content should be encouraged, including red meat, egg yolk, leafy vegetables, and fortified cereals. Vitamin C enhances iron absorption.

Extreme physiologic stress

Following severe trauma or injury, the body goes into shock, characterized by reduced blood pressure, heart rate, oxygen consumption, and temperature. The body experiences a decrease in blood volume and decreased blood flow to bodily tissues.

Shock lasts briefly, and then the body begins to mobilize its defenses to combat the stressor. This mobilization phase can last several weeks or longer, and is characterized by a state of hypermetabolism and hypercatabolism that enables the body to heal. Increases in basal energy expenditure may range from 10% for bone fractures to 100% for extensive burns. Glycogen stores are depleted and the hormone cortisol mobilizes amino acids from muscle to be used in gluconeogenesis. Lean body mass is lost throughout the healing process, with some amino acids used for energy, some for rebuilding tissue, and some for counteracting lactic acidosis. Fatty acids are metabolized quickly, but ketosis does not develop because of stimulation of the nervous system. Insulin levels are blocked, leading to a diabetic-like state of high blood glucose.

Extensive burns

Extensive burns can increase basal energy expenditure by 100% or more. Protein catabolism and nitrogen excretion are increased, and protein is also lost through the wound itself. Fluid and electrolyte losses from the wound can be severe, and the initial treatment period should focus on replacing fluid and electrolytes and maintaining balance. Calculation of kcal requirements can be determined by various formulas that consider kcal/kg and total body surface area burned. Additional energy is required to meet the demands of wound healing, fever, infection, weight loss, and surgery. Protein needs are increased and may be determined by monitoring the patient's wound status and nitrogen balance. Vitamin C supplementation is helpful for the collagen formation needed in wound healing. Magnesium can be lost from wounds in large levels; supplementation may be necessary. Zinc is recommended for those receiving parenteral nutrition or for those with deficiencies to enhance wound healing.

Burn Management

3 Phases of Burn Management
The duration of the emergent phase (resuscitative) is 24-48 hours, but it can last up to 5 (or more) days. Fluid loss and edema formation signal onset, and this phase and continues until fluid motorization and diuresis begin. Basal metabolic rate (BMR) increases 50% to 100%. Other complications: Arrhythmias, hypovolemic shock, Impairment of circulation to limbs (caused by circumferential burns, and then the edema formation), escharotomies (incisions through eschar) are done to restore circulation to compromised extremities.

Acute Phase: Fluid motorization and dieresis signal the onset of this phase. This phase ends when the burn wound has healed, or when the affected area is completely covered.

Rehabilitative: This phase may take weeks or months. Patient is no longer grossly edematous because of fluid mobilization, full and partial thickness burns more evident, bowel sounds return, patient more aware of pain and condition. Needs high levels of protein, vitamin K and C, and zinc.

Accidental injury

Nutritional support for accident victims should begin as soon as the patient's vital signs are stable. Although positive nitrogen balance may not be achieved in the first days following trauma, further loss of lean body tissue may be prevented. Introduction of oral feeding may be delayed because of shock, pain, injury complications, or depression. Enteral nutrition is routinely given to avoid complications of protein loss that include hypoalbuminemia, infection, slow wound healing, skin breakdown, and reduced immune function. The degree of trauma determines the amount of carbohydrate and protein needed. Most patients' needs are satisfied by 35 to 45 kcal/kg. Lipid should provide approximately 30% of kcal, and protein needs vary from 1 to 2 g/kg, depending on severity of injury.

Surgery

Individuals recovering from surgery generally delay oral feeding for 24 to 48 hours, to wait for normal peristalsis to return. Fluid and electrolyte balance should be monitored postoperatively and maintained intravenously as needed. Positive nitrogen balance enhances wound healing and reduces infection; most patients can meet their energy and protein needs on the standard diet provided.

Cancer

Some research shows a link between the amount of fat intake and the development of cancers of the breast, colon, and prostate. The composition of the fat may be more important than total intake: ingestion of longer chain polyunsaturated fatty acids and monounsaturated fats found in olive oil have been associated with lower cancer incidence. Fiber intake has been researched extensively as it pertains to the development of colon and rectal cancer. It is thought that the protective effects stem from increased transit time of foodstuffs, lessening the exposure of the bowel to toxins in food. Vitamins A, C, and E have demonstrated activity as cancer inhibitors, perhaps because of their antioxidant activity. Alcohol consumption is linked to several cancers, including mouth, pharynx, and esophagus. The link may be the result of depression of the immune system, malnutrition from alcoholism, or directly caused cell toxicity.

Radiation therapy
Radiation therapy is a local treatment, so side effects are limited to the area being treated. In radiation therapy to the abdominal area, side effects may include nausea, vomiting, or diarrhea. If the bowel is damaged, the absorption of carbohydrate, fat, and electrolytes may be adversely affected. Radiation enteritis is a long-term side effect that results from damage to the small bowel, and side effects include abdominal pain, steatorrhea, nausea, diarrhea, and vomiting. Avoiding greasy foods or foods with strong odors is advised. Frequent small, bland meals may be well tolerated. Choosing foods with a high nutrient density can help to combat the weight loss that accompanies radiation to the bowel.

Radiation to the head and neck area can damage salivary glands, leading to chronic dry mouth (xerostomia) and severe dental decay. Difficulty swallowing and taste alterations may compound a patient's low appetite. Soft, bland, high-protein foods are advised. Supplementation with OTC nutritional drinks may help keep energy intake up.

Cachexia
Cancer cachexia is a syndrome of malnutrition unique to cancer patients. It is characterized by weight loss, anemia, weakness, and anorexia. A variety of problems may contribute to the development of this syndrome, including increased energy needs, abnormal metabolism, acid-base imbalance, and loss of normal immune and endocrine function. Because of the complex nature of the syndrome, an increase in energy intake alone will not cause reversal of the syndrome; only successful treatment of the underlying malignancy will cause the cachexia to diminish.

Although cancer patients typically exhibit reduced food intake, associated with a decrease in basal metabolic rate (BMR), cancer patients have an increase in BMR. This is theorized to be due to factors beyond the increased energy needed for tumor growth; metabolic aberrations are assumed to exist as well. Cancerous tissue requires a great deal of glucose and protein for growth, with lean body mass providing much of the needed protein to the cancerous cell.

Vanillylmandelic acid test

A test for catecholamine-secreting tumors performed on a 24-hour urine specimen and based on the fact that vanillylmandelic acid is the major urinary metabolite of norepinephrine and epinephrine.

The test is to measure catecholamines and can help diagnose a tumor in the adrenal glands called a pheochromocytoma. Symptoms of a pheochromocytoma include sudden episodes of high blood pressure, excessive sweating, headaches, periods of abnormally fast heartbeats (palpitations), tremors, and anxiety. The amount of catecholamines produced by such a pheochromocytoma can vary greatly.
There is a special diet for 2 to 3 days before and during the test.

The diet usually excludes:
Caffeine (found in coffee, tea, cocoa, and chocolate)
Amines (nitrogen-containing substances found in bananas, walnuts, avocados, fava beans, cheese, beer, and red wine)
Any foods or fluids containing vanilla
Licorice
Aspirin

Kwashiorkor

Kwashiorkor comes from a phrase that means "the disease of the displaced baby when the next one comes." Young children in developing countries are at greatest risk of this disease of protein malnutrition, and the decline often begins when the child is weaned from the breast so that the next born may begin to breastfeed. People in impoverished areas often consume low-nutrient, protein-poor diets that lead to extreme protein deficiency characterized by low albumin, pitting edema, wasting, weakness, and an enlarged liver. Children are especially at risk because of their higher requirements for protein.

Marasmus

Marasmus is a state of semi-starvation that occurs when a child receives inadequate energy from the diet over a period of time. This disease is also associated with weaning, and is characterized by wasting, absence of body fat, weakness, and stunted growth.

Iatrogenic malnutrition

Iatrogenic malnutrition refers to malnutrition that occurs in the hospital setting because of adverse treatment effects, dislike of food, poor communication between dietitian and food service staff, or other factors related to hospitalization.

Anorexia nervosa

Anorexia nervosa is most prevalent in teenage girls from middle-class backgrounds, although the incidence is rising in males. The disorder is characterized by inadequate intake of food, and may include excessive exercise and/or voluntary vomiting that causes the patient to lose 25% or more of their body weight. Physical signs may include fat depletion and loss of lean body tissue, cessation of menstruation in females, hair loss, dry skin, fingernail deformities, edema, and heart rhythm disturbances due to electrolyte imbalances.

Patients are resistant to therapy, and successful treatment integrates psychological treatment with nutritional support. Electrolyte imbalances or dehydration should be addressed promptly, followed by a moderate diet planned in conjunction with the patient. Energy intake of 30 to 40 kcal/kg is a reasonable goal to help achieve normal weight gain, but follow-up care and monitoring is important, as the relapse rate is high.

Obesity

The body mass index (BMI = W/H^2, weight in kg and height in m) is the preferred measure for determining whether an individual is overweight or obese. A BMI of 30 or greater classifies an individual as obese. A BMI of 25 to 29.9 classifies one as overweight. A variety of factors may contribute to the condition of obesity, including environment, culture, heredity, and internal physiological differences. Many variables that determine the individual regulation of body weight are genetically determined, such as resting metabolic rate, amount and size of fat cells, and subtle hormonal and neurological factors that control the feeling of satiety. The set point theory argues that people have a predetermined weight that is governed by fat stores in the body, and individuals will achieve homeostasis by returning to this weight over time regardless of feeding habits. Obesity is associated with a range of diseases and disorders, including hypertension, diabetes, heart disease, gallstones, and arthritis.

Nutritional care

Treatment of overweight patients may be viewed as caring for a chronic disease, as few individuals maintain their weight. Weight cycling refers to the trait of obese persons to lose weight and regain it several times over their life. Typically, more weight is regained than was lost, and the composition of weight regained tends to be higher in adipose tissue and lower in lean muscle mass. Successful weight-loss programs usually integrate diet, exercise, and behavior change. Many dieting individuals experience a "plateau effect," where weight reduction slows or stops completely. Loss of muscle used to support fatty tissue contributes to a reduction of resting metabolic rate.

Steady weight loss over a long period of time helps to conserve lean body mass and reduce fat stores. Achievement of ideal body weight may not be possible for individuals with a BMI of greater than 40, so final goals should be individualized. A diet that provides 500 kcal/day less than required for maintenance should provide weight loss of approximately 1 lb. a week.

Obesity and Native Americans

Being overweight or obese increases a Native American's risk of heart disease, type 2 diabetes, high blood pressure, stroke, breathing problems, arthritis, gallbladder disease, sleep apnea (breathing problems while sleeping), and some cancers, such as renal cell cancer. In one specific population in Arizona, a study found that 80% of American Indians were overweight.

Chemotherapy

Chemotherapy is a systemic treatment, and side effects vary according to the drugs and dosage used. Chemotherapy kills rapidly dividing cells, so the entire GI tract may be affected, leading to nausea, vomiting, diarrhea, mouth sores, and inflammation of the esophagus.

The patient can become severely anorectic because of taste aversions caused by metallic taste and nausea. Patients may associate eating with pain, nausea, and vomiting to such an extent that formerly favorite foods are rejected, and cooking odors alone can trigger GI upset. Food service workers may be instructed not to remove tray lids in the patient's room in the hospital setting, as the subsequent release of food odors leads to rejection. Meat aversion is especially common, so protein sources may need to come from bland dairy foods, such as cottage cheese. Serving foods cold or at room temperature can increase their appeal. If malnutrition becomes severe or the gut loses function, temporary enteral or parenteral nutrition may be required.

Esophagitis

Esophagitis is an inflammation of the lower part of the esophagus due to irritation of the lining caused by gastric acids. Less common causes include inflammation due to intubation, chronic vomiting, or viral infection. The function of the lower esophageal sphincter is one factor that affects reflux, and periodic reflux can be caused by hormonal changes that weaken the muscle, such as pregnancy or oral contraceptives. Medications for esophagitis include antacids, drugs that decrease gastric production, or medications that increase lower esophageal sphincter pressure. Nutritional management includes weight loss to decrease intragastric pressure, and avoiding foods that reduce esophageal sphincter competency such as fatty foods, alcohol, and caffeine.

Dysphagia

Dysphagia, or difficulty in swallowing, is usually due to neurological disease. Swallowing thin liquids presents the highest risk of aspiration into the lungs. Thickening substances may be added to beverages to ease swallowing. Moist foods that form a good bolus are usually better tolerated; sticky foods such as peanut butter or bulky foods such as raw carrots are poorly tolerated.

Dental caries

Dental caries form when bacteria in the mouth ferment dietary carbohydrates, especially sucrose, causing the formation of acids. The acids decalcify the surface of the tooth until salivary flow clears food debris from the mouth and the buffering action provided by the lower pH of saliva neutralizes the acids. Saliva also contains calcium and phosphorus, which help to remineralize eroded areas after a meal. If the acid is trapped in plaque formations on the teeth, the acid production may continue for an hour after the meal. When pH drops below 5.5, the acid is able to destroy tooth enamel.

The frequency of consumption of cariogenic food affects caries formation. Eating a large portion of dessert is less damaging than snacking throughout the day. Sticky foods that adhere to the tooth are more cariogenic. The amount of time the food is in the mouth provides opportunities for bacteria to act, so liquids are less cariogenic than solid foods. Cheddar cheese and sugarless gum have been shown to prevent the drop of pH in the mouth.

Pregnancy-induced hypertension

Pregnancy-induced hypertension (PIH) is characterized by hypertension, edema, low blood volume, low albumin count, and excessive protein excretion in the urine. It usually presents toward the end of pregnancy, especially in very young patients of low socioeconomic status who are pregnant for the first time. The cause is unknown, but it is associated with lack of prenatal care and poor calcium and protein status. PIH is usually defined as a systolic blood pressure of greater than 140 and/or diastolic pressure of greater than 90. Protein in the urine greater than 500 mg defines preeclampsia, the precursor to eclampsia, which is characterized by seizure close to the time of delivery.

At one time, sodium restriction was advocated for treatment of PIH; however, this has not been shown to be effective. Receiving standard prenatal care and following recommended prenatal nutrition guidelines is advised to detect and prevent complications.

Hyperemesis gravidarum

Hyperemesis gravidarum is a severe and intractable form of nausea and vomiting in pregnancy. It is a diagnosis of exclusion and may result in weight loss; nutritional deficiencies; and abnormalities in fluids, electrolyte levels, and acid-base balance. The peak incidence is at 8 and 12 weeks of pregnancy, and symptoms usually resolve by week 16. Interestingly, nausea and vomiting of pregnancy is generally associated with a lower rate of miscarriage. Extreme nausea and vomiting may be related to elevated levels of estrogens or human chorionic gonadotropin.

Signs/Symptoms:
Weight loss
Dehydration
Decreased skin turgor
Postural changes in BP and pulse

Recommend carbohydrates in small amounts

AIDS

AIDS is caused by the bloodborne virus HIV, which destroys T lymphocyte function and therefore causes severe immune deficiency. The virus is also transmitted through breast milk, so HIV-positive mothers should not breastfeed. The disease is associated with susceptibility to various opportunistic infections, lymphoma, Kaposi sarcoma, and encephalopathy. Organs affected by the complications of AIDS can include the liver, kidneys, GI tract, and pancreas. Oral candidiasis is common in AIDS patients, which makes eating painful. Energy needs are increased in patients with infections or febrile illness, yet oral intake can be poor because of nausea, vomiting, or fatigue. The protein malnutrition common to AIDS patients can further increase their susceptibility to infections. However, protein intake may be restricted for those with renal disease.

Goals of nutritional care include preservation of protein stores, prevention of vitamin or mineral deficiencies that reduce immune status, and treatment of complications that compromise nutritional status.

COPD

Chronic obstructive pulmonary disease (COPD) is the airway obstruction that develops as a result of chronic bronchitis and/or emphysema. Chronic bronchitis is characterized by a productive cough that may come and go but never resolves. Emphysema is a condition characterized by enlarged alveoli (air sacs) that exhibit degraded walls and a loss of elasticity. Patients with severe COPD are at risk for cor pulmonale, a condition in which the right ventricle of the heart is enlarged because of increased pressure in the pulmonary arteries.

The malnourished state common to COPD patients is thought to be a result of increased energy needs, anorexia, and increased oxygen consumption. The goals of nutritional support include maintaining ideal body weight, managing medication side effects, and managing the edema of patients with cor pulmonale. Edema can mask weight loss, so assessment should account for this. Some edematous patients can achieve control with sodium and fluid restriction; others need diuretics. Energy requirements may approach 150% of resting energy expenditure. High-calorie liquid supplements may help patients reach their energy intake goals.

Acute respiratory distress syndrome

Acute respiratory failure can occur in patients with chronic obstructive pulmonary disease when the respiratory muscle is no longer strong enough to enable the lungs to exchange enough gases to keep blood oxygen at functioning levels. Patients with this condition usually have poor nutritional status and are at risk for worsening their status during hospitalization. Patients who can improve their protein levels have a better chance of weaning from mechanical ventilation. Goals include preserving lean body mass, preventing further weight loss, and maintaining fluid balance, while taking into account the patient's impaired ability to clear carbon dioxide from the body. Increased carbohydrate in the diet is associated with increased carbon dioxide production, so 50% of the nonprotein calories provided should come from fat. Enteral feedings are recommended for patients with a functional gut, but care in tube placement should be taken to avoid the risk of aspiration.

Morbidity, mortality, and focus group

Morbidity rate

↗ new cases   ↗ all cases

Can refer either to the incidence rate or to the prevalence rate of a disease.

Mortality rate
The number of people dying from a particular disease during a given time interval.

Focus group
A small group selected from a wider population and sampled, as by open discussion, for its members' opinions about or emotional response to a particular subject or area, used especially in market research or political analysis.

Planning and Intervention

Nutrition intervention

Nutrition intervention encompasses those actions or steps a dietitian takes to change a behavior, counter a risk factor, or improve a condition he or she encounters in the individual or community being assessed.

Formula Selection

When selecting an appropriate enteral formulation, both formula characteristics and patient-specific factors should be considered. Formula variables include: digestibility/availability of the nutrients, nutritional adequacy, viscosity, osmolality, ease of use, and cost. Patient variables include: nutritional status and requirements, electrolyte balance, digestive and absorptive capacity, disease state, renal function, medical or drug therapy, and possible routes available for administration. Adult enteral formula products fall into one of the following categories: general use, high nitrogen, high nitrogen and high calorie, fiber enriched, semi-elemental, fat modified, and specialty.

Evidence-based dietetics practice

tools used in nutrition care to prevent disease and enhance health in patients. This type of practice uses the ability to glean what is most important in the medical literature and combine that information with patient values and professional knowledge in order to provide effective treatment to individuals. The tool adds credibility to the profession of dietetics in that not only must the dietitian be able to find the best evidence to support his or her clinical decisions, the dietitian must also view the data through a critical lens in order to choose the best course of action.

Types of diets

Vegetarianism → no meat, egg & dairy

Some vegetable protein sources lack in 1 or more "essential" amino acids. For example, grains and nuts are low in lysine and legumes are low in methionine. A vegetarian diet does not include fish, a major source of omega-3 fatty acids, though some plant-based sources of it exist such as soy, hempseed, pumpkin seeds, canola oil, and, especially, walnuts and flaxseed. Some suggest that vegetarians have higher rates of deficiencies in those nutrients, which are found in high concentrations in meat. Surprisingly, studies endorsed by the American Dietetic Association found that vegetarians were not deficient in iron or calcium. On the other hand, vitamin B_{12} and zinc from vegetarian sources other than dairy products and eggs are not readily absorbed by the body and a vegan diet usually needs supplements. Vegetarians may be low in vitamin D, zinc, B_{12}, and iron.

Combo PK

→ no meat & egg

Lacto-vegetarianism: Do not eat meat or eggs but do consume dairy products. Most vegetarians in India and those in the classical Mediterranean lands, such as Pythagoreans, are or were lacto-vegetarian.

→ no meat

Lacto-ovo vegetarianism: Do not eat meat but do consume dairy products and eggs. This is currently the most common variety in the Western world.

→ no meat & dairy

Ovo-vegetarianism: Do not eat meat or dairy products but do eat eggs.

→ no animal products

Veganism: Those who avoid eating any animal products, including eggs, milk, cheese, and sometimes honey, are known specifically as dietary vegans. Most also avoid using animal products, such as leather and some cosmetics, and are called vegans.

Raw food diet
A raw food diet involves food (usually vegan) that is not heated above 46.7°C (116°F); it may be warmed slightly or raw, but never cooked. Raw foodists argue that cooking destroys enzymes and/or portions of each nutrient. However, some raw foodists believe certain foods become more bio-available when warmed slightly as the process softens them, which more than negates the destruction of nutrients and enzymes. Other raw foodists, called "living foodists," activate the enzymes through soaking the food in water before consumption. Some spiritual raw foodists are also fruitarians, and many eat only organic foods.

Macrobiotic diet
A macrobiotic diet involves a diet consisting mostly of whole grains and beans and is usually spiritually based, such as fruitarianism.

Natural Hygiene
Natural Hygiene, in its classic form, involves a diet made up principally of raw vegan foods.

Fruitarianism
Fruitarianism involves a diet of only fruit, nuts, seeds, and other plant matter that can be gathered without harming the plant. Some fruitarians eat only plant matter that has already fallen off the plant. This typically arises out of a holistic philosophy. Thus, a fruitarian will eat beans, tomatoes, cucumbers, pumpkins, and the like, but will refuse to eat potatoes or spinach. It is disputed whether it is possible to avoid malnutrition with a fruitarian diet, which is rarer than other types of vegetarian or vegan diets.

Freeganism
Freegans practice a lifestyle based on concerns about the exploitation of animals, the earth, and human beings in the production of consumer goods. Many tend towards veganism, but this is not an inherent practice. Those that eat meat generally support the arguments for vegetarianism, but as freeganism is concerned about waste, freegans prefer to make use of discarded commodities than to allow them to go to waste and consume landfill space.

Pesco/pollo vegetarianism (semi-vegetarianism)
Some people choose to avoid certain types of meat for many of the same reasons that others choose vegetarianism (e.g., health, ethical beliefs). For example, some people will not eat "red meat" (e.g., mammal meat [beef, lamb, pork]) while still consuming poultry and seafood. It may also be used as an interim diet by individuals who are on a path to becoming fully vegetarian.

Flexitarianism
Flexitarians adhere to a diet that is mostly vegetarian but they occasionally consume meat. Some, for instance, may regard the suffering of animals in factory farm conditions as their sole reason for avoiding meat or meat-based foods and will eat meat or meat products from animals raised under more humane conditions or hunted in the wild.

Ketogenic diet

The ketogenic diet gets its name because the high fat content of the diet results in conversion of fat-to-ketones that are utilized as an energy source in place of glucose. If carbohydrates (which are composed of sugars) are eliminated from the diet, and a diet very high in fat is substituted, the body has no dietary sources of glucose. As a result, ketones are made from the available sources and these are used as fuel instead. It is necessary to be scrupulous in the restriction of carbohydrates because even a very small amount of sugar can cause the body to shift to glucose production and use, which it prefers to ketones.

For example, this restriction is such that children on the diet have to be careful to take sugarless daily multivitamins. Supplements of folate, B_6, B_{12}, vitamin D, and Ca are required with this diet. The ketogenic diet is often used in the treatment of epilepsy or seizure disorders.

Hemodialysis diet

The hemodialysis diet is an eating plan tailored to patients who are in stage 5 of chronic kidney disease (CKD), also known as end-stage renal disease (ESRD). These patients have very little or no kidney function and must undergo dialysis to clean their blood of waste and excess fluids. Hemodialysis is one type of dialysis. The procedure is done several times a week, usually for 3 to 4 hours at a time. The hemodialysis diet is designed to reduce the amount of fluid and waste that builds up between hemodialysis treatments. The hemodialysis diet will restrict foods that contain high amounts of sodium, phosphorus, and potassium. The hemodialysis diet will introduce a higher amount of protein into the eating plan. Certain fruits, vegetables, dairy products, and other foods that are very high in potassium will need to be restricted on the hemodialysis diet. Recommended 1.2 g protein/kg.

Peritoneal dialysis diet

The peritoneal dialysis (PD) diet is designed for patients who choose PD instead of hemodialysis. It is a slightly different diet than the hemodialysis diet, because of the differences in the dialysis treatments. Unlike hemodialysis, PD is performed daily. As a result, the body does not buildup as much potassium, sodium, and fluid, so the diet is more liberal. Protein requirements are higher, because protein is lost through the peritoneal membrane. Patients on PD are at risk for infection, so a diet with adequate protein is needed to keep the body strong. Unlike hemodialysis patients, PD patients are likely to keep normal or low potassium levels. Patients may be encouraged to eat potassium-rich foods such as tomatoes, orange juice, and bananas if their blood test levels are too low. The peritoneal dialysis diet is not as restricted in sodium and fluid compared with the diet for hemodialysis, because dialysis is performed daily. Recommend 1.2 to 1.3 g protein/kg.

Drug - nutrient interactions

Alcohols/Ethanol
Reduced absorption of fat, retinol, thiamin, cobalamin and folate; impaired utilization and storage of retinol; increased urinary excretion of zinc and magnesium.

Analgesics/Aspirin
Increased urinary excretion of ascorbic acid; may cause GI bleeding and subsequent iron deficiency; increased folate and vitamin D requirements.

Antacids/Aluminum- or Calcium-Containing
Reduced iron, copper, phosphate and magnesium absorption.

Antibiotics/Penicillins, Aminoglycosides, Chloramphenicol
Increased urinary excretion of amino acids; reduced intestinal vitamin K and cobalamin synthesis; possible malabsorption of fat, cobalamin, calcium, magnesium, and carotenoids.

Anticoagulants/Coumadin
Vitamin K decreases and tocopherol increases drug effect.

Anticonvulsants/Phenobarbital, Phenytoin
Folate antagonists; increased vitamin D, vitamin K, and pyridoxine requirements; impaired vitamin D metabolism leading to hypomagnesemia, hypocalcemia, and hypophosphatemia.

Antidepressants/Imipramine
May induce riboflavin deficiency; increased appetite.

Antihypertensives/Hydralazine
Pyridoxine antagonist; increased urinary excretion of manganese and pyridoxine.

Antimalarials/Pyrimethamine, Sulfadoxine
Folate antagonists.

Antineoplastics/Methotrexate
Folate antagonist; may impair fat, calcium, cobalamin, lactose, folate, and carotene absorption.

Antitubercular/Isoniazid
Accelerated metabolism of pyridoxine; subsequent pyridoxine deficiency blocks conversion of tryptophan to niacin, leading to niacin deficiency; reduced calcium absorption; reduced conversion of vitamin D by the liver.

Antiulcer/Cimetidine
Impaired cobalamin absorption.

Cardiac Glycosides/Digoxin
Increased urinary excretion of calcium, magnesium, and zinc. Anorexia.

Corticosteroids/Hydrocortisone, Prednisone, Dexamethasone
Reduced calcium and phosphate absorption; increased urinary calcium, potassium, ascorbic acid, zinc, and nitrogen excretion; increased pyridoxine and vitamin D metabolic requirements.

Diuretics/Furosemide, Thiazides, Spironolactone
Increased urinary potassium, sodium, chloride, magnesium, zinc, and iodine excretion; reduced calcium excretion leading to hypercalcemia and hypophosphatemia with thiazides, increased calcium excretion with furosemide; increased urinary sodium and chloride; reduced urinary potassium excretion.

Hypocholesterolemic Agents/Cholestyramine, Colestipol
Reduced absorption of fat, fat-soluble vitamins, calcium, cobalamin, folate.

<u>Laxatives/Bisacodyl, Phenolphthalein, Mineral Oil</u>
Abuse leads to general malabsorption, steatorrhea, and dehydration. Malabsorption of fat-soluble vitamins, electrolytes, calcium.

<u>Oral Contraceptives/Conjugated estrogens, Ethinyl estradiol, Mestranol</u>
Increased folic acid and possibly pyridoxine and ascorbic acid requirements; reduced calcium excretion, altered tryptophan metabolism.

<u>Stimulants/Caffeine</u>
Increased urinary calcium excretion.

Calculating Basal Energy Expenditure

BEE refers to the metabolic activity necessary to sustain life (i.e., respiration, pulse, body temperature) and can be estimated using the following equation:
Harris-Benedict equation: BEE (kcal/day):
Males = 66.5 + (13.7 X W) + (5 X H) - (6.8 X A)
Females = 655 + (9.6 X W) + (1.7 X H) - (4.7 X A)
where:
W = usual or adjusted weight in kilograms
H = height in centimeters
A = age in years

Calculating Total Energy Expenditure

TEE can be estimated by multiplying the BEE by a factor that accounts for physical activity and clinical status. Only one factor should be used (i.e., do not add multiple factors). Select the factor that corresponds to the patient's dominant situation. Most patients will require 1.3 to 1.7 times the BEE in total caloric intake or between 30 and 35 kcal/kg.

Only rarely do calorie requirements exceed 2 x BEE or 40 kcal/kg in any patient. The TEE is adjusted as illness progresses and recovery proceeds to avoid complications of under- or overfeeding.

Adjusted body weight

If the patient is severely underweight (less than 80% of ideal body weight [IBW]), then use Current Weight for nutrient calculations. If the patient is obese, use:
Adjusted Body Weight = IBW + 0.25 (Usual Weight – IBW).

* IBW can be used for nutritional assessment purposes.

Fluid requirements for adults

A healthy adult ingests approximately 1 mL of free water/kcal of energy, or 35 to 50 mL/kg body weight/day. Hospitalized patients usually require 30 to 35 mL/kg/day. Fluid needs may also be approximated as 1,500 mL per m² BSA. However, wide variations in fluid intake are normally well tolerated without producing hypo- or hypernatremia or fluid overload. Patients with liver disease, renal failure, cardiac or pulmonary diseases, or closed head injuries may require restricted fluid intakes while patients with nasogastric output, diarrhea, hypovolemia secondary to burns or trauma, diuresis, fistulae, and insensible losses may require additional fluids. Insensible losses are the result of respiration, fecal loss, evaporation, and fever. Volume-depleted patients should be rehydrated and electrolytes repleted before initiating PN (i.e., fluid deficits should not be corrected with amino acid and dextrose solutions). PN solutions are extremely hyperosmolar and cannot be converted to an equivalent iso-osmolar volume or volume of free water.

Electrolyte requirements

Electrolyte needs are adjusted daily based on lab results and current clinical status of the patient. The typical adult baseline electrolyte requirements during nutritional repletion are:

Sodium (chloride, acetate, or phosphate) 60 to 150 mEq
- Potassium (chloride, acetate, or phosphate) 70 to 150 mEq chloride (sodium or potassium) 60 to 150 mEq
- Magnesium (sulfate) 8 to 24 mEq
- Phosphate (sodium or potassium) 7 to 10 mmol per 1000 kcal

Nutritional repletion therapy increases electrolyte requirements. During the first 3 to 5 days of refeeding, patients typically pass through 3 phases of electrolyte utilization. During the first 24 to 48 hours, total body deficits must be replaced. In the second phase, which may last for several days, anabolic processes are induced, which result in increased intracellular uptake of potassium and phosphate. After approximately 1 week of providing nutritional therapy, electrolyte requirements become relatively stable.

Fat requirements

A wide range of fat intake is generally well tolerated by most individuals. Current national guidelines recommend limiting fat intake to less than 30% of total kcals. A higher percent fat intake may be desired for patients with poor appetites/limited food intake to increase caloric density of foods (fat contains 9 kcal/g vs. 4 kcal/g in carbohydrates and protein). A minimum of 2% to 4% kcals as linoleic acid is required daily to prevent essential fatty acid deficiency.   └→ min = 2-4%
max = 30%

Protein requirements

Protein needs may vary greatly with the metabolic status of the patient. The average patient receiving nutritional intervention requires 0.8 to 2 g protein/kg usual body weight. The obese patient is unusual. Use of usual body weight can result in overfeeding. It is recommended to use adjusted body weight (ABW) for reasonable estimation of nutrient requirements. The goals of nutrition support are to minimize protein breakdown, preserve lean body mass, promote protein synthesis, and optimize immune responses.

Neonates

Protein requirements   → 40 wks
- Term infants need 1.8 to 2.2 g/kg/day.   → < 36 wks
- Preterm (very low birth weight [VLBW]) infants need 3 to 3.5 g/kg/day (IV or enteral). Start early: VLBW neonates may need 1.5 to 2 g/kg/day by 72 hours.
- Restrict stressed infants or infants with cholestasis to 1.5 g/kg/day.

- Very high protein intakes (greater than 5 to 6 g/kg/day) may be dangerous.
- Maintain NP Calorie/Protein ratio (at least 25 to 30:1).

Types of baby formulas
- Soy formula: Not recommended for premature babies: impaired mineral and protein absorption; low vitamin content. Used if galactosemia, cow milk protein intolerance (CMPI), secondary lactose intolerance following gastroenteritis.
- Pregestimil: (Alimentum is similar, but with sucrose.) Hydrolyzed casein; 50% MCT; glucose polymers. Used if malabsorption or short bowel syndrome.
- Portagen: Casein; 75% glucose polymers + 25% sucrose; 85% MCT. Useful for persistent chylothorax. Can cause EFA def.
- Similac PM 60/40: Low sodium and phosphate; high Ca/PO4 ratio. Used in renal failure, hypoparathyroidism.
- Similac 27: High energy with more protein, Ca/Po4, lytes.
- Used for fluid-restricted infants: CHF, bronchopulmonary dysplasia.
- Nutramigen: Hypoallergenic, lactose and sucrose free.
- Used for protein allergies, lactose intolerance.
- Note: Medium chain triglyceride (MCT) is a special nutritional supplement that helps digest and absorb fats.

Carbohydrate requirements
Carbohydrate Enteral: Human milk/ 20 Cal/oz formula = 67 Cal per 100 cc. Lactose is carbohydrate in human milk and term formula. Soy and lactose-free formula have sucrose, maltodextrins, and glucose polymers. Preterm formula has 50% lactose and 50% glucose polymers (lactase level lower in premature babies, but glycosidases active). Lactose provides 40% to 45% of calories in human milk and term formula.

Energy requirements for neonates
Stressed and sick infants need more energy (e.g., sepsis, surgery). Babies on parenteral nutrition need less energy (less fecal loss of nutrients, no loss for absorption): 70 to 90 Cal/kg/day+ 2.4 to 2.8 g/kg/day protein adequate for growth. Count nonprotein calories only. Protein preferred to be used for growth, not energy.
- 65% from carbohydrates, 35% from lipids ideal.
- Greater than 165 to 180 Cal/kg/day not useful.

Enteral feeding

Indications for EN:
Patients with adequate GI function, inadequate oral intake, at significant risk for clinical malnutrition, and who are likely to benefit from nutrition support.

Contraindications (absolute or relative) for enteral EN
- Complete bowel obstruction or severe bowel ileus.
- Intractable vomiting or major upper GI hemorrhage.
- Complete inability to absorb nutrients through the GI tract.
- Severe hemodynamic instability, severe postprandial pain, GI ischemia, diffuse peritonitis.
- Inability to obtain safe or proper enteral access or maintain desirable body positioning.

- GI abscesses, fistulas, or lymphatic (chylous) injury that seriously impair feeding integrity.
- No outcome benefit expected or risk is greater than expected benefit.
- Patient refuses.

Routes of administration

Continuous feeding with a pump is the most common and preferred method of providing enteral feedings to hospitalized patients. For patients administering their own feedings at home, or for patients in settings where a pump is not available, bolus feedings may be offered. Slow introduction of feedings allows the patient to adjust to the osmolarity of the solution. Osmolarity refers to how many particles are suspended in the solution. High osmolarity formulas can cause cramping or diarrhea as water is drawn into the gut. 40 to 60 ml/h can be given over a period of 18 to 24 hours, with monitoring for tolerance. After 24 hours, formula should be discarded to avoid contamination.

Bolus feedings should be calculated by dividing the patient's daily needs into several small meals. High osmolarity formulas should be started at half-strength; low osmolarity formulas can be started at full strength. Fluid needs are not always met by formula, and 1 mL water/kcal should be offered after feeding to prevent dehydration, especially with nutrient-dense formulas.

Nasoenteric Feeding Tubes

Tubes are passed through the nose to various points in the GI tract and are named with reference to the location of the terminal end of the feeding tube. Examples include nasogastric, nasoduodenal, and nasojejunal tubes.

Advantages: These avoid general anesthesia or surgical procedure, and there is a low incidence of complications.

Disadvantages: There is a risk of aspiration (may be less with nasoduodenal and nasojejunal tube), x-ray confirmation of correct tube placement is required, and it is suited only to short-term (less than 6 weeks) use.

Tube Enterostomy

Tubes are placed either laparoscopically, operatively, or percutaneously. Examples include esophagostomy, gastrostomy (PEG), percutaneous endoscopic jejunostomy (PEJ), needle catheter jejunostomy (NCJ), operative laparoscopic gastrostomy, and operative laparoscopic jejunostomy.

Advantages:
- May be used immediately or within hours of placement.
- May be used for long-term support.
- May be used in presence of significant disease of upper GI tract (esophagus, stomach and duodenum).
- Percutaneously placed tubes avoid risks of surgery and general anesthesia.
- Laparoscopic feeding tubes allow patients to return home the same day after procedure.

Disadvantages: may require endoscopy, abdominal ultrasound, or radiologic procedure with contrast media; endoscopy may be difficult or impossible in presence of tumor or stricture, altered anatomy or severe obesity; laparoscopically or operatively placed tubes require general anesthesia; potential for chronic wound complications

Free water requirements

Most patients on enteral nutrition therapy will require additional fluid to meet minimum fluid requirements. To calculate additional fluid requirements, begin by determining the patient's total fluid needs. Then determine the amount of free water provided by the tube feeding formula by multiplying the percent free water content (information available in diet manual, on enteral formulary cards, or by contacting a dietitian) by the total volume of tube feeding formula to be administered each day. Subtract the free water supplied by the formula from the calculated total free water requirement, which equals remaining volume of free water, and divide the remaining into 3 or 4 boluses per day.

Example: A 50-year-old woman weighing 55 kg requires full-strength Isosource HN at 55 mL/h to meet her energy and protein requirements and 1,800 to 2,000 mL fluid/d. Isosource HN is 82% free water. Then 55 mL/h x 24 hr x 0.82 = 1,082 mL free water/d provided by the enteral formula. Her additional fluid needs are 1,800 – 1,082 = 718 mL/d or about 3 boluses of 250 mL each.

Formulas

Enteral feeding may be the choice for those unable to maintain nutrition orally because of surgery, dysphagia, coma, or esophageal obstruction. The GI tract must still be functional, with more than 2 feet of working small intestine. Formulas may be commercially prepared, which offers convenience, consistency, and reduced expense, but individually prepared solutions may better meet the needs of some patients. Modular formulas are composed from varying amounts of carbohydrate, fat, protein, vitamins, minerals, and water. Enteral feedings can also be made from whole foods that have been pureed and strained. Advantages of this method include reduced cost and presence of trace nutrients; disadvantages include increased chance of contamination and the need for a larger feeding tube. Patients with malabsorption from short-bowel syndrome or other diseases may need defined formulas, which are easier to digest because of the simpler energy forms they contain. Glucose or dextrins provide carbohydrates, amino acids provide protein, and monoglycerides and diglycerides provide lipids. Most enteral formulas provide 1 to 1.5 kcal/cc.

Transition to cyclic or bolus feedings

Enteral nutrition therapy is usually the first course of transition. An intermitten infusion schedule follows.

Intermitten infusion (Bolus feedings): administered by gravity dip or syringe bolus if needed (for example, for a patient with gastric feeding tubes).

Cyclic feeding: can be administered by infusing the formula for a specific amount of time, when the patient desires time without using the pump. This is especially good for patients with intestinal feeding tube sites

Complications

If a patient has more than 3 episodes of diarrhea a day, several feeding-related problems may be at fault. Patients should be assessed for lactose intolerance, and offered lactose-free formula if needed. Formula should be discarded every 24 hours to avoid diarrhea from bacterial contamination. If formula has high osmolarity or is being infused too rapidly, continuous drip may be appropriate. If nausea or vomiting occurs, this may indicate that the GI tract is not functioning.

Repositioning the tube into the duodenum may help, or parenteral feeding may be necessary. If patient is aspirating the formula after feeding, there is a risk of pneumonia. This may be prevented by elevating the patient's head during feeding, changing to a lower bore (smaller) tube, or placing the tube in the duodenum. Obstruction of the feeding tube may be suspected if the patient does not receive more than 12 hours of a feeding. Frequent flushing of the tube or changing to a large bore tube can help prevent this.

Parenteral nutrition

Parenteral nutrition refers to the infusion of nutrients directly into the circulation. This is to be used as a last resort when the GI tract is not functional. If the patient is expected to resume oral nutrition shortly, peripheral veins may be used to provide glucose and fluid for a brief duration. For total nutrition provided over a longer period of time, central vein feeding is used, usually via the superior vena cava. Significant amounts of calories can be provided this way, up to 4,000 kcal to promote anabolism, as the large volume of blood quickly dilutes the hypertonic (concentrated) solution. Total parenteral nutrition is an option when the GI tract is not working because of surgery, organ failure, short-bowel syndrome, or bowel obstruction. It is also needed when patients have aspiration problems, extreme anorexia or cachexia, or liver and kidney failure with special amino acid requirements.

Fat emulsion is used as a concentrated calorie source and to prevent essential fatty acid deficiency in patients receiving PN. When used as a source of calories for critically ill patients, 15% to 50% of total calories may be supplied as fat. However, to avoid the fat overload syndrome, maximum intravenous fat intake should not exceed 2.5 g/kg/day. The fat overload syndrome is a potentially lethal syndrome, consisting of lipemic serum, massive fat deposition in the lungs and liver, spleen and reticuloendothelial blockade, sepsis, and thrombocytopenia. In order to prevent fatty acid deficiency, linoleic acid must be provided as 2% to 4% of total caloric intake (500 mL of 10% lipid emulsion 2 to 3 times/week will supply adequate linoleic acid for most patients). The following maximum infusion rates are recommended: 500 cc of 10% lipids over 8 to 12 hours; 500 cc of 20% lipids over 12 to 16 hours. For critically ill patients with respiratory compromise, continuous 24-hour fat infusion provides stable energy intake. Fat emulsion should be used cautiously in patients with severe liver disease or dysfunction, or history of hyperlipidemia (e.g., AIDS), as these patients have a decreased capacity to clear the infused fat.

Indications for PN
Severely malnourished or at significant risk, unable to obtain more than 50% of nutritional needs from oral or enteral nutrition, and likely to benefit from nutrition support. Massive small bowel resection, GI ischemia or postprandial pain, intractable vomiting, prolonged bowel obstruction/ileus, diffuse peritonitis, severe radiation enteritis, some GI abscesses or fistulas, moderately to severely malnourished, planned elective surgery, and unable to feed enterally.

Clinical Conditions Warranting Very Cautious Use of PN:
- Hyperglycemia (> 150 to 200 mg/dL) or Hyperosmolality (> 350 mOsm/L).
- Severe azotemia (BUN > 100 mg/dL).
- Serum deficit or excess in Na, K, Phos, Cl.
- High risk for fluid overload (risk can be minimized by decreasing previously ordered IVF).

Composition of formula
For protein synthesis and anabolism to take place, the total parenteral nutrition (TPN) solution can provide 1 g of protein for every 150 calories. For severely stressed patients, the solution may be adjusted to provide 1 g of protein per 100 calories. Protein is provided by crystalline amino acids. Common solutions range from 5% to 15% amino acids. The types of amino acids can be adjusted according to the disease state. For example, branched-chain amino acids can be used in solutions

for patients with liver failure, and essential amino acid–rich formulas are given to patients with kidney failure. Carbohydrate is usually provided in the form of dextrose, which has a higher osmolality than glucose. No more than 4 or 5 mg/kg/min should be given to prevent hyperglycemia and excessive carbon dioxide production. Lipids provide 25% to 35% of calories to avoid essential fatty acid deficiency. Potassium may be increased in high anabolic states to balance the movement of potassium into the cells. Phosphorus is important when high calorie solutions are given to prevent hypophosphatemia.

Standard Parenteral Electrolyte Package
The standard electrolyte package available provides the following:
- Sodium 25 mEq
- Potassium 40.6 mEq
- Calcium 5 mEq
- Magnesium 8 mEq
- Acetate 33.5 mEq
- Gluconate 5 mEq
- Chloride 40.6 mEq

Phosphorus is NOT included in the standard electrolyte package and must be added separately. PN solutions typically contain more phosphate than calcium (as great as 6:1 molar ratio). Cramps may result from excessive phosphate administration. The solubility of calcium in PN solutions is limited by formation of calcium phosphate and carbonate, as well as magnesium salts. Unfortunately, calcium solubility is unpredictable because it depends upon factors such as the commercial sources of the PN components, the order of mixing the PN components, the solution pH, and temperature and storage conditions.

Trace element requirements
The trace elements zinc, copper, chromium, manganese, iodine, iron, and selenium must be provided in PN to prevent clinical deficiency. It is recommended that all adult PN patients be supplemented daily with a standard trace element package. The standard trace element package available provides the following:
- Zinc 5 mg
- Copper 1 mg
- Manganese 0.5 mg
- Chromium 10 mcg
- Selenium 60 mcg
- Iodide 75 mcg

Iron is not included in the standard trace element package. Iron is not routinely added to PN solutions because it may alter the stability of other PN components.

Medications
Administration of medications via PN may be beneficial when there is limited venous access and/or the patient is fluid restricted. The major problem associated with the addition of medications to PN is the potential for incompatibilities. The following issues should be considered if a medication is to be added to PN. Certain medications should not be mixed with any PN if intermittent infusion is necessary to achieve therapeutic serum levels (i.e., antibiotics). Medications that require a precise rate of infusion (i.e., cardiovascular agents) are not recommended to be added to PN solution. Doses of a medication cannot be readily adjusted once combined with the PN. Adding alkaline medications

to PN admixtures may increase the potential for calcium-phosphate incompatibilities. Medication must be chemically stable in PN solution for over 24 hours. Medications routinely added to PN solutions include: H₂ antagonists (e.g., ranitidine) and insulin. The use of Y-site or piggyback drug delivery has helped prevent or avoid drug compatibility problems.

Transitional feeding

Transitional feeding refers to the period when a patient switches from parenteral to enteral or oral feeding, or from enteral to oral feeding. Patients are at risk for hypophosphatemia during this time, and must be monitored closely. When patients have been without food for a period of time, aggressive refeeding causes phosphorus to rapidly leave the plasma and enter the cell in order to take part in the manufacture of adenosine triphosphate. The risk is increased in alcoholics, diabetics, and patients with kidney disease. Phosphate supplementation may be necessary to prevent severe metabolic and hematological side effects. Patients may also experience low levels of potassium as cellular needs increase, so monitoring and supplementation as necessary should occur. Intestinal enzyme counts are low after a period of no food, and patients may not tolerate lactose at first. First meals should be lactose-free, low in sodium and carbohydrate, and supplemented with electrolytes as needed.

phos & potas.

Refeeding Syndrome

low phosphate   low magnesium   low calcium

This syndrome of hypophosphataemia, hypomagnesaemia, hypocalcaemia, and fluid retention is seen in severely malnourished patients when they are started on enteral or parenteral nutrition. Thiamine deficiency may also be a feature.

Life-threatening dysrhythmias and congestive cardiac failure can result. During starvation, total body loss of these minerals is compensated for by movement of ions out from the cells into plasma, which maintains normal, or near normal plasma levels. When feeding is started, the increase in insulin level encourages ions to move intracellularly and plasma concentrations fall.

Risk Factors:
- Anorexia nervosa
- Classic kwashiorkor
- Classic marasmus
- Chronic alcoholism
- Chronic malnutrition-underfeeding
- Prolonged IV hydration
- Prolonged fasting
- Morbid obesity with massive weight loss, prolonged fasting

Types of diets

- Clear liquid diet: supplies fluid, sugar, and salt (from broth). It is often ordered before or after surgery, or after prolonged fasting. This diet is inadequate in nutrients: 600 kcal, 150 g CHO, and negligible protein and fat.
- Full liquid diet: may be used when solid foods are contraindicated. Adequate in most nutrients (especially if a high protein supplement is added...p.16-17). Because milk-based foods constitute a large portion of this diet, patients with milk/lactose intolerance may need a substitution for milk.

- <u>Blenderized liquids:</u> <u>contains shakes, other liquids, and baby foods</u> for patients with a wired jaw. Pureed diet is <u>for significant problems chewing or swallowing,</u> but is too thick for wired jaw.
- <u>Mechanical soft diet:</u> is appropriate for many patients having difficulty with solid foods because of <u>mild difficulty chewing, mild dysphagia, or weakness.</u>
- <u>Soft postsurgical diet</u> is modified for <u>ostomy patients and general GI postop patients,</u> but requires <u>normal ability to chew.</u>
- <u>Postgastrectomy diet</u> has <u>snacks, and limits simple sugars, size of meals, and liquids at meals.</u> Dysphagia diets and restrictions in fluid viscosity are only recommended by speech pathology.
- <u>Diabetic, cardiac, and renal diets</u> <u>restrict the type and amount of food provided</u>, therefore, they may not be appropriate in patients who are eating poorly. If only a Na restriction is desired, order a 2 g Na diet, not a cardiac prudent diet that also restricts fat/chol.

Liquid supplements

Nutrient-dense liquid supplement 3 times daily, such as Boost Plus, resulted in wt gain, and in the most poorly nourished patients was associated with improved function and reduced mortality.
- <u>Resource Fruit Beverage:</u> 8 oz, clear liquid, high sugar, some protein, fat free, lactose free. Berry, Peach, Orange. 250 kcal (14% protein), 9 g Protein, 53 g CHO, 0 g Fat, < 80 mg Na, < 20 mg K, 160 mg Phos, 10 mg Ca, 1 mg Mg.
- <u>Ensure High Protein:</u> 8 oz, high protein, moderately high Kcal, low residue, lactose free. Vanilla, Chocolate, Berry. 230 kcal (21 % protein), 12 g Protein, 31 g CHO, 6 g Fat, 290 mg Na, 500 mg K, 250 mg Phos, 300 mg Ca, 100 mg Mg.
- <u>Boost Plus:</u> 8 oz, high Kcal, moderate protein, low residue, lactose-free. Vanilla, Chocolate, Strawberry. 360 kcal (16% protein), 14 g Protein, 45 g CHO, 14 g Fat, 170 mg Na, 380 mg K, 310 mg Phos, 330 mg Ca, 105 mg Mg.
- <u>Carnation Instant Breakfast:</u> Mix powder packet with 8 oz milk for high kcal, moderate protein dairy shake, high in lactose. Vanilla flavor. Mixed w/ 8 oz whole milk = 280 kcal (17% protein), 12 g protein, 39 g CHO, 8 g fat, 200 mg Na, 610 mg K, 480 mg Phos, 550 mg Ca, 110 mg Mg.
- <u>Carnation Instant Breakfast, No Sugar Added:</u> Mix with 8 oz milk for high protein, high kcal dairy shake, high in lactose. Box has Vanilla, Chocolate, and Strawberry flavors. Mix with 8 oz whole milk = 220 kcal (22% protein), 12 g protein, 24 g CHO, 8 to 9 g fat, 220 mg Na, 630 mg K, 480 mg Phos, 540 mg Ca, 110 mg Mg.
- <u>Scandishake:</u> Mix powder packet with 8 oz milk (or substitute) for very high kcal, lower protein shake, no added vitamins or minerals. Vanilla and Chocolate. Mix with 8 oz whole milk: 600 kcal (9% protein), 13 g Protein, 69 g CHO, 29 g Fat, 215 to 240 mg Na, 650 to 970 mg K, no other specific nutrient info.
- <u>MightyShake:</u> 4 oz, high kcal, moderate protein, dairy, contains lactose. Vanilla, Chocolate, Strawberry. 200 kcal (12% protein), 6 g Protein, 30 g CHO, 6 g Fat, 60 mg Na, 150 to 210 mg K, 100 to 150 mg Phos, 150 mg Ca, 24 mg Mg.
- <u>Nepro:</u> 8 oz, renal, high kcal, moderate protein, low in K, Phos, Mg, and water, lactose-free. Vanilla and Butter Pecan. 475 kcal (14% protein), 16.7 g Protein, 53 g CHO, 23 g Fat, 200 mg Na, 250 mg K, 165 mg Phos, 325 mg Ca, 50 mg Mg.
- <u>Boost Pudding:</u> 5 oz, high kcal, low volume, moderate protein, lactose-free. Vanilla and Chocolate. 280 kcal (12% protein), 7 g protein, 33 g CHO, 9 g fat, 125 mg Na, 250 mg K, 200 mg Phos, 250 mg Ca, 60 mg Mg.

Modular Enteral/Oral Additives

- **ProMod:** Whey protein powder. 1 scoop = 5 g protein, 28 kcal. Mix 1 scoop with 50 to 100 mL of lukewarm water for bolus administration into enteral tube (or mix with oral liquids or pureed foods). Addition to the enteral feeding bag is not recommended. Whey is a high-quality protein.
- **GlutaSolve:** Glutamine powder. 1 pkg = 15 g glutamine, 90 kcal. Mix with 80 mL water for bolus administration into enteral tube (or mix with oral liquids or pureed foods). Give 1 to 3 times/day (see dosing below). Giving it mixed in the enteral feeding formula/bag is not recommended.
- **Polycose Powder:** Glucose polymers. 1 tbsp powder = 23 kcal. May be added to most tube feeding formulas and most foods and beverages to add carb kcal.
- **Microlipid:** 50% safflower oil/50% water emulsion. 1 mL = 4.5 kcal. For use in oral or tube-feeding formulas as a source of linoleic acid and fat kcal.
- **Medium Chain Triglyceride (MCT) Oil:** 15 ml (1 tbsp) = 115 kcal. Does not require bile acids. Can be absorbed in colon. Adheres to feeding tube lumen. Does not provide essential fatty acids.
- **Instant Food Thickener:** modifying liquids to a nectar-, honey-, or pudding-like consistency, as recommended by speech pathology. Poor patient acceptance.

Hypocaloric and hypercaloric feeding

↗ low cal

Hypocaloric feeding with adequate protein can be justified by obesity, poorly controlled glucose, or when starting to feed malnourished or highly stressed patients.

↗ high cal

Hypercaloric feeding (mild) can be justified in underweight preoperative patients and during unstressed convalescence. Excess Kcal can increase the risk of hyperglycemia, hypercapnea, hepatic steatosis, hypertriglyceridemia, and volume overload.

Percutaneous endoscopic gastrostomy

Percutaneous endoscopic gastrostomy (PEG) is the most popular. Complications include tube dislodgment, bleeding, infection, leakage, and gastric fistula. PEG tubes with a jejunal extension (PEG/J) may be beneficial when a patient requiring long-term EN cannot tolerate gastric feeding short-term. PEG feeding has not shown positive outcomes in advanced dementia.

Jejunostomy

Jejunostomy is usually placed surgically for short- or long-term intestinal EN. Indications: prolonged gastric ileus or obstruction, gastroparesis, reflux/aspiration, severe pancreatitis, or need for multiple surgeries (e.g., trauma wounds [no need to stop J-tube EN for surgery]).

J-tube vs. G-tube
A J-tube feeds directly into the jejunum and a G-tube goes directly to the stomach. Note: The J-tube allows feeding without involving the stomach.

NJ (nasojejunum)-tube
This is similar to the nasogastric (NG) tube except once in the stomach it continues through the pyloric valve, duodenum (first part of the small bowel), and into the jejunum (second part of the

- 123 -

small bowel). NJ tubes have the same drawbacks of the NG tube but because the end of the tube is in the jejunum instead of the stomach, NJ tubes can help reduce vomiting associated with reflux.

NG-tube
This is a long thin tube that is inserted through the child's nose, throat, and esophagus down into the stomach. A pump or gravity feed may be used to supply the food through the tube. Feeds can be given in bolus or continuous amounts. Bolus means large amounts over a short period of time. For example, mealtimes can be mimicked by giving 3 large meals a day through the tube.

Community nutrition program

When developing a nutrition program geared toward a specific population, the first step is to develop a mission statement, or the guiding philosophy of the program. Defining the needs of the population is central in forming this philosophy. Next, one should define some broad goals that the program is meant to achieve. The next step is to hone in on the goals to formulate some measurable objectives that give meaning and purpose to the program; these should be written as concrete action statements. Then one should define the focus of the program by setting priorities; this may mean that some goals will need to be set aside. With prioritized goals in place, one can develop a plan of action, which should include all of the alternative ways of achieving the goals. A budget can then be developed, and implementation of the plan follows. Depending on the scope of the program, implementation may include small-scale outreach efforts such as health fairs or may involve lobbying to pass new legislation.

Dietary Reference Intakes

Dietary Reference Intakes (DRI) are meant to replace the Recommended Dietary Allowances that have long provided reference values to help people know how much of what nutrient they should be getting in an adequate diet. Rather than providing one catchall value for all individuals, this reference includes the estimated average requirement (EAR), adequate intake (AI), and tolerable upper intake levels (UL). While the RDA shares values that would meet the nutritional needs of most individuals when consumed daily, DRI shares goals that are meant to be achieved over time. EAR provides the intake that would meet the needs of half the population using median rather than average to determine which 50% is included in the reference group. If not enough data are available to determine EAR, then AI is an estimate that assumes an adequate value in healthy people. UL levels should not be exceeded, or nutrient toxicity may occur.

Dietary guidelines

USDA guideline changes
The United States Department of Agriculture began issuing nutrition guidelines in 1894, and in 1943 the department began promoting the Basic 7 food groups. In 1956, Basic 7 was replaced with the Basic Four food groups. These were fruits and vegetables, cereals and breads, milk, and meat. Basic Four lasted until 1992, when it was replaced with the Food Pyramid, which divided food into six groups: 1) Bread, cereal, rice, pasta 2) Fruit 3) Vegetables 4) Meat, poultry, fish, dry beans, eggs, nuts 5) Milk, yogurt, cheese 6) Fats, oils, sweets. The Food Pyramid also provided recommendations for the number of daily servings from each group.

The Food Pyramid and MyPlate
The USDA's Food Pyramid was heavily criticized for being vague and confusing, and in 2011 it was replaced with MyPlate. MyPlate is much easier to understand, as it consists of a picture of a dinner

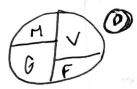

plate divided into four sections, visually illustrating how our daily diet should be distributed among the various food groups. Vegetables and grains each take up 30% of the plate, while fruits and proteins each constitute 20% of the plate. There is also a representation of a cup, marked Dairy, alongside the plate. The idea behind MyPlate is that it's much easier for people to grasp the idea that half of a meal should consist of fruits and vegetables than it is for them to understand serving sizes for all the different kinds of foods they eat on a regular basis.

Most experts consider MyPlate to be a great improvement over the Food Pyramid, but it has still come under criticism from some quarters. Many believe too much emphasis is placed on protein, and some say the dairy recommendation should be eliminated altogether. The Harvard School of Public Health created its own Healthy Eating Plate to address what it sees as shortcomings in MyPlate. Harvard's guide adds healthy plant-based oils to the mix, stresses whole grains instead of merely grains, recommends drinking water or unsweetened coffee or tea instead of milk, and adds a reminder that physical activity is important.

Retailer labeling

The FDA created a voluntary program to promote retailer labeling of the top 20 most commonly sold fruits, vegetables, and fish, as well as the 45 best-selling cuts of raw meat and poultry. The nutrient information needs to be available as a brochure, leaflet, notebook, or stickers in the appropriate grocery department.

Labels for fruits, veggies, and raw fish include the following:
- Name of the fruit, vegetable, or fish.
- Serving size.
- Calories per serving.
- Amount of protein, carbohydrates, fat, and sodium per serving.
- Percent of the Recommended Daily Allowances (RDA) for iron, calcium, and vitamins A and C per serving.

Healthy People 2020

In January 2010, the Department of Health and Human Services launched a comprehensive, nationwide health promotion and disease prevention agenda. Healthy People 2020 contains hundreds of specific objectives designed to serve as a road map for improving the health of all people in the United States. Healthy People 2020 builds on similar initiatives pursued over the past several decades. Two overarching goals—increase quality and years of healthy life, and eliminate health disparities—served as a guide for developing objectives that will actually measure progress. The objectives are organized in 42 topic areas, each representing an important public health area. Each objective has a target for improvements to be achieved by the year 2020. A limited set of the objectives, known as the Leading Health Indicators, are intended to help everyone more easily understand the importance of health promotion and disease prevention, and to encourage wide participation in improving health in the next decade.

These Indicators were chosen based on their ability to motivate action, the availability of data to measure their progress, and their relevance as broad public health issues. National Center for Health Statistics (NCHS) is responsible for coordinating the effort to monitor the nation's progress toward the objectives.

USDA Healthy Eating Index

USDA Healthy Eating Index is a summary measure of overall diet quality. It provides a picture of the type and quantity of foods people eat and the degree to which diets comply with specific recommendations in the Dietary Guidelines and the USDA's MyPlate.

Bowes & Church's Food Values of Portions Commonly Used

One of the most comprehensive print versions of nutrient composition tables is *Bowes & Church's Food Values of Portions Commonly Used*, by Jean A. T. Pennington, Ph.D. Some 8,500 foods are listed according to food group with analysis results for 30 nutrients, but they are not in "Nutrition Facts" label format.

Agencies providing nutrition assistance

The Food and Agriculture Organization of the United Nations provides a place where nations can peacefully interact to combat hunger and malnutrition worldwide. The organization focuses on helping developing nations, particularly by helping them to develop agriculture policy, providing expertise to help them stretch limited dollars, and developing data to help development.

The World Health Organization (WHO) is the public health branch of the United Nations and seeks to help all people attain the highest level of health possible. Nutrition activities of the WHO include its recently developed "Global Strategy on Diet, Physical Activity, and Diet."

Voluntary health agencies that promote nutrition include non-profit agencies such as the American Heart Association, which engages in initiatives such as publishing diet and lifestyle recommendations. Professional organizations such as the American Dietetic Association reach out to the public with activities such as National Nutrition Month and by engaging in advocacy to promote the nutritional status of people worldwide.

Food and Drug Administration

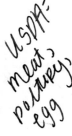

The FDA ensures the safety and wholesomeness of almost 80% of the United States' food supply, all foods except meat, poultry, and some egg products, which are regulated by the USDA. The FDA does the job so well that American food is as safe as any in the world, but changing tastes and other developments keep presenting the agency with new challenges. For example, Americans today eat a greater variety of imported foods than ever, and they are relying more and more on commercially prepared food products. The growing numbers of senior Americans have increased the proportion of the US population considered at risk for developing foodborne illness to 25%.

Scientists have identified more than 5 times as many foodborne pathogens than were known 50 years ago; in addition, the FDA has recently confronted such potentially serious food safety hazards as transmissible spongiform encephalopathies (TSEs), chemical contaminants, pesticides, and food allergens.

Food, Drug, and Cosmetic Act

Prohibits adulteration
Prohibits misbranded information
Regulates food additives/generally recognized as safe (GRAS)

Monitors carcinogenic effects
Calls for extensive testing
Does not cover fish, meat, poultry, and eggs
Does monitor shellfish transport with interstate regulations

Joint Commission

The Joint Commission evaluates and accredits more than 15,000 health care organizations and programs in the United States. An independent, not-for-profit organization, the Joint Commission is the nation's predominant standards setting and accrediting body in health care. Since 1951, the Joint Commission has maintained state-of-the-art standards that focus on improving the quality and safety of care provided by health care organizations. The Joint Commission's comprehensive accreditation process evaluates an organization's compliance with these standards and other accreditation requirements.

Federal Nursing Home Reform Act

The Federal Nursing Home Reform Act or OBRA '87 created a national minimum set of standards of care and rights for people living in certified nursing facilities. The legislation has the following benefits: emphasis on a resident's quality of life as well as the quality of care; new expectations that each resident's ability to walk, bathe, and perform other activities of daily living will be maintained or improved absent medical reasons; a resident assessment process leading to development of an individualized care plan; 75 hours of training and testing of paraprofessional staff; rights to remain in the nursing home absent non-payment, dangerous resident behaviors, or significant changes in a resident's medical condition; new opportunities for potential and current residents with intellectual disability or mental illnesses to receive services inside and outside a nursing home; a right to safely maintain or bank personal funds with the nursing home; rights to return to the nursing home after a hospital stay or an overnight visit with family and friends; the right to choose a personal physician and to access medical records; the right to organize and participate in a resident or family council; the right to be free of unnecessary and inappropriate physical and chemical restraints.

Food and Agriculture Organization

The Food and Agriculture Organization (FAO) of the United Nations leads international efforts to defeat hunger. Serving both developed and developing countries, FAO acts as a neutral forum where all nations meet as equals to negotiate agreements and debate policy. FAO's activities comprise 4 main areas:
- Putting information within reach.
- Sharing policy expertise.
- Providing a meeting place for nations.
- Bringing knowledge to the field.

Nutrition Education and Training Program

The Nutrition Education and Training Program (NET) provides educational and support opportunities for child nutrition programs' personnel, teachers, and students in public or private schools, child care centers, and other institutions. NET focuses on integrating concepts about the basic nutritional value of food and the relationships between proper nutrition and physical, mental, and emotional health into existing curricula in order to encourage the selection and consumption of well-balanced meals. NET typically sponsors programs and activities such as developing nutrition resource guides to be used statewide in conjunction with the "Healthy Lifestyles" Core Curricula for preschool, elementary, and secondary levels and a separate nutrition guide for food service personnel; coordinating a statewide network of people to provide training to school food service personnel, educators, students, and the community at large; circulating nutrition curriculum materials and conducting workshops for all program audiences.

National School Lunch Program

Since 1946, the National School Lunch Program (NSLP) has made it possible for schools throughout the nation to serve wholesome lunches to children to help meet their nutritional needs. These lunches make a vital contribution to children's mental and physical development. School lunch programs help students by making healthy eating choices available. In recent years, recipes have been modified to reduce the fat, salt, and sugar content of school lunches. Items purchased are reviewed and, where possible, selected to improve the nutritional quality of the meals. Classroom instruction is reinforced by using the meals and dining areas as learning laboratories. Students now have more menu choices, including entrees, vegetables, fruits, and alternatives such as salad, potato, and pasta bars. By increasing awareness of the federal "Dietary Guidelines for Americans," the program promotes health and helps reduce the risk of chronic disease.

All lunches must meet the nutritional requirements outlined in the "Dietary Guidelines for Americans," published jointly by the USDA and the US Department of Health and Human Services, and must provide one-third of the children's nutritional requirements for the day.

Food Distribution Program

Through the Food Distribution Program (FDP), the USDA makes a variety of donated foods (referred to as commodities) available to institutions and programs that provide nutritional services to eligible persons. These institutions and programs include the National School Lunch Program, the Child and Adult Care Food Program, and the Summer Food Service Program. The Emergency Food Assistance Program (TEFAP) provides commodities to soup kitchens and food banks. Other charitable institutions also occasionally receive food. Depending on market conditions, as many as 40 to 60 different commodities may be supplied to participants during the year. The commodities may be frozen, canned, fresh, or dry, and include meats, poultry, vegetables, fruits, grains, and dairy products. Not all commodities are available in every setting. In some situations, commodities are offered in addition to cash assistance for meal services. The commodities are acquired through 3 congressionally authorized agricultural support programs: price support, surplus removal, and the National School Lunch Program.

Child and Adult Care Food Program

The USDA works to ensure a healthy, well-balanced variety of nourishing foods for children and adults in day care away from home. The program offers reimbursement for meal service expenses and other aid to eligible childcare centers, family and group day care homes, adult day care centers, and outside-school-hours care programs that serve meals to children and adults. Monthly reimbursements to participating centers and day care homes assist caregivers in providing more nutritious, healthful meals. Reimbursements are based on the number of meals claimed and the family incomes of the children and adults served. Participating facilities may be reimbursed for up to 3 meals per child per day: breakfast, lunch, dinner, and supplements (snacks). Outside-school-hours care centers may receive reimbursement for breakfast, an afternoon snack, and dinner, as well as for lunch and additional snacks on weekends, holidays, during school vacations, and off-track periods.

National School Breakfast Program

Children who come to school hungry because they got up too late to spend time eating breakfast, weren't hungry before leaving home, didn't have an adult to encourage them to eat, or didn't have food in the home find it difficult to stay alert and learn. The SBP provides children with nutritious foods before their school day begins, thus improving their diets and encouraging the learning process. Schools operating the SBP report increases in test scores, decreases in absenteeism, and an overall improvement in student behavior when children eat breakfast. All students may eat breakfast if the program is offered at their school. Students who qualify for free or reduced-price school lunch are eligible for the same benefits in the breakfast program. A school breakfast is designed to satisfy one-quarter of a child's recommended daily dietary needs and must meet the nutritional requirements outlined in the "Dietary Guidelines for Americans." Local schools have information about eligibility and applications to receive these benefits.

Summer Food Service Program

USDA is designed to offer nutritionally balanced, high-quality meals to children during summer vacations, interim, and off-track periods. The program is particularly targeted to low-income children who may not have adequate nutrition when schools are not in session. The SFSP provides meals to children 18 years of age and younger at approved sponsored sites. Meals served include breakfast, lunch, supplements, and dinner, depending on the type of service site. A program sponsor may be any of the following types of organizations and may provide the program in 1 or more places:
- A public or private nonprofit School Food Authority;
- A public or private nonprofit residential summer camp;
- A unit of local (municipal or county) government; or
- A private nonprofit organization that regularly serves the public.

Private nonprofit organizations may only sponsor the SFSP in areas where a School Food Authority or local government will not do so.

Food Stamp Program

The Food Stamp Program (USDA, 1964) serves as the first line of defense against hunger. It enables low-income families to buy nutritious food with coupons and Electronic Benefits Transfer (EBT) cards. Food stamp recipients spend their benefits to buy eligible food in authorized retail food stores. The Program is the cornerstone of the federal food assistance programs, and provides crucial support to needy households and to those making the transition from welfare to work. Food stamp benefits are based on figures from the Thrifty Food Plan for June of the previous year. This program has monthly benefits for recipients.

Expanded Food and Nutrition Education Program

The EFNEP is federally funded and conducted through the Cooperative Extension Service in every state and US territory. For more than 30 years, EFNEP has been helping families with children learn how to eat healthier meals and snacks, stretch their food dollars, and reduce the risk of foodborne illness. Adults are faced with the challenges of paying rent, utilities, day care, and other daily expenses, and families experience the stress of trying to provide a variety of nutritious foods and maintain healthy diets on limited budgets. EFNEP provides a variety of tools and ideas to help families cut food costs and provide healthy meals and snacks for family members.

Adults enrolled in EFNEP learn how to:
- Plan low-cost nutritious meals.
- Prepare quick and healthy meals and snacks.
- Shop for the best food buys.
- Keep foods safe to eat.
- Eat right and light to control sugar, salt, fat, and calories.

National Research Council

The NRC is part of the National Academies, which also comprises the National Academy of Sciences, National Academy of Engineering, and Institute of Medicine. These are private, nonprofit institutions that provide science, technology, and health policy advice under a congressional charter. The Research Council was organized by the National Academy of Sciences in 1916 to associate the broad community of science and technology with the Academy's purposes of furthering knowledge and advising the federal government. The NRC has a policy of fortification and enrichment with foods.

Healthy Start

Healthy Start was initiated in 1991 with the goal of improving the health of pregnant women and reducing infant mortality for populations affected by a higher than average infant mortality rate. Clinics provide free prenatal care to women within their community, using mobile clinics when necessary. The period between pregnancies is targeted as an ideal time when women can be counseled or treated for problems that may affect future pregnancies, such as substance abuse, obesity, or diabetes.

Special Milk Program

The USDA encourages consumption of milk by children who do not participate in other child nutrition programs. For example, children attending split-session kindergartens who do not have access to the breakfast and lunch programs may participate in the SMP. The SMP is also available to other private nonprofit institutions devoted to the care and training of children. The federal government sets a reimbursement rate annually for each half-pint of milk. This rate is always less than the cost of the milk. Children should be charged a price equal to the difference between the reimbursement rate and the actual cost of the milk. In some settings, milk is served free of charge to eligible children, and the reimbursement covers the full cost.

After School Snack Program

Children who participate in the snack program will benefit from a nutritional boost they might not otherwise get. Organizations can use the after school snack as one more enticement to encourage children to participate in educational and enrichment activity during a time of day when many young people are unsupervised.

Nutrition Services Incentive Program

NSIP, formerly the Nutrition Program for the Elderly (NPE), is administered by the US Department of Health and Human Service's (DHHS) Administration on Aging, but receives commodity foods and financial support from the US Department of Agriculture's Food and Nutrition Service (FNS).

WIC Program

WIC is for low-income women, infants, and children up to age 5 who are at nutritional risk. The program provides nutritious foods to supplement diets, information on healthy eating, and referrals to health care. WIC is a federal grant program. WIC is administered at the federal level by FNS. The following individuals are considered categorically eligible for WIC: Women who are pregnant (during pregnancy and up to 6 weeks after the birth of an infant or the end of the pregnancy), postpartum (up to 6 months after the birth of the infant or the end of the pregnancy), breastfeeding (up to the infant's first birthday); infants (up to the infant's first birthday); children (up to the child's fifth birthday). To be eligible for WIC, applicants must have income at or below an income level or standard set by the state agency or be determined automatically income-eligible based on participation in certain programs. The state agency's income standard must be at or below 185% of the federal poverty guidelines (issued each year by the Department of Health and Human Services). Applicants must be seen by a health care provider such as a physician, nurse, or nutritionist.

Union and collective bargaining

Union
A union is an organization that represents employee interests and rights to management on issues such as wages, work hours, and working conditions.

Collective bargaining
Collective bargaining is a system in which unions and management negotiate with each other to develop the work rules under which union members will work for a stipulated period of time.

Unemployment insurance and worker's compensation

Unemployment Insurance
This is a mandatory program that provides a subsistence payment to employees between jobs. This program is funded primarily by employers.

Worker's Compensation
This is a state insurance program that protects workers in case of a work-related injury or disease that results from employment.
It is funded by a payroll tax that is paid to an insurance company or state fund based on experience.

USDA's School Breakfast Program, Special Milk Program, and Summer Food Program

The USDA's Food and Nutrition Service has been in operation since 1975, providing cash reimbursement to schools that provide free or low-cost breakfasts to qualifying low-income students. The meal provides one-fourth of the daily requirements for nutrients, and the USDA's Team Nutrition helps the food service staff of schools with menu planning and other training and educational efforts.

The USDA's Special Milk Program provides milk to children who do not participate in other federal meal programs. The program is meant to encourage consumption of milk among children, and schools are reimbursed for the milk they provide. The program also contributes to the nourishment of children who attend abbreviated schedule classes where meal programs are not available.

The USDA's Summer Food Program helps fill the gap when school ends for summer break. This program combines wholesome meals with summer activities in sites such as camps or community centers. Children may receive up to 3 meals a day if enrolled in residential camps.

USDA's National School Lunch Program

Established by President Truman in 1946, the National School Lunch Program works to ensure the health of the nation's children by providing free or reduced cost lunches to public schools, nonprofit private schools, and residential child care facilities. Qualifying schools receive federal subsidies in turn for providing nutritionally balanced meals to students who meet income guidelines. Children from families with incomes between 130% and 185% of the poverty level receive lunches for free or reduced prices, and non-qualifying children must pay full price, although the programs must not operate for profit. The foodservice program decides what food is served, but lunches must provide one-third of the nutrients specified by the Dietary Guidelines for Americans. Schools get additional support in the form of commodity foods available from local surplus stock. Team Nutrition USDA further supports schools by providing nutrition training, recipes and menus, and other educational assistance.

USDA's Child and Adult Care Food Program (CACFP)

CACFP provides meals and snacks to low-income children and impaired elderly individuals enrolled in day care settings. The program also provides snacks to low-income children enrolled in after-school care. Those in day care may receive up to 2 meals and 1 snack; after-school participants younger than age 18 can receive 1 snack per day. An exception is homeless shelters, which can provide 3 meals a day to children residing there. The program covers both public and private care settings, including personal residents providing in-home day care.

Reimbursement varies, and may be calculated as a percentage, per meal count, or blended per meal rates. Additional funds are provided to centers to cover costs incurred in the planning and implementing of the program. The USDA provides recipes and purchased commodities to assist those after-school care facilities with limited food preparation areas.

USDA Commodity Food Distribution Program

The USDA's Food and Nutrition Sciences Service is charged with administering the Food Distribution Program. Through the Food Distribution Program, USDA purchases foods through direct appropriations from Congress, and under surplus-removal and price-support activities. The foods are distributed to state agencies for use by eligible local outlets, including schools. Schools participating in the National School Lunch Program and the School Breakfast Program may receive USDA commodity meats, vegetables, fruits, grains, and dairy products. Who is Eligible to Apply: Public and nonprofit private schools, child care institutions, Summer Food Service Program Sponsors, as well as Elderly Nutrition Programs, Commodity Supplemental Food Programs, Food Distribution on Indian Reservations, and The Emergency Food Assistance Program. Amount of funds available: Funding is received in the way of entitlement dollars to be spent on the purchase of the donated foods.

Dietary guidelines

The 2005 Dietary Guidelines for Americans
Nine areas are addressed, such as physical activity, fat and carbohydrates. There are 23 key recommendations for the general population as well as guidelines for specific groups, such as women of childbearing age. Recommended amounts of food to eat in one day are provided for 12 different calorie levels based on energy needs. Recommendations below are for the 2,000 calorie reference level.
Grains: 3 or more servings of whole grains per day (the first time for a specific number of servings of whole grains).

Fruits and Vegetables: 9 servings (or 4 1/2 cups) per day and suggests at least three cups per week of legumes (the first time for a specific amount of legumes).
Milk: 3 cups (or milk equivalents) per day for all adults.
Meat: 5 1/2 ounces per day, a slight decrease
Fats: Limit trans fatty acids (the first time trans fatty acids are mentioned).

Healthy people program

Healthy People is a program that was first developed by the US Department of Health and Human Services in 1979. It is designed to deal with the preventable causes of disease, disability, and premature death with the goals of increasing the quality of life, increasing the length of life, and eliminating gaps and inequality in the healthcare system. The current iteration of the program, Healthy People 2020, has a targeted timeframe for reaching the goals in 2020 (hence the name). The program is divided into 42 focus areas, with each focus having specific goals. There are around 1200 objectives in the current program, an increase of almost 200% over the previous version. The overarching emphasis of the Healthy People program is health education, promotion, and protection.

5 A Day for Better Health Program

5 A Day for Better Health Program is one of the most widely recognized health promotion messages in the world. More than 35 countries have developed programs to increase fruit and vegetable consumption using the 5 A Day for Better Health Program as a model. The program, a noteworthy example of government agencies working together with private industry, voluntary health organizations, and advocacy groups, is the largest public-private partnership for nutrition in the United States. The Department of Health and Human Services (HHS), including the National Cancer Institute and the Centers for Disease Control and Prevention, and the USDA recently signed an agreement to formalize and expand their commitment to promote the 5 A Day message nationwide, and, particularly, in American schools. USDA has made a substantial contribution to help increase the amount and choices of fruits and vegetables in school cafeterias. The 5 a Day for Better Health Survey looks at those 18 years of age and older.

Adverse effects of medications

- Bleeding in the GI tract is a common side effect of aspirin, and this causes the body to lose iron even in the absence of obvious symptoms such as blood in the stool. Aspirin can also decrease the uptake of ascorbic acid and alter the distribution of ascorbic acid in the body, leading to decreased amounts in the body and increased excretion in the urine.
- Diuretics such as thiazide can increase bone resorption or increase intestinal calcium absorption, resulting in the excretion of potassium, sodium, and magnesium through the urine.
- Corticosteroids can increase protein breakdown, decrease calcium absorption, and decrease protein synthesis. The result can be decreased bone formation, increased excretion of potassium and nitrogen, and increased need for vitamin D.
- The antidepressant lithium carbonate can cause changes in sodium distribution in the body or excessive excretion. Monoamine oxidase inhibitors (MAOIs) can increase the appetite, leading to weight gain.

Monitoring and Evaluation

Nutrition monitoring

Nutrition monitoring refers to the ongoing process of surveillance of a patient's status by gathering information about the patient's status in relation to their diagnosis, treatment plan, and outcome. Monitoring is important to ascertain whether the patient is improving, or whether corrective action needs to be taken based on lack of progress or failure to meet desired outcomes. Monitoring data should be collected from the initiation of the intervention, and should be reviewed regularly to determine that the activities of the intervention are being transformed into results that meet some specified standard.

Nutrition protocol

Nutrition protocols may be developed by a profession or an organization to assist the professionals in making the best decisions for patient care. They may be included in the policy and procedure manual of an organization, so that each clinician follows the same principles of care and service delivery for patients with a particular diagnosis. The protocol reads like a set of instructions, and may include timelines for delivering treatments, monitoring procedures, doing appropriate lab work, and deciding to seek consultations.

Nutrition evaluation

Nutrition evaluation is a tool used to measure the efficacy of the nutrition intervention on a patient. The evaluation process measures objective outcomes that show that the patient's behavior or health has improved as a result of the service or intervention. An example would be demonstrating that the diabetic patient can monitor his or her own blood glucose and adjust insulin doses as needed.

Indicators

Indicators are used in the quality assurance process as a marker to direct attention to processes or outcomes that need additional investigation. In other words, indicators serve as monitoring tools that allow the professional to monitor the quality of care and make adjustments.

Rate-based indicators: Rate-based indicators use data to evaluate what would happen if the best possible care was provided. The indicator is expressed as a rate or proportion. For example, this indicator might ask, "What would happen if 95% of the patients in ABC Nursing Home maintained ideal body weight for a six-month period?" A tolerable threshold would be developed for this nursing home, and any number below the acceptable threshold would be a reason to initiate a plan of action.

Sentinel event indicators: A sentinel indicator refers to a serious event or incident that would always provide a reason for further action or investigation. The threshold for these incidents is always 0% or 100%. For example, 0% of patients in the nursing home will acquire *Salmonella*.

Guarding consumers against fraudulent care

National Council against Health Fraud

The National Council against Health Fraud is a private, voluntary agency that advocates for the consumer by focusing on and identifying the public health problems of quackery and misinformation. They argue that nutrition products and services should be safe and effective, and they believe in the importance of the scientific process for validating claims. They lobby for consumer health laws, investigate claims of dubious health products and services, and educate the public about health fraud through various mechanisms.

Federal Trade Commission
The Federal Trade Commission (FTC) is the government's agency for protecting consumers. Consumers can file a complaint with the FTC or get free information on issues to help consumers spot and avoid bogus products. They advise that a healthy amount of skepticism be used when evaluating nutritional products such as those that promise easy weight loss.

HIPAA
HIPAA guidelines state the medical documentation entered by a health care provider is considered to be a permanent legal document; as such notes should be typed or written in black ink. Enter notes in the medical chart during or immediately following the visit. All entries should be signed and dated. If an entry has to be made after the interaction with the patient, the time of the interaction and the time the entry was made should be noted.

If diet orders are incorrect in the chart, the dietitian should contact the doctor who wrote the order rather than making the change him or herself. If the dietitian needs to make a correction, the proper procedure is to draw a single line through the text and initial and date the change. If the change is to be made after documentation is complete, an addendum can be added to the chart. Corrections are not to be made by obliterating the original note or by removing pages from the chart.

Behavior modification

Operant conditioning
The psychologist B.F. Skinner argued that the environment was more important in shaping behavior than one's thought processes. He said that people's behavior can be predicted through the observation of stimuli and responses. Skinner said that because the stimulus is not always present to cause a behavior, the result of the behavior is more important than the presence of the stimulus. If an individual expects a positive result, he or she will engage in the behavior. If a negative result is expected, the behavior will be avoided. When the positive result is achieved repeatedly, this provides positive reinforcement.

Modeling
Modeling refers to the behavior change that occurs when an individual copies the behavior displayed by another person, the model. If the model possess characteristics the observer values, such as power or intelligence, the observer will be more likely to imitate the behavior. Targeting highly respected members of a population can prepare them to serve as models for the rest of the population.

Avoidance learning
Avoidance learning occurs when an individual learns to behave in a certain way in order to avoid unpleasant consequences. The behavior is reinforced by the individual's desire to avoid the punishment. An example of this is in a case of nutritional counseling in which an individual is chastised by a health care professional because he or she is not following his or her prescribed renal diet, resulting in further kidney problems. The individual follows the diet, not because of the kidney problems, but because he or she wants to avoid further criticism.

Extinction

Extinction learning is often discussed in the context of fear conditioning. If an unpleasant stimulus is paired with a neutral stimulus, eventually the neutral stimulus will elicit a response. Then, when the neutral stimulus is presented alone, eventually the fear response will be eliminated.

Punishment

Punishment involves trying to change behavior by providing an unpleasant consequence as a result of the behavior. If the punishment occurs repeatedly, learned helplessness occurs, in which the individual feels the problem has no solution.

Formative and summative assessments

Formative assessment is conducted throughout the educational process. The goal of formative assessment is to discover what the target group knows and what they do not understand, so that teaching methods can be tailored throughout the duration of teaching. Encouraging frequent discussion among participants can give the instructor cues that reveal which topics are still unclear to the individual. Breaking into small groups for discussion, and then sharing those thoughts with the larger group can also provide insight to the instructor. Frequent, brief quizzes may also communicate where learning gaps lie.

Summative assessments include the typical final exams or tests that evaluate how well one has learned the material as a whole. This kind of assessment is more formalized, as opposed to the informal discussions that can characterize formative assessments. Although summative assessments cannot help the instructor change the learning that has already taken place, they may help identify areas for improvement in future educational endeavors.

Feedback systems

Negative feedback system:
"The output reverses the input." The result is to reverse the original change to the controlled condition; if original input was a decrease in activity, then output will be to increase it. Conversely, if original input was an increase in activity, then output will be to decrease it. Another way of stating it is that there is an opposite directional change with negative feedback systems. The result of a negative feedback system should be to maintain the controlled condition within its very narrow, ideal range.

Positive feedback system:
"The output reinforces the input." The result is to strengthen/reinforce the original change to the controlled condition. Since the original input is an increase in activity, then the output will be to increase that activity even further. Another way of stating it is that there is a same directional change with a positive feedback system. The result of a negative feedback system is to make the controlled condition progressively increase.

Performance evaluations

Performance evaluations are used by the manager to examine the contribution of each employee to the foodservice operation. The evaluation is a standardized form that allows each employee to be objectively judged against the same criteria. The form can be used as a training tool to let each employee know what the expectations of the position are, and the form can be used as a way to provide regular feedback to the employee about his or her performance in key areas. Employees can also use the evaluation process as an opportunity to give individual and private feedback to their supervisor. Positive or negative evaluations can be used to initiate disciplinary procedures or promotions. Evaluations can be formatted as checklists (yes or no) or scales with assigned point values (on a level of 1 to 5, the employee meets this criterion). Managers need to be aware of the possibility of the halo effect, when an employee's excellent or poor execution of one skill biases the reviewer in the rest of the evaluation.

Test-retest, parallel forms, split-half reliability

Test-retest: A measure at 2 different times with no treatment in between will yield the same results.
Parallel-forms: Two tests of different forms that supposedly test the same material will give the same results.
Split-half reliability: If the items are divided in half (e.g., odd vs. even questions), the 2 halves give the same results.

Duo Trio Test

1. Prepare three samples, two of which are the same.
2. Using one of the two identical samples as a control, decide which of the other samples is the same as the control.
3. Record the tasters' responses.

Descriptive Flavor Analysis Panel

DFAP helps identify and quantify specific flavor attributes. Panel of experts.

RACE

Rescue
Activate alarm
Confine the fire
Evacuate/Extinguish (NFPA/OSHA fire safety)

Assume all fire drills are the real thing

Management of Food and Nutrition Programs and Services

Functions of Management

Management planning

The short-range or operational planning encompasses the budgeting activities that will take place over the course of a year. The operational plan allocates resources toward the achievement of goals that may bring an organization closer to meeting long-term goals. A sound operational plan can be used as a rationale for the ensuing year's operating budget.

The combination of several years of operational planning can help managers meet their long-term goals, usually defined by time periods of five years or more. Long-term goals are defined by their mission and vision statements, which provide the answers to such questions as, "Who are we, where are we now, where do we want to be, and how do we get there?"

Strategic planning also focuses on finding long-range solutions. Strategic planning considers the purpose of the foodservice operation in making decisions that will affect long-term allocation of resources such as expansions, equipment acquisition, or other capital outlay.

Managerial skills

The management skills required to some degree by all dietetics professionals include technical skills, human skills, and conceptual skills. Technical skills would include those that involve knowing the mechanics of the equipment in the kitchen, or knowing how to prepare all of the menu items in a foodservice operation. These types of skills are highly desirable in a kitchen line manager, who needs to be proficient enough in these areas to both train employees and act as a fill-in worker when necessary. Human skills include the ability to positively interact with others and build trust and motivation through excellent communication skills.

These skills are necessary at all levels of management: lower levels of management need them to interact with dozens of people throughout the day, and upper level managers need them to provide a positive trickle-down effect. Conceptual skills include those analytical skills that allow upper management to carry out the mission of the organization.

Success of the organization
In addition to possessing excellent communication skills, managers should be very action-oriented. A good manager should work alongside his or her employees on a daily basis, and be able to describe his or her day with action verbs: fixing, repairing, regulating, solving, developing, and coaching. Keeping in mind the adage, "The customer's always right," managers should listen and learn from the people they serve every day.

Managers should also be internally motivated and autonomous, possessing the skills and confidence to go out on a limb to solve problems. Managers in successful organizations take risks when confronted with unique problems, and explore new avenues to getting the job done.

Successful managers recognize the value of their employees, and therefore invest a great deal of time and effort in developing, teaching, and supporting their employees.

Productivity can only be increased and maintained through the recruiting and retention of motivated, informed staff.

Strategic planning

Practical Guidelines for Effective Strategic Planning:
1. Involve everyone you need to carry out your plan.
2. Work collaboratively with those whose help you need.
3. Schedule a full-day retreat.
4. Document your plan.
5. Make it as simple as possible.
6. Develop an action plan for each strategic objective.
7. Keep the process alive by updating it continuously.
8. Make sure that your plan fits senior management's goals.
9. Don't undertake too much—prioritize your objectives.
10. Keep your plan visual.
11. Communicate the plan down the line.
12. Create an accountability document.

SWOT

SWOT stands for strengths, weaknesses, opportunities, threats. The first two components (Strengths and Weaknesses) generally deal with elements found within the company, and the last two (Opportunities and Threats) examine the environment outside the company. SWOT profiles, along with a corporation's mission and major goals, make up the tools you'll need to develop and form strategies. They are the components of the Strategic Management Model. These game plans reflect in broad terms how, where, and why the company should compete as well as against whom.

Disaster preparation

Managers should maintain an updated employee roster that lists names and phone numbers, and employees should be required to wear photo identification badges when working. Only authorized personnel should be allowed in the foodservice department, and visitors should check in with a supervisor before entering the premises. Receiving clerks should become familiar with regular delivery persons and suspicious persons or activities in the receiving area should be reported. Employees should become familiar with emergency procedures during training, and drills should be conducted regularly to maintain awareness. Evacuation routes and emergency phone numbers should be clearly posted. Personal items such as purses and meal containers brought from home should be kept out of the food production area to prevent the malicious introduction of a contaminant. Doors and windows in receiving areas should remain closed and locked unless deliveries are being made. Keep hazardous chemicals in a locked storage area, and maintain strict policies over the possession and use of keys for all secured areas.

Determining staffing needs

Foodservice managers must decide on staffing that will be adequate to cover the production, serving, and cleaning needs of the operation. It may be helpful to rely on industry standards available for the type of operation to determine the staffing needs.

For example, in the dietary department of extended care facilities, the expected production norm is five meals per labor hour. School foodservice workers are expected to produce 13 to 15 meals per labor hour. Managers can calculate the number of meals to be served to determine how many employees should man each shift. Staffing levels can then be adjusted to account for employee skill and meal complexity.

An FTE or full-time equivalent can be used to determine the right mix of full- and part-time workers for a facility. The total number of hours worked divided by 40 yields the FTE count. The budget will allow for a given number of FTEs to be hired in a foodservice operation.

Employee motivation

Herzberg's theory
In the 1950s, Herzberg conducted a study in which he asked employees to recall a time when they felt particularly good or bad about their job. He asked them what made them feel this way, and based on their responses developed his theory of motivation and hygiene. He classified hygiene elements as those present in the work environment, such as pay, supervision, and working conditions. Herzberg argued that hygiene elements could not be used to motivate employees, but could prevent motivation from occurring if the elements were believed to be inferior. In this theory, motivating elements are those that relate to a sense of achievement, growth, opportunity, and personal satisfaction. All hygiene elements must be perceived to be satisfactory to the employees before motivation can occur. According to this theory, the recognition and esteem that one gains from a promotion is more motivating than the salary increase.

McClelland's achievement-affiliation theory
McClelland's theory of motivation argues that employees need a sense of achievement, a feeling of power, and a desire for affiliation. The level of these needs varies among individuals, and an understanding of these varying needs can be used by managers to motivate employees and place them in a position that best utilizes their skills. Achievement-motivated employees are motivated when they are allowed to strive toward moderately difficult goals. They feel rewarded by the process of problem-solving, and enjoy comparing their progress to their peers.

Employees with a high need for power enjoy directing the actions of others, and taking charge of activities. A low-ranking employee with a high need for power may be perceived as being "bossy."

Employees with a high need for affiliation are motivated by their desire to be liked and accepted by others. They appreciate feedback from their peers and managers about how cooperative and pleasant to work with they are.

Vroom's expectancy theory
Vroom argues that employees will be motivated to perform on the job when they feel that the extra effort they put forth will lead to better performance, and this improved performance will result in the achievement of a desired outcome or reward. The three components of this theory are expectancy, instrumentality, and valence. If the person expects their effort to result in an increased performance, they will be motivated to put forth the extra effort. An employee may not expend additional effort in organizing the stock room if he or she knows it will not be maintained in the following shift. Instrumentality means that the person believes their performance will be rewarded, and valence refers to the value the employee places on the rewards or outcomes. Managers should link better performance to rewards, and determine which rewards employees value the most.

Leadership styles

An autocratic leader acts in a solo fashion, making decisions without consulting others. This style of leadership causes the highest levels of dissatisfaction among employees, but it may be effective in some applications, such as a decision that will not be affected by the input of others.

Bureaucratic leaders value organizational norms and the hierarchy present in the chain of command, and expect their employees to respect the manager based on his or her position as a leader.

Participative leadership involves a continuum of participation by the employees or team working with a leader to solve problems. A trend in this style of management is the use of quality circles, which allow small groups of employees that meet regularly to brainstorm.

Managers that practice a laissez-faire style of leadership allow workers to make decisions with little or no guidance from management. Employees under this type of leadership tend to suffer from a lack of coherence and motivation in their work.

Drucker's management by objectives theory

Peter Drucker argued that in order to function effectively, every member of an organization should have a set of goals and objectives to work towards, ideally to be accomplished within a specific time frame. The objectives each employee is to accomplish are matched to the goals of the organization, so that when all employees are performing according to the standards set by the manager, the organization will be meeting its goals as well. The goals should be developed with the SMART acronym in mind: they should be specific, measurable, achievable, realistic, and time-related. The goals should be developed in conjunction with the employees, so management by objectives can be thought of as a form of participative leadership. In addition to goal development, the manager's tasks include the provision of support to employees as they strive to meet their goals and the joint evaluation of results with employees.

Problem-solving

The nominal group technique advocated by Delbecq is a problem-solving method similar in style to brainstorming, with added structure and control. In this process, a facilitator or leader convenes a group of individuals who silently record their ideas and thoughts regarding the problem at hand for several minutes. The ideas are then gathered by the facilitator, and compiled onto a wipe board or flip chart. Each idea is discussed and clarified for the group. The group members anonymously rank the ideas, and a vote is cast for the most popular idea.

The Delphi technique solicits the opinions of experts on the matter at hand, without the requirement for a face-to-face meeting. Web-based survey tools or email may be used. This methodology utilizes the benefit of complete anonymity, allowing participants to change their minds with impunity. Results are compiled, and an agreement is reached. A second survey may be conducted if no consensus is made.

The fishbone diagram is a way of using brainstorming to determine the cause of a problem in the organization or department, and then identifying and categorizing possible solutions. The spine or leading line of the skeleton is the problem statement phrased as a question. For example, a fishbone analysis may be conducted to address the question, "Why are the meal carts delivered late at every noon meal?" Each possible cause should be drawn as a line attached to the problem statement, and may fall into such categories as equipment, policy, or employees. Possible solutions are then discussed and added to the diagram as additional "bones."

Pareto charts graphically illustrate the causes behind a recurring problem in the department in bar chart form. This is useful when data exists that allow precise analysis of contributing causes. A popular use of the chart is discerning which 20% of causes are contributing to 80% of the problems in the department.

Conflict-resolution methods

Conflict in the workplace is unavoidable. It can stem from misunderstandings, personality differences, organizational change, or other sources. Conflict can result in lowered employee morale, increased employee turnover, and lowered productivity. Managers cannot eliminate conflict, but they should expect to act as mediators and facilitators in conflict resolution.

Managers with a dominating or suppressing style may try to resolve conflict by aggressively exercising their power of authority or passively pretending the problem does not exist. Either way results in a winning situation for the manager and a losing situation for the employees.

Compromising managers try to find a middle ground that the conflicting parties can agree upon. This strategy does little to help the organization or prevent future conflicts.

Managers with an integrative problem-solving style create a culture of cooperation rather than competition, so that all parties participate in the problem-solving. The result is that concessions are made without anyone feeling like the loser.

Decision matrix

A matrix used by teams to evaluate possible solutions to problems. Each solution is listed. Criteria are selected and listed on the top row to rate the possible solutions. Each possible solution is rated on a scale from 1 to 5 for each criterion and the rating is recorded in the corresponding grid. The ratings of all the criteria for each possible solution are added to determine each solution's score. The scores are then used to help decide which solution deserves the most attention.

Organization

Organization Chart:
Graphic display of reporting relationship that provide a general framework of the organization.

Organizational Breakdown Structure (OBS):
Tool used to show the work units or work packages that are assigned to specific organizational units.

Outsourcing:
Outsourcing is paying a second party to perform one or more of your internal processes or functions. Business process outsourcing of certain functions is an increasingly popular way to improve basic services while allowing professionals time to play a more strategic role in their organizations. Frequently outsourced: payroll, 401(k) administration, employee assistance, and retirement planning.

An organizational chart provides a visual reference that shows where employees fit into an organization in terms of rank and functional relationship with one another. A typical chart depicts the owner or department head at the top of the chart, followed by lines of authority leading to the next person in charge, with each succeeding level including the next in line in authority. Chart placement is based on formal titles, and may not be a reliable indicator of where the real power lies in an organization. The chain of command also shows the delineation of authority from the highest- to the lowest-ranked worker. However, placement high in the chain of command does not necessarily entitle one to give orders to one lower in the chain. For example, the director of nursing would not commonly issue orders to a foodservice employee.

The concentric model of organization does away with the hierarchy system, and invites all organizational members to contribute equally to problem solving.

Myers-Briggs Indicator

Test developed by Katharine C. Briggs and Isabel Briggs Myers to categorize people according to where they lie on four scales, each reflecting a different dimension of human behavior: extrovert-introvert, sensing-intuitive, thinking-feeling, and judging-perceiving. These scales comprise 16 different psychological types, each associated with a number of well-documented behavioral traits.

Objectives:
Similar to goals, a good faith effort to meet numerical goals through modifications in employment procedures and practice. Goals and objectives are set after careful external and internal labor analysis.

Hierarchal Management, High-Performance Work Teams

Hierarchical Management:
Traditional functional, or line, management in which areas and sub areas of expertise are created and staffed with human resources. Organizations so established are ongoing in nature.

High-Performance Work Teams:
Group of people who work together in an interdependent manner such that their collective performance exceeds that which would be achieved by simply adding together their individual contributions. Characteristics of such a team include strong group identify, collaboration, anticipating and acting on other team members needs, and a laser-like focus on project objectives.

Goals and guidelines

Goals:
Good faith quantitative objectives an employer voluntarily sets as the minimum progress that can be achieved within a certain time period through all-out efforts at outreach recruitment, validating selection criteria, creation of trainee positions, career ladders, etc.

Guideline:
Document that recommends methods and procedures to be used to accomplish an objective.

Discrimination

The act of distinguishing between and among different things. It is also a charge brought by people alleging the operation of prejudice. When an individual is discriminated against because of an accident, birth, or condition, it is unlawful. Thus discrimination may also be a conclusion of the courts when plaintiffs have shown an adverse impact with regard to the employment of protected class persons and employers have failed to demonstrate business necessity.

Competency, Cost-of-Living Adjustment (COLA), and Collective Bargaining

Competency:
Critical skill, or in some cases personality characteristics, required of an individual to complete an activity or project, or otherwise required for a certain position. For example, the ability to think strategically is considered by some to be a critical competency for a person who will be the manager of a large and complex project.

Cost-of-Living Adjustment (COLA):
An increase in pension benefits after retirement that offsets the effects of inflation in the economy.

Collective Bargaining:
Statutory mechanism for employees to participate collectively in the determination of their terms and conditions of employment. Through meetings between their elected representatives and their employer, the employee's terms and conditions of employment are negotiated. Also used to resolve labor disputes.

SWOT

Strengths
Weaknesses
Opportunities
Threats

The first two components (Strengths and Weaknesses) generally deal with elements found within the company, and the last two (Opportunities and Threats) examine the environment outside the company. SWOT profiles, along with a corporation's mission and major goals, make up the tools you'll need to develop and form strategies. They are the components of the Strategic Management Model. These game plans reflect in broad terms how, where, and why the company should compete as well as against whom.

Theory X Management

Theory X Assumptions
People inherently dislike work. People must be coerced or controlled to do work to achieve objectives. People prefer to be directed.

Theory X Management
Approach to managing people described by Douglas McGregor. Based on the philosophy that people dislike work, will avoid it if they can, and are interested only in monetary gain from their labor. Accordingly, the Theory X manager will act in an authoritarian manner, directing each activity of his or her staff.

Theory Y Management

Theory Y Assumptions
People view work as being as natural as play and rest. People will exercise self-direction and self-control towards achieving objectives they are committed to. People learn to accept and seek responsibility.

Theory Y Management
Approach to managing people described by McGregor. Based on the philosophy that people will work best when they are properly rewarded and motivated, and that work is as natural as play or rest. Accordingly, the Theory Y manager will act in a generally supportive and understanding manner, providing encouragement and rewards to his or her staff.

Theory Z Management

Theory Z Management:
Approach to managing people developed by Ouchi. Based on the philosophy that people need goals and objectives, motivation, standards, the right to make mistakes, and the right to participate in goal setting. More specifically, describes a Japanese system of management characterized by the employee's heavy involvement in management, which has been shown to result in higher productivity levels when compared to United States or Western counterparts. Successful implementation requires a comprehensive system of organizational and sociological rewards. Its developers assert that it can be used in any situation with equal success. Also called participative management style.

Threshold:
Time, monetary unit, or resource level, placed on something, which is used as a guideline that, if exceeded, causes some type of management review to occur.

Plan-Do-Check-Act

Plan-Do-Check-Act (PDCA) cycle
A four-step improvement process originally conceived of by Walter A. Shewhart.
The first step involves planning for the necessary improvement.
The second step is the implementation of the plan.
The third step is to check the results of the plan.
The last step is to act upon the results of the plan.

It is also known as the Shewhart cycle, the Deming cycle, and the PDCA cycle.

Authoritarian Management Style and Autocratic Management Style

Authoritarian Management Style:
Management approach in which the manager tells team members what is expected of them, provides specific guidance on what should be done, makes his or her role within the team understood, schedules work, and directs team members to follow standard rules and regulations.

Autocratic Management Style:
Management approach in which the manager makes all decisions and exercises tight control over the team. This style is characterized by communications from the manager downward to the team and not vice versa.

Maslow's Hierarchy of Needs

Theory of motivation developed by Abraham Maslow in which a person's needs arise in an ordered sequence in the following five categories:
Physical needs
Safety needs
Love needs
Esteem needs
Self-actualization needs

Herzberg's Theory of Motivation

Theory of motivation developed by Fredrick Herzberg in which he asserts that individuals are affected by two opposing forms of motivation: hygiene factors and motivators. Hygiene factors such as pay, attitude of supervisor, and working conditions serve only to demotivate people if they are not provided in the type or amount required by the person. Improving hygiene factors under normal circumstances is not likely to increase motivation. Factors such as greater freedom, more responsibility, and more recognition serve to enhance self-esteem and are considered the motivators that energize and stimulate the person to enhance performance.

Decision-making

Change model
Although individuals may understand the need to adopt healthier lifestyle choices, successful long-term change is difficult to achieve. The stages of change model argues that behavior change does not happen as a single event; rather, it occurs gradually over time in a recognizable series of steps. In the pre-contemplation stage, the person is not interested in change, and may be in denial regarding serious health issues. When contemplation occurs, the person begins to consider making a change, weighing the pros and cons.

During the preparation phase, patients become determined to change, and may try the new behavior in small doses to test the waters. When the action stage is reached, adopt the desired behavior. In maintenance, the new behavior becomes ingrained over the long term as a habit. Occasional slip-ups may characterize the maintenance stage. Recognizing which stage an individual is in can help the health professional plan an intervention to help that person move on to the next stage.

Health belief model
The health belief model attempts to explain why individuals choose not to take part in healthy lifestyle changes or programs designed to improve their health, even when the person knows he or she is at risk for illness or disability because of health status. The model presents several belief and value continuums that predict whether change will occur. Perceived susceptibility describes how likely a person feels he or she is to experience disease or adverse effects. Perceived seriousness refers to the extent the person believes the disease or problem would affect his or her life. A perceived benefit of action implies that the person recognizes the disease possibility as serious, and

is weighing the benefits of change. Barriers to taking action may include negative beliefs about change or physical or social impediments to change. Cues to action may be external, from a family member or health professional, or internal messages prompting change.

Decision-making styles

<u>The Directive Style</u>
- Prefers simple, clear solutions
- Makes decisions rapidly
- Does not consider many alternatives
- Relies on existing rules

<u>The Analytical Style</u>
- Prefers complex problems
- Carefully analyzes alternatives
- Enjoys solving problems
- Willing to use innovative methods

<u>The Conceptual Style</u>
- Socially oriented
- Humanistic and artistic approach
- Solves problems creatively
- Enjoys new ideas

<u>The Behavioral Style</u>
- Concern for their organization
- Interest in helping others
- Open to suggestions
- Relies on meetings

Quality practice

The Standards of Practice in Nutrition Care (SOP), Standards of Professional Performance (SOPP), and the Scope of Dietetic Practice Framework (SODPF) all work together to support quality dietetic practice according to the philosophy set forth by the Nutrition Care Process and Model – Complex Conditions and Model. The SODPF is not a list of services that one is or is not authorized to perform; rather, it is a dynamic framework that encompasses the knowledge base, ethics, research, education, and standards of care that make up the profession of dietetics. SOP includes the range of services that a dietitian might provide in a safe, sanctioned setting. SOPP describes the satisfactory behavior one should execute when acting in the professional role of dietitian. It can be used within the profession to evaluate one's own performance, by administrators to determine if patient needs are being met, or by human resources departments to make hiring and employment decisions.

Human Resources

Foodservice job design

The goal of job design is to organize the tasks contained in one job so that the employee is able to complete the work safely, efficiently, and with a measure of personal satisfaction. The first step is to conduct a job analysis, which consists of an overall study of the nature of the job. The supervisor should seek the input of the employee in this information gathering process. This information can then be used to create the job description. The description is the formal compilation of all duties and skills needed to perform the job. This description can be used to match employees with pertinent skills to a matching job. The job breakdown takes each duty listed in the description, and details exactly how the task is to be performed. Job enlargement adds variety to assigned tasks to prevent boredom. Job enrichment builds additional responsibility and independence into a job to add to employee satisfaction.

Selecting foodservice employees

Recruiting

Successful recruiting can be done from in-house candidates, or can be done outside of the organization. In-house recruiting has the advantages of selecting someone who has shown that he or she fits into the culture of the organization, and retaining skilled employees who might otherwise look for opportunities elsewhere. External recruiting can be done with the aid of advertising, placement services, or college career services.

Interviewing

Employee interviews can be structured or unstructured. Structured interviews are conducted from a predetermined list of questions used for each applicant. Advantages include consistency in information gathering among applicants. Disadvantages include insufficient information gathered from ill-prepared questions. Unstructured interviews use open-ended, unplanned questions and conversations to elicit information. Inexperienced interviewers need to be aware of the possibility of including questions that are not permissible in the interview process, such as those relating to age or marital status.

Illegal interview questions:
- Where were you born?
- Where are your parents from?
- What's your heritage?
- What religion are you?
- Are you married?
- Is this your maiden or married name?
- With whom do you live?
- How many kids do you have?
- Do you plan to have children?
- How old are you?
- What year were you born?
- When did you graduate from high school?
- Which religious holidays will you be taking off from work?
- Do you attend church regularly?
- Have you ever been arrested?

- Have you ever spent a night in jail?
- Do you have any disabilities?
- What's your medical history?
- How does your condition affect your abilities?

<u>Temp to Perm</u>
A worker is sent out as a temporary employee for a prescribed period of time, with the understanding that the person may eventually be hired directly as a full-time or contract employee by the client company. At the end of the pre-agreed trial period, if the employee decides that he or she wishes to continue working here, and the client in turn decides that they would like for this employee to stay, then an employment agreement becomes possible.

<u>Unions</u>
A union is a group of employees who use the power of their numbers to negotiate for better benefits, wages, or working conditions in an organization. If the organization is union shop, the employee must be a member of the union as a condition of employment. In an open shop, the employee can decide whether or not to join the union. Closed shop unions are ones in which the employer can hire only union members, which is an illegal practice.

Employers of unionized workers shall not be subject to secondary boycotts, such that the workers refuse to negotiate with the employer via a neutral third party unless union demands are met. Union members may not demand to be paid for services not rendered. Employers may not interfere with the activities of the union by coercing employees or inquiring about union activities. Employers cannot discriminate against union members in hiring, nor can employers refuse to engage in the collective bargaining process.

Bona fide occupational qualification

A minimum qualification requirement needed as a prerequisite to being able to do a particular job. BFOQs, if challenged, must be demonstrated to be valid by the employer. The courts have interpreted BFOQs very narrowly, especially with regard to sex. Each applicant must be treated as an individual in comparing his or her skills to the skills required to perform the job.

Productivity management

Productivity management analyzes the data that illustrate how inputs, such as labor and inventory, are converted into outputs, such as meals sold or consultations delivered. If one wishes to increase productivity, one must find ways to either increase outputs or decrease inputs. The ratio considers only one input and one output at a time. To calculate how many meals were produced per labor hour for one eight-hour day, and 12 full time employees were on shift, the number of meals served for that day would be divided by 96 hours (12 x 8).

Work simplification techniques involve examining each step involved in a worker's task, and eliminating those unnecessary steps that reduce productivity and contribute to fatigue. The charts and diagrams produced for the purpose of work simplification can also be used in the training of new employees, allowing a new worker to quickly reach the same level of efficiency as a seasoned employee. Examples include process charts and worker flow diagrams.

Increasing worker productivity

The Hawthorne studies were carried out in a number of series by the General Electric Company, who initially wanted to discover a way to increase worker production by utilizing more effective lighting techniques. In the first study, one group of workers was exposed to diminishing light, while the lighting of the control group was held constant. Production went up in both groups, even though the experimental group was subjected to lighting so dim they could barely see. In the second study, researchers provided the supervision to the two groups of workers, and gave each group varying amounts of work and break times. Once again, productivity increased regardless of variable manipulation. This led researchers to conclude that the special attention given the groups caused the increased productivity. The term "Hawthorne effect" was coined to describe the increase in productivity seen in workers who are singled out. This supports the notion of providing individual attention and support to employees in order to maximize performance.

Maslow's hierarchy of needs

Maslow's hierarchy of needs compiled research on the factors that motivate human behavior, and then organized this research into a tiered level of progression so that one could understand and predict an individual's efforts to meet internal goals. At the base of the needs pyramid are physiological goals, which satisfy the basic requirements of life such as food, water, and shelter. These needs must be met before one can progress to the next tier, which encompasses safety needs. From a workplace standpoint, this would include the need for a safe working environment. The next tier describes an individual's need to belong, which can be satisfied by the camaraderie found between employees. When these needs are met, an individual strives to meet esteem needs, which managers can offer through recognition of good work. When all lower tier levels are met, one can strive for self-actualization, where one gains the satisfaction of fulfilling his or her potential for growth.

Operant conditioning

The Operant Conditioning Process:
1. Stimulus (S) or Antecedent (A) – A signal, cue, or specific context.
2. Response (R) or Behavior (B) – The target behavior that you want to change.
3. Consequences (C) – Outcomes that occur based on a behavior.

Increasing desired behaviors

Guidelines for Increasing Desired Employee Behaviors:
- Make sure that you understand the S-R-C linkage.
- Make sure that the consequence is positively valued by the employee.
- Link positive consequences with the desired behavior more frequently to facilitate acquisition of behavior.
- Vary the frequency of using positive consequences to maintain the desired behavior.
- Vary the type of positive consequences used.
- Watch the costs associated with administering positive consequences.

Willful Misconduct

The employee's burden in attempting to prove a case of "serious and willful misconduct" can be very difficult. First, the employee must show that the misconduct was "serious"; that is, that the injury reasonably to be expected to result from exposing an employee to a recognizable hazard will be severe. Second, he or she must also show that the conduct was "willful"; that is, that the employer actually knew of the dangerous condition, yet deliberately failed to take corrective action. This requirement has been interpreted by the courts to mean conduct that is something more than even gross negligence.

Disciplinary action

Foodservice operations should include a formal disciplinary process in their policy and procedure manual that acts as a guide both for the supervisor and the employees. Well-defined discipline procedures enable the supervisor to respond consistently to infractions, and reduce the possibility of paying unemployment compensation to workers terminated for misconduct. Having a detailed plan of action before meeting with the employee can help the supervisor avoid waffling or backing down in the event of an emotional confrontation. A common sequence of disciplinary action would include an oral warning, a written warning, suspension, and termination. Each step should be accompanied by thorough documentation and placed in the employee's file. All disciplinary matters should be dealt with in a private setting, and should focus on how the employee can correct or improve his or her behavior. Using positive coaching, exercising patience, and teaching by modeling correct behaviors may salvage difficult employees.

Performance Measures

Performance measures should identify the population to be measured, the method of the measurement, and the data source and time period for the measurement. Each measure should also be:

- Objective
- Easy to understand
- Controllable by minimizing outside influences
- Timely
- Accurate
- Cost-effective
- Useful
- Motivating
- Trackable

Performance measures are quantitative or qualitative ways to characterize and define performance. They provide a tool for organizations to manage progress towards achieving predetermined goals, defining key indicators of organizational performance and customer satisfaction.

Protection for foodservice employees

As it pertains to employment, the Civil Rights Act prevents the use of discriminating hiring practices based on race, color, sex, or national origin. Furthermore, employers cannot segregate or classify their employees based on these characteristics. Employers should be careful to exclude thinly veiled discriminatory questions on the application that could be used as a basis for filing a discrimination suit, such as questions about a woman's pregnancy or maiden name. The Equal Employment Opportunity Act amended the Civil Rights Act, adding more specific language that defines discriminatory hiring practices, and including political affiliation as a characteristic one may not consider in making hiring decisions.

The Fair Labor Standards Act sets guidelines for minimum wage and overtime pay for more than 40 hours worked. The act also sets guidelines for child labor, specifying that children younger than 14 years of age may not be employed by foodservice operations. Children younger than 18 may not operate hazardous power-driven food preparation machines.

Protections and benefits for employees

The Worker Investment Act of 1998 seeks to meet the needs of both employers and employees by setting guidelines for education and training that will help employers succeed in their jobs. Individuals seeking employment will be able to utilize employment centers that measure the aptitude of the applicant and match the skills to available jobs. This also enables employers to easily find qualified applicants for open positions.

The Family and Medical Leave Act requires employers to provide eligible employees with up to 12 weeks of unpaid leave to care for a new baby or to recover from a serious health issue or assist an immediate family member with a serious health issue. The act applies to organizations with more than 50 workers, and employees must have 12 months of service and 1,250 hours of service with that employer to qualify.

The Americans with Disabilities Act requires employers with 15 or more employees to make reasonable accommodations to allow disabled individuals to perform their job duties.

Collective bargaining

The collective bargaining process is a method of negotiating between unionized employees and their employer in order to settle a grievance. The goal of the process is to reach a mutually satisfactory agreement that will define the terms and conditions of employment in the organization for a defined period of time. The parties involved in the process may include the owner and management of the organization; the union steward, who acts as the union representative; and the bargaining unit, a group of employees chosen to negotiate because of their communication skills or interest in the grievance. A neutral third party may also be involved in the process. A conciliator may offer suggestions and advice in a nonbinding mediation hearing. An arbiter may be asked to step in and make a binding decision in an arbitration hearing if the two sides reach an impasse.

Occupational Safety and Health Act

The Occupational Safety and Health Act (1970) – Employee Rights
- The right to safety and health on the job.
- The right to accompany an inspection.
- The right to be informed of workplace hazards.
- The right to request inspections.
- The right to file a complaint.

The Occupational Safety and Health Act (1970) – Employer Responsibilities
- Meet the general duty responsibilities to provide a safe and healthful workplace.
- Notify employees of their rights under OSHA.
- Provide training mandated under OSHA.
- Comply with all industry-specific standards.

- Maintain accurate records (e.g., OSHA no. 200 log) of work-related injuries, accidents, and deaths.
- Abate cited violations within the period prescribed by OSHA.
- Provide employees with protective equipment needed for a job.
- Maintain records of employee exposures to workplace hazards.

Age Discrimination in Employment Act

Age Discrimination in Employment Act of 1967:
- Prohibits discrimination against individuals who are 40 years of age or older.
- Guidelines for overcoming or preventing age discrimination include:
- Audit organizational culture.
- Rethink and change attitudes about older workers.
- Assess and modify practices that may discriminate against older workers.
- Include older workers in diversity task forces.

Pregnancy Discrimination Act

Pregnancy Discrimination Act of 1978:
- Protects pregnant employees from discrimination in employment.
- Employers must allow pregnant employees to work until it affects their performance and the disability is at a level that is comparable to other conditions where workers could not continue.
- Employers must allow women to return to work after childbirth on the same basis as for other disabilities.

Employers may not do the following:
- Refuse to hire a pregnant employee.
- Terminate an employee after discovering the employee's pregnancy.
- Fail to permit the employee to be part of the normal cycle of office culture.
- Refuse to provide lighter duty, if the employee needs it.

Sexual harassment

Behaviors that may constitute sexual harassment include:
- Touching.
- Telling sexually oriented jokes.
- "Elevator Eyes."
- Allowing pin-up calendars, or other sexually oriented images in the workplace.
- Making sexually oriented comments.
- Repeatedly making unwanted sexual advances toward another employee.
- Making conditions of employment based on "sexual favors."
- Physical assaults (e.g., grabbing).

Fair labor standards act

The Fair Labor Standards Act of 1938 was enacted to establish a minimum wage, to limit work hours, and to discourage oppressive child labor. Referred to as the Wage Hour Act because it ensures fair treatment of employees with respect to wages and hours. Act defines exempt and nonexempt employees.

Equal employment opportunity commission

Federal agency responsible for administration of several statutes that prohibit discrimination; has power to subpoena witnesses, issue guidelines that have the force of law, render decisions, provide technical assistance to employers, provide legal assistance to complainants, etc.

Equal pay act

The Equal Pay Act of 1963 makes it unlawful to pay wages to members of one sex at a rate lower than paid to members of the other sex for equal jobs that require equal skill, effort, and responsibility. Jobs must be substantially equal based on job content.

Consolidated Omnibus Budget Reconciliation Act

The federal Consolidated Omnibus Budget Reconciliation Act (COBRA) requires that most employers sponsoring group health plans offer employees and their families the opportunity for a temporary extension of health care and union Employee Benefit Fund coverage called "continuation coverage" at group rates in certain instances in which coverage under the program would otherwise end.

Whistleblower Protection Act

The Whistleblower Protection Act of 1989 is to strengthen and improve protection for the rights of federal employees, to prevent reprisals, and to help eliminate wrongdoing within the government by:
- Mandating that employees should not suffer adverse consequences as a result of prohibited personnel practices.
- Establishing:
  - That the primary role of the Office of Special Counsel is to protect employees, especially whistleblowers, from prohibited personnel practices.
  - That the Office of Special Counsel shall act in the interests of employees who seek assistance from the Office of Special Counsel.
  - That while disciplining those who commit prohibited personnel practices may be used as a means by which to help accomplish that goal, the protection of individuals who are the subject of prohibited personnel practices remains the paramount consideration.

Financial Management

Business plan

A business plan is appropriate for new facilities establishing goals and objectives for operations, and it is also helpful for existing facilities to help them continue with their development. Plans can vary, but most plans describe the operation, and use mission statements, vision statements, or corporate philosophies to articulate what is meaningful to the organization. The product or service offered should be described in a way that sets it apart from its competitors. Marketing strategies should be outlined.

The management team and organizational structure should be described. The lending institution and the owner will want to see a financial plan that includes projected cash flow, projected profit and loss, and a projected balance sheet. An operational plan should include the timeline for accomplishing tasks, the production methods that will be used, and the type and amount of labor that will be required. Your bank will be interested in:
- How you intend to repay a loan/overdraft.
- What you are going to do with the money.
- How the loan will help the business to grow.
- What other loan or debt commitments you have.

Most lenders operate a credit-scoring system. Information is logged into a computer program, which recommends whether a loan should be given or not. Make sure you give up-to-date and relevant information. A good relationship with your bank manager will not influence the credit score.

Common reasons why business plans and loan applications fail include:
- A weak management team.
- A flawed marketing plan.
- Unrealistic forecasts.
- Incomplete and poor presentations.

Budgets

Good budgeting practices empower foodservice managers with the information they need to analyze the financial status of the operation and make buying decisions.
- An operating budget itemizes revenue, expenses, debt, and cash flow for the accounting period. This information is used to estimate the profitability of the operation. The operating budget shows the manager how much revenue is required to continue with the operation of the establishment, with wiggle room built in to accommodate unexpected expenses.
- The cash budget projects the difference between sales and expenses. The cash budget helps the manager predict if additional funds will be available in the event of a crisis. A sound cash budget may also be a requirement of obtaining credit for the purpose of purchasing new equipment.
- A capital budget is a plan for large acquisitions or facility improvements whose benefits are expected to be realized over a period of years. An example is the planning and financing of a dining room expansion.
- Traditional or incremental budgeting uses the budget from the previous accounting period as the basis for planning the current accounting period. An incremental amount is added to

- 156 -

each subsequent budget to plan for inflation. This method assumes that expenses will remain the same from one accounting period to the next, and may encourage unnecessary spending in order to maintain the budget into the next period.

- Zero-based budgeting ignores what happened in previous accounting periods and requires each expense to be justified. This is a time-consuming but useful method for institutions that have wide variations in their expenses.
- Flexible budgets are prepared at the end of the accounting period to accommodate varying levels of revenue. This type of budget correlates varying expenses to varying levels of production in order to predict future expenses and revenue.
- Performance budgets focus on the expenses necessary to achieve a performance goal, such as the money it takes to feed all children in a school district's summer lunch program.

Costs

- Indirect costs incurred by foodservice operations are fixed, and remain the same regardless of how much revenue is generated. Examples include the mortgage payment for the facility or fire insurance.
- Direct, variable, flexible costs vary according to the sales and production of the operation. Examples include food and paper products.
- Semi-variable costs have both fixed and variable components. For example, the electricity necessary to illuminate the establishment is a set cost, but electricity usage rises as cookware is used more frequently to serve larger crowds.
- Sunk costs are those purchases that have already been made and cannot be reversed or altered. For example, if a consultant was hired to educate the management team on ways to prevent harassment in the workplace, and the training was complete, this would be a sunk cost.
- Differential cost is the difference in cost between two comparable alternatives.

Prepaid expenses

It is quite common to pay for goods and services in advance. You have probably purchased your automobile insurance this way, perhaps prepaying for an annual or semi-annual policy. Or, rent on a building may be paid ahead of its intended use (e.g., most landlords require monthly rent to be paid at the beginning of each month). Another example of prepaid expense relates to supplies that are purchased and stored in advance of actually needing them.

Cost-saving measures

Food costs make up the largest part of a foodservice operation's budget, but food costs can also be manipulated by savvy managers in order to meet budget requirements. There are many opportunities for food waste to occur between receiving and serving. Using (first-in-first-out) FIFO storage methods to reduce spoilage and teaching cooks the proper way to trim meat reduces waste.

Overproduction is common in industries such as catering, where large quantities of food are often discarded after an event. Software programs can help managers track waste and determine how much food should be prepared. Combining buying power with other operations allows managers to negotiate lower prices with vendors. Supervising the receiving process prevents "short" orders or substitution of inferior products.

Labor costs are not as flexible as food costs, but investing in quality equipment that reduces food preparation time can result in long-term savings.

Operating costs such as utilities usually account for approximately 15% of the budget, and are not susceptible to a great deal of control.

Accounting methods

Accrual-basis
Generally accepted accounting principles (GAAP) require that a business should use the "accrual basis."

Cash-basis accounting
An alternative method in use by some small businesses (small businesses may not be required to apply GAAP) is the "cash-basis." It is much simpler, but its financial statement results can be very misleading in the short run. Under this easy approach, revenue is recorded when cash is received (no matter when it is "earned"), and expenses are recognized when paid (no matter when "incurred").

Straight Line Depreciation

A method of computing amortization (depreciation) by dividing the difference between an asset's cost and its expected salvage value by the number of years it is expected to be used. Depreciation is used in accounting to try and match the expense of an asset to the income that the asset helps the company earn. For example, if a company bought a piece of equipment for $1 million and expected it would have a useful life of 10 years, it would be depreciated over the 10 years. Every accounting year the company would expense $100,000 (assuming straight line depreciation), and this would be matched with the money that the equipment helps to make each year.

Inventory methods

Average cost
LIFO: Last in first out
FIFO: First in first out
Types of depreciation:
Declining Balance
Straight Line
Sum of the year's digits

Financial status

Liquidity ratios
Liquidity ratios can be used to demonstrate to creditors that a foodservice operation is able to meet its short-term debts. The liquidity ratio is calculated by dividing the operation's current assets by its current liabilities. A high ratio tells creditors that the business is fully capable of covering its short-term debts. A low ratio tells the owners that assets are being used to build business.

Net worth ratios
A net worth ratio is used to demonstrate to creditors that long-term debts can be fulfilled over the course of 12 months. This ratio is calculated by dividing current liabilities by net worth. Companies

with a small net worth and a large amount of liabilities may have difficulty securing additional credit.

Turnover ratios

Turnover ratios divide the cost of goods sold by the average cost of the inventory. If the ratio is too low, the manager may not have enough stock on hand. If the ratio is high, the operation's cash is tied up in excess inventory or inventory may be stagnant.

Daily food cost report

The daily food cost report reveals what percent of income was spent on food by dividing daily food cost by daily income. This figure is useful in calculating menu prices for individual items, which usually are priced three times above the cost in order to achieve an acceptable profit margin.

Profit margin

The profit margin is calculated by dividing the net profit by the revenue. The net profit is the amount of money remaining after all expenses have been deducted, including supplies, labor, taxes, and utilities. A negative profit margin indicates that revenues need to be increased or expenses need to be reduced.

Food cost per meal

Food cost per meal is calculated by dividing the food cost per month by the number of meals served per month. This figure can be compared with the meal cost for other meals or days to ascertain if the plate cost is reasonable. A high plate cost for one meal should be balanced out by lower priced meals on the menu.

Program evaluation tools

Cost-effectiveness analyses

Cost-effectiveness analyses are conducted when the outcome of a nutrition intervention has already been determined to be worthwhile, but the methods by which the outcome will be achieved are in dispute. In this evaluation tool, both the costs of each method and the potential consequences need to be studied.

The analysis is helpful when deciding between a method that is more expensive and more helpful, and a method that is a lower cost alternative, yet also less helpful. The difference between the two methods may be marginal and difficult to discern without extensive review of previously published data.

Value analyses

Value analysis is a way of exploring whether the expense of a new service, technology, or alteration in practice can be justified by the positive outcomes it will bring. In other words, managers want to get the most utility out of an investment for the least expense. For example, this analysis may be used to determine if the savings in labor justify the savings achieved by a new dishwashing system.

Cost-benefit analyses

The cost-benefit analysis is a way to objectively assess whether a nutrition intervention program is desirable by comparing the cost of the effort, as expressed in a dollar amount, to the benefits of the program, expressed in some quantitatively measurable unit. This quantitative analysis can be beneficial in securing grants or approvals to proceed with a planned intervention. The benefits of the program may be analyzed in terms of lives saved, positive dietary changes made, disease status improved, or reduction in the length of hospital stay. The benefits must be expressed as a dollar amount, so that comparison against cost can be made. Therein lies one of the principle drawbacks of cost-benefit analysis; it is not possible to place a dollar amount on a human life. However, it is not possible to execute every program that may save a life, so the benefit may be rephrased as "reducing the risk of death."

Spearman's rho, ANOVA, and t-test

Spearman's rho is a measure of the linear relationship between 2 variables.

Analysis of variance (ANOVA) performs comparisons like the t-test, but for an arbitrary number of factors. Each factor can have an arbitrary number of levels. Furthermore each factor combination can have any number of replicates. ANOVA works on a single dependent variable. The factors must be discrete. The ANOVA can be thought of in a practical sense as an extension of the t-test to an arbitrary number of factors and levels. It can also be thought of as a linear regression model whose independent variables are restricted to a discrete set.

When more than two groups or populations are being studied, using analysis of variance can help to evaluate the validity of the study. The overarching rationale for analysis of variance is to determine whether differences between groups are statistically significant, or due to chance. This computation involves dividing the variance between groups by the variance within groups. The "between groups variance" is calculated by using sample group means, and the "within groups variance" is the average of the variances within each sample group being examined. If there are no differences between the group means, the variance will be small; the variance grows larger as the difference between the means grows larger. The test is useful when comparing studies with unequal sample sizes. Analysis of variance can also be used when researchers want to economize by sampling one time and answering many questions about the data gathered, rather than running several studies on each variable separately.

The t-test is typically used to compare the means of 2 populations. Specifically, this java applet can be used to determine whether or not the means in 2 sample populations are significantly different. Nothing is assumed of the sample populations in this implementation.

Mean, median, and mode

The arithmetic mean, commonly referred to as the average, consists of a set of scores divided by the number of scores. So, in the number group 10, 11, 12, 12, 13, the mean is 11.6. The mean must be used with caution, because a small number of outlying scores can make the mean less representative of the population. The median is the score that appears in the middle of an ordered list of scores. So, in the previous example, the median is 12. If an even number of scores is present, the median is calculated by taking the average of the two scores in the middle of the list. The mode is the score that occurs with the most frequency in a list. The mode in the example provided is 12. If two modes are present, the data are called bimodal. If many modes are present, mode may not provide the researcher with a meaningful measure.

Distribution forms

In the mathematically perfect standard normal curve, the mean, median, and mode are the same. In most real distribution forms, the data can take on several different patterns or "skews." When the distribution is skewed left, or negatively skewed, the tail of the curve extends to the left and the data hump is located on the right. If the skew is positive, or skewed to the right, the tail of the curve extends to the right and the data hump is on the left.

In either type of skew, the mean is located closest to the tail, the mode is located closest to the data hump, and the median is in between. A bimodal curve will have two data humps, and the mean and median will be located between the humps.

P-value

The P value is used to help researchers determine whether or not to reject the null hypothesis. By rejecting the null hypothesis, researchers are saying in effect that "nothing" is not going on. In other words, the data points to a relationship between the variables being studied, and the hypothesis may be tenable. The p value can be thought of as the likelihood of seeing results more significant than what the study achieved if the null hypothesis were true. If the P value is small, or less than 0.05, research standards state that the findings of the study are statistically significant. The smaller the P value, the higher the researcher's confidence that the results are not due to chance, but are caused by a relationship that exists between the variables.

Chi-square test

The chi-square test can be used when researchers want to compare a set of observed data with a set of expected data to see if a statistically significant pattern exists. In a hypothetical example, a clinician observes that 2% of the individuals in his or her city are managing a diagnosis of celiac disease. However, in a class the clinician is conducting, a large number of the participants have been diagnosed with celiac disease. Theory would lead the clinician to expect that 2 out of every 100 individuals in this population would have celiac disease. However, 8 out of 64 members of the class have celiac disease. The observed number of celiac cases does not meet the expected number of celiac cases in the class. The chi formula provides the researcher with a figure that can be analyzed by looking at a critical chi value chart. If the figure falls into the critical region, the null hypothesis is rejected.

Gantt chart

A Gantt Chart is a horizontal bar chart used in management as a tool for graphically representing the schedule of a set of specific activities or tasks. The horizontal bars indicate the length of time allocated to each activity, so the x-axis of a Gantt chart is subdivided into equal units of time (e.g., days, weeks, months). The y-axis of a Gantt chart, on the other hand, simply lists all the activities or tasks being monitored by the Gantt chart. A simple look at a Gantt chart should enable its user to determine which tasks take the longest time to complete, which tasks are overlapping with each other, etc.

General ledger, profit and loss statement, and balance sheet

A general ledger contains the history of a foodservice operation's financial dealings throughout the lifecycle of the business. When a new ledger is created for a fledgling business, the assets will include any equipment, property, or inventory on hand, and the liability section will list all loans that were obtained to start the business. As the business progresses, the ledger will be further divided into cash, accounts payable, and accounts receivable sections.

The profit and loss statement is derived from information contained in the ledger sheet. This statement lists the income and expenses for each accounting period, and tallies the profit, loss, or break-even status of the organization.

The balance sheet contains two sections that, when compared, must be equal to one another. On one side of the sheet is a list of all of the organization's assets, such as inventory, cash, and equipment. The other side of the sheet lists liabilities combined with equity. Liabilities include account payable items; equity represents the amount of money invested in the business.

Debit and credit

Debit
An item of debt as recorded in an account.
The left-hand side of an account or accounting ledger where bookkeeping entries are made.
An entry of a sum in the left-hand side of an account.
The sum of such entries.

Credit
The deduction of a payment made by a debtor from an amount due.
The right-hand side of an account on which such amounts are entered.
An entry or the sum of the entries on this side.
The positive balance or amount remaining in a person's account.
A credit line.

Cost, Expense, Liability, and Income

Cost
An amount paid or required in payment for a purchase; a price.

Expense
An expenditure of money; a cost.

Liability
A financial obligation, debt, claim, or potential loss.

Income
The amount of money or its equivalent received during a period of time in exchange for labor or services, from the sale of goods or property, or as profit from financial investments.

Marketing and Public Relations

Marketing

The elements that make up the marketing mix of a product include the product, price, place, and promotion.

- In foodservice, the product can be the menu item or the way it is served. Managers should consider the qualities of the product that set it apart from its competitors and allow it to meet the needs and wants of the customer.
- Pricing strategy needs to be carefully considered to avoid undercharging practices that lead to lower profit margins, or overpricing practices that lead to stagnant inventory and loss of customer base. Pricing considerations include daily specials or discounts.
- Place includes distribution considerations. Cell phones and the internet have provided new ways for customers to access menus and place orders from remote locations.
- Promotion may be the most important marketing element in the mix. Advertising, press releases, on-site radio broadcasts, or any other way to increase visibility of the establishment can build and retain the customer base.

4 P's of marketing
- Product
- Price
- Promotion
- Place

Product: What is it? What "need" does it address? The functional specs? What are its Features and benefits?

Price: What is Price? (vs. cost?) Channel Pricing? Strategies: markup, perceived value, skimming, going rate. Tactics: Discounts, terms, currency.

Place (i.e., distribution): The Path to the Buyer! Channels, cost (price) tradeoffs, control issues

Promotion: advertising, events, press releases, trade shows, direct vs. indirect, brand awareness, brochures, datasheets, freebies.

Networking

Networking is a powerful and indispensable tool for marketing your business. The more you put into your networking efforts the more you will get out. By exchanging information, ideas, contacts, and business referrals, you increase your client and referral base. You will also find yourself privy to information about industry trends, trade associations, and key people in particular industries.

Trade associations, chambers of commerce, trade fairs, and business conferences offer networking opportunities. Join and become active in those groups that best fit your business goals or match your personal interests.

Arrow diagramming method
Network diagramming technique in which activities are represented by arrows. The tail of the arrow represents the start of the activity; the head of the arrow represents the finish of the activity.

The length of the arrow does not represent the expected duration of the activity. Activities are connected at points called nodes (usually drawn as circles) to illustrate the sequence in which activities are expected to be performed (also called activity-on-arrow).

Queuing theory

The study of how systems with limited resources distribute those resources to elements waiting in line, and how those elements waiting in line respond. Examples include the distribution of cars on highways (including traffic jams), data through computer networks, and waiting in a lunch line.

Here are details of three queuing disciplines:
First In First Out – This principle states that customers are served one at a time and that the customer that has been waiting the longest is served first.

Last In First Out – This principle also serves customers one at a time; however, the customer with the shortest waiting time will be served first.

Processor Sharing – Customers are served equally. Network capacity is shared between customers and they all effectively experience the same delay

Word-of-mouth

Word-of-mouth is extremely important and is also a very powerful promotional tool. Customers talking about you to friends, family, and acquaintances have much more influence and credibility than any other kind of advertisement.

Remember: bad word-of-mouth travels and multiplies at least four times faster than good word-of-mouth, so make sure your customer service is spot on right from the start. Many small businesses have not only survived (without a huge advertising budget), but grown with good word-of-mouth working for them.

Pricing strategies

Breakeven point
Breakeven analysis is a calculation used to determine the point at which sales volume covers fixed costs and variable costs. The fixed cost of a product includes the total cost required to produce the first product item, and this cost does not vary unless new equipment must be purchased. Fixed costs are high, often in the tens of thousands of dollars. Variable costs are those that are added on after the first item is produced, such as labor and additional inventory that must be purchased to produce each additional product. Variable costs should be below the menu price. Breakeven analysis can be used to answer the question, "At what point will the production of this product stop costing us money and start making profits?" The answer to this question can help management determine menu prices. The formula for determining breakeven point is calculated by dividing fixed costs by the selling price minus the variable cost.

Determining selling price
Factor method: The factor method is the traditional way of determining menu pricing strategies, although this method focuses on food costs to the exclusion of labor and other contributing costs. The factor method is determined by first calculating the mark-up factor, which is the figure derived

by dividing 100 over the food cost percentage. The mark-up factor multiplied by the raw food cost yields the selling price.

Prime cost method: The prime cost method considers both food costs and labor, and is appropriate for calculating costs for menu items that require a great deal of skill to prepare. The selling price is determined by multiplying the prime cost by the mark-up factor, where prime cost equals raw food cost plus labor cost. Mark-up is calculated by dividing 100 by food cost percentage plus labor cost percentage.

Cost of profit: Cost of profit pricing is used when the menu price must be calculated in a way so that it ensures a specific percentage of profit. It is calculated by dividing total food cost by desired food cost percentage.

Partnerships

A business owned by two or more people, who agree to share in its profits, is considered a partnership. Like the sole proprietorship, it is easy to start and the red tape involved is usually minimal. The tax structure is the same as proprietorship except the profits and losses of the partnership are divided by an agreed percentage by the partners.

Advantages
The main advantages of the partnership form are that the business can:
1. Draw on the skills and abilities of each partner,
2. Offer employees the opportunity to become partners, and
3. Utilize the partners' combined financial resources.

However, for your own protection, it is advisable to have a written partnership agreement that will spell out the specifics of the agreement.

Corporations

A corporation differs from the other legal forms of business in that the law regards it as an artificial being that possesses the same rights and responsibilities as a person. This means that, unlike sole proprietorships or partnerships, it has an existence separate from its owners. It has all the legal rights of an individual in regards to conducting commercial activity—it can sue, be sued, own property, sell property, and sell the rights of ownership in the form of exchanging stock for money. Benefits of a corporation include:
1. Limited liability: owners are not personally responsible for the debts of the business,
2. The ability to raise capital by selling shares of stock, and
3. Easy transfer of ownership from one individual to another.

Advantages:
Stockholders have limited liability. Corporations can raise the most investment capital. Corporations have unlimited life. Ownership is easily transferable. Corporations utilize specialists.

Disadvantages:
Corporations are taxed twice. Corporations must pay capital stock tax. Starting a corporation is expensive. Corporations are closely regulated by government agencies.

Sole proprietorships

A business owned by one person, who is entitled to all of its profits and responsible for all of its debts, is considered a sole proprietorship. This legal form is the simplest, providing maximum control and minimum government interference. Currently used by more than 75% of all businesses, it is often the suggested way for a new business that does not carry great personal liability threats. The owner needs to secure the necessary licenses, tax identification numbers, and certifications in his or her name, to be in business. The main advantages that differentiate the sole proprietorship from the other legal forms are:
1. The ease with which it can be started
2. The owner's freedom to make decisions
3. The distribution of profits (owner takes all)

Advantages
You're the boss. It's easy to get started. You keep all profits. Income from business is taxed as personal income. You can discontinue your business at will.

Disadvantages
You assume unlimited liability. The amount of investment capital you can raise is limited. You need to be a generalist. Retaining high-caliber employees is difficult. The life of the business is dependent on the owner's.

Principles of Management

There is an organization called the Taylor Society that has collected 13 principles of Taylorism, but more briefly, the idea of scientific management boils down to 4 basic principles:
- Scientific research and analysis of work, its elements, standards, and rates.
- Scientific selection, training, and development of first-class workers.
- Intimate, friendly, and hearty cooperation for scientific work principles (anti-unionism).
- Equal division of responsibility among managers in functional areas (not just over people).

F.W. Taylor's contributions to management
F.W. Taylor is known as the "Father of Scientific Management" and was nicknamed "Speedy" Taylor for his reputation as an efficiency expert. His techniques were:
- To initiate a time study rate system.
- Create functional foremen.
- Establish cost accounting.
- Devise a system of pay for the person and not the position.

Management styles

Laissez-faire management style
Management approach in which team members are not directed by management. Little information flows from the team to the manager, or vice versa. This style is appropriate if the team is highly skilled and knowledgeable and wants no interference by the manager.

Open-door policy
Management approach that encourages employees to speak freely and regularly to management regarding any aspect of the business or product. Adopted to promote the open flow of

communication and to increase the success of business operations or project performance by soliciting the ideas of employees. Tends to minimize personnel problems and employee dissatisfaction.

Authoritarian Management Style

Management approach in which the manager tells team members what is expected of them, provides specific guidance on what should be done, makes his or her role within the team understood, schedules work, and directs team members to follow standard rules and regulations.

Autocratic Management Style

Management approach in which the manager makes all decisions and exercises tight control over the team. This style is characterized by communications from the manager downward to the team and not vice versa.

Blake and Mouton managerial grid

The managerial grid describes a manager's style based on where he or she falls on a grid with two axes: the vertical axis shows the manager's concern for people, and the horizontal axis shows the manager's concern for production. A manager who ranks high on concern for people but low on concern for production will be viewed as an ineffectual pushover more concerned about acceptance than results. A manager who ranks high on concern for production but low on concern for people tends to exercise an autocratic style of leadership, and is concerned with matters of domination and control. The most effective managers rank high or equally moderate on both concerns. These managers value employee morale and utilize teamwork to accomplish their goals.

Traditional or classical approach

The classical management school of thought is characterized by the traditional bureaucratic structure of top-down authority. This management style places value in the hierarchy, and depends on rational guidelines to lend structure to the organization. Classical management embraces the scalar principle, which shares that authority flows in a vertical line from the highest to the lowest position in an organization. This school of thought originated early in the twentieth century and is criticized for being too simplistic and not considering the dynamics of small groups.

Systems approach

The systems approach argues that an organization is composed of interdependent components, so that an event that affects one part of the organization will in turn affect other parts of the organization. The systems approach characterizes an organization as open and interactive, so that the organization can affect and be affected by the environment. The environment could include any entity outside of the foodservice operation that has dealings with the facility, such as vendors or regulatory agencies.

Leadership style

Contingency or situational

Contingency and situational leadership models argue that there is no one right way to manage, and methods that are effective for one situation may be inappropriate in other situations. This theory explains why sometimes formerly successful managers suddenly become inept when faced with a new situation. The manager applies the same techniques that worked in the past, but the results are different because the situation is different. The path-goal theory of leadership provides an example in that a manager may tailor his or her approach to the situation at hand. A strong leader will clarify the path to success for his or her employees, removing barriers and providing rewards along the way. The kind of rewards provided will by tailored to the skill and motivation level of each individual employee.

Transactional and transformational
Transactional and transformational leadership are two distinct ways of motivating and influencing employees, and each style is grounded in a distinct value set and way of thinking.

Transactional leaders focus on the bottom line, and seek ways to manipulate employees so that short-term goals will be achieved, possibly even at the expense of long-term job satisfaction. Transactional leaders have a limited amount of tools with which to problem-solve, but they remain focused on carrying out the prescribed roles the current system has given them, and they are not reform-oriented.

Transformational leaders are concerned with motivating employees by incorporating meaning and purpose into the tasks to be achieved. These types of leaders recognize the importance of building an organizational culture that appreciates the long view. Short-term goals are not accomplished at the expense of employee morale, and managers do not become so mired in daily activities that they lose sight of the mission of the organization.

Power

Reward power is based on the ability to reward someone for following orders or the ability to remove negative consequences for following orders. Coercive power is available to managers who use their ability to punish subordinates who do not carry out orders. Managers who use this power exclusively will never realize the full potential of their staff. Legitimate power is the influence the manager is able to exert due to the authority of his or her position. Legitimate power is weak as a stand-alone type of power; managers need another type of power to back it up or employees will eventually disregard the power conferred by the manager's position. Expert power may be wielded by one who demonstrates expertise in an area the other employees do not. Lower-level managers with high levels of technical skills, such as kitchen line managers, commonly possess this kind of power. Referent power is based on personality and respect; employees voluntarily follow a manager with this type of power because they wish to model this person.

Worker - manager relationship

Scientific management
Before Taylor's scientific management, managers rarely came into contact with their workers, and the enforcement of job performance was carried out by factory foremen. In the early 1900s, Taylor developed a notion that every task to be accomplished by an employee could be distilled down to an exact science, so that each person would be trained in this most efficient way of carrying out a task instead of trying to figure out best practices. Taylor viewed the worker as a machine, and thought that workers were motivated by money alone.

Human relations theory
Human relations theory proponents argue that employees get satisfaction from the social aspects of work, and benefit when they can function in a team-oriented setting. Individuals are motivated by more than money, and managers should connect with the emotions and individual needs of employees. Theory Z is a human relations theory that argues that employees are the lifeblood of a company, and should be rewarded with lifelong tenure and benefits.

HACCP

Hazard Analysis and Critical Control Point (HACCP) involves seven principles:
- Analyze hazards. Potential hazards associated with a food and measures to control those hazards are identified. The hazard could be biological, such as a microbe.
- Identify critical control points. These are points in a food's production—from its raw state through processing and shipping to consumption by the consumer—at which the potential hazard can be controlled or eliminated.
- Establish preventive measures with critical limits for each control point.
- Establish procedures to monitor the critical control points. Such procedures might include determining how and by whom cooking time and temperature should be monitored.
- Establish corrective actions to be taken when monitoring shows that a critical limit has not been met.
- Establish procedures to verify that the system is working properly, for example, testing time-and-temperature recording devices to verify that a cooking unit is working properly.
- Establish effective record keeping to document the HACCP system.

*Each of these principles must be backed by sound scientific knowledge.

Communication

Importance of communication
- It's not just WHAT you say, but also HOW you say it that matters.
- If you can't communicate, don't expect others to do what you want them to do.
- Communication skills are one of the best predictors of "success" in the business world.

Communication process
- The Sender: Idea, Encoding of an Idea: Taking an idea and translating it into an appropriate message.
- The Receiver: Decoding, Idea Received: Interpreting a message and receiving it.

Effective Upward Communication
General guidelines for effective upward communication:
- Always keep your boss informed of the situation.
- Focus on solutions, not problems.
- Follow the chain of command.
- If you have a pressing issue, make an appointment with your boss.
- Be sure to state your objective and the amount of time needed.
- Play close attention to how you frame your message.
- If you are unsure of how your boss will respond to an issue, run it by him/her in writing first.
- When presenting information, be sure to provide written documentation.
- Be as concise as possible.

Change

Several models and theories have been developed that address the need for, methods of, and barriers to ushering in organizational change. It is human nature to resist change, and this includes change in the workplace. Employees may be resistant to change because they are more focused on how the change will affect them than with how it might improve the organization. People appreciate the feelings of security and sameness they derive from their jobs, and may fear that the change will make their tasks unpleasant in some way.

The manager should approach organizational change by giving employees ample time to adjust to the change and voice their concerns. Managers may devote one or more employee meetings to discussions about the change. Verbal communication should be accompanied by printed literature, to reduce the chance for misunderstanding. If possible, employees should be included in the decision-making process involving the transition, so that employees feel ownership of the change.

Conflict

Likert's four-system concept
Likert argues that every organization can be characterized by four management styles. Exploitative-autocratic systems feature autocratic leadership, threats used as motivators, and an absence of teamwork. Benevolent-autocratic leaders have a patronizing "I know what's best for you" attitude. Consultative systems are characterized by some teamwork and a moderate amount of trust between supervisor and subordinate. Participative systems are ideal, and are characterized by high levels of teamwork and communication.

Johari window
The Johari window provides a tool to compare the self we know with the self others see. The open arena consists of facts readily known to the self and others. The façade contains facts known to the self but hidden from others. This includes attitudes and biases that may be sources of conflict. The blind spot contains facts others know about the individual, but not known to the individual. An example of this is a person who thinks of him or herself as a hard worker but is viewed by others as lazy. The unknown area contains characteristics hidden to the self and others.

Project management

Critical path method
In management, a critical path is the sequence of project network terminal elements with the longest overall duration, determining the shortest time to complete the project. The duration of the critical path determines the duration of the entire project. Any delay of a terminal element on the critical path directly impacts the planned project completion date (i.e., there is no float on the critical path).

A project can have several, parallel critical paths. An additional parallel path through the network with the total durations just shorter than the critical path is called a subcritical path. Originally, the critical path method considered only logical dependencies among terminal elements. A related concept is the critical chain, which adds resource dependencies.

Quality Improvement

Quality improvement activities

<u>Joint Commission standards</u>
The mission of the Joint Commission is to help health care organizations continuously improve the quality and safety of the care they provide. They do this through the administration of accreditation and certification programs that allow organization to demonstrate that they meet quality standards for patient safety. The Periodic Performance Review is an annual assessment that organizations submit to the Commission to show compliance with National Patient Safety Goals, and to identify problem areas needing improvement. If a Joint Commission Survey identifies any standards that are categorized as "not compliant," the organization shall file an Evidence of Standards Compliance report that details the plan of action to correct the deficiencies. The plan of action will use quantifiable criteria called Measures of Success to resolve any identified problem areas. If an organization is not compliant with the patient safety standards in the Joint Commission manual, they will be assigned a Requirement for Improvement (RFI). Failure to resolve an RFI can result in loss of accreditation.

Evaluations

Part of a foodservice manager's role is to evaluate the operation on an ongoing basis to determine if the performance of the operation meets the standards set by the management team. The benefits of evaluation include the revelation of the strengths and weaknesses of the operation and the ability to engage in problem-solving before issues grow out of control. It is important that the manager document both the evaluative process and the outcome, as the manager is responsible for the quality the department or facility provides. The evaluation may be outcome-evaluated, comparing the end results to the standards developed: Did health status improve? Were savings realized? Alternatively, the evaluation may be process-oriented: Did the process result in the accomplishment of the objectives?

Measurement types may include norm-referenced, comparing the learner against the group average; criterion-referenced, comparing the learner against what should have been learned; or comparative, looking for similarities or differences between learners.

Quality control and quality assurance

Quality Control refers to quality-related activities associated with the creation of project deliverables. Quality control is used to verify that deliverables are of acceptable quality and that they are complete and correct. Examples of quality control activities include deliverable peer reviews and the testing process.

Quality assurance refers to the process used to create the deliverables, and can be performed by a manager, client, or even a third-party reviewer. An example of quality assurance includes process checklists. Quality assurance is outcome oriented and deals with patient care.

Continuous Quality Improvement and Total Quality Management

Definitions of CQI and TQM vary. While CQI focuses on industrial methods and TQM on management philosophy, the terms often are used interchangeably because of their shared history and assumptions. CQI and TQM are based on the work of pioneers in industrial management such as W. Edwards Deming, Joseph Juran, Armand Fiegenbaum, and Kaoru Ishikawa. CQI focuses on the system and uses outcome assessments.

Total quality management

Total quality management (TQM) is an approach that uses all of an organization's resources to produce high-quality products and services. Organizations that practice TQM have the attitude that getting the job done right the first time and every time reduces waste and results in satisfied customers. The three elements that comprise TQM can be remembered as the three C's: customers/clients, culture, and counting. The customer ultimately decides what quality standards the organization should strive for.

The workplace culture emphasizes quality in all processes and tasks. Counting means accurate measurement and evaluation tools are utilized to review the efficacy of current practices. The PDCA commitment of managers in TQM means: plan what is to be done, do it, check the results, and act on the results.

Continuous improvement is an important tenet of TQM practices. Continuous improvement is the recognition that one should always be working to improve work processes for better future results.

Typical Elements of an Effective TQM Program:

1. Process Orientation
   - Cross-Functional Teams
   - Customer Focus
   - Benchmarking
   - Investment in Employee Training
   - Data-Based Decision Making

2. Employee Empowerment
   - Continuous Improvement
   - Open Communication
   - Quality-Driven Culture

Outcomes of Total Quality Management:
   - Reduced costs
   - Increased productivity
   - Higher customer satisfaction and retention
   - Fewer defects in products and services
   - Shorter product development cycles
   - Greater profitability

Juran's steps for quality planning

Juran provides a roadmap for quality planning. This roadmap consists of 10 steps, with one overriding principle. The overall principle requires us to apply measurements to each step. The steps are:
   - Customers
   - Discover Customers' Needs
   - Translate the Customers' Needs into our Language

- Establish Units of Measure
- Establish Measurement
- Develop Product
- Optimize Product Design
- Develop the Process
- Optimize: Prove the Process Capability
- Transfer to Operations

PDCA cycle

<u>Plan</u> to improve your operations first by finding out what things are going wrong (that is, identify the problems faced), and come up with ideas for solving these problems.

<u>Do</u> changes designed to solve the problems on a small or experimental scale first. This minimizes disruption to routine activity while testing whether the changes will work.

<u>Check</u> whether the small scale or experimental changes are achieving the desired result. Also, continuously check nominated key activities (regardless of any experimentation going on) to ensure that you know what the quality of the output is at all times to identify any new problems when they crop up.

<u>Act</u> to implement changes on a larger scale if the experiment is successful. This means making the changes a routine part of your activity. Also act to involve other persons (other departments, suppliers, or customers) affected by the changes and whose cooperation you need to implement them on a larger scale, or those who may simply benefit from what you have learned (you may, of course, already have involved these people in the Do or trial stage).

Outcome management systems

Outcome management systems gather data that allow the professional to evaluate the efficacy of an entire process in a timely manner, so that improvements can be made. The data may be compiled in such a way that it is accessible to a number of organizational stakeholders, such as patients, taxpayers, accrediting bodies, or the media. Statistical sampling may be used to evaluate the treatment of large numbers of patients, and results are compared with previous findings or benchmarks of other model organizations.

Revenue-generating services

For revenue-generating services to be effective, others must know about them. This requires internal and external marketing and advertising. Some advertising methods that may be effective include: print media, such as posters, banners, fliers, and signs, in and outside of the organization; promotions, to include taste-tests, open houses, raffles/drawings/contests, discounts; fairs targeting the appropriate audiences; radio and television commercials; web-based advertising. The most effective marketing of any service is done through word-of-mouth, as it is based upon recommendations from previous customers. Offer customers future discounts for referrals. Ask for letters of reference from satisfied customers and add these to the marketing portfolio.

Additionally, if revenue will be used towards new programming and/or philanthropic goals, be sure to mention this in advertising. Customers often prefer giving business to a worthy cause versus someone's pockets.

Important terms

Balance Sheet: A statement of a business or institution that lists the assets, debts, and owners' investment as of a specified date.

Base Annual Salary: The base salary before the addition of overtime pay or of any temporary or "emergency" increases approved for a limited period or purpose, or any extra service compensation or additional stipend or pay for other services.

Check Sheet: A data recording tool designed by the user to facilitate the interpretation of results.

Compensation: Remuneration for services rendered or for damages incurred. Includes pay, incentives, and benefits provided to employees.

Cost of Good Sold: On an income statement, the cost of purchasing raw materials and manufacturing finished products. Equal to the beginning inventory plus the cost of goods purchased during some period minus the ending inventory.

Cost: An amount paid or required in payment for a purchase; a price.

Defined Benefit Plan: A retirement program under which the retirement benefit to be paid is some percentage of final salary rather than simply the return on investment of the retirement fund.

Defined Contribution Plan: A retirement program under which an employee contributes a percentage of salary and the return on investment determines the retirement benefit.

Delphi Estimating: The Delphi estimating technique uses a group of subject matter experts who develop estimates independently, discuss differences and assumptions, and go through one or more revision cycles, until a single estimate is agreed upon.

Delphi Technique: Form or participative expert judgment; an iterative, anonymous, interactive technique using survey methods to derive consensus on work estimates, approaches, and issues.

Democratic Management Style: Participative management approach in which the manager and team make decisions jointly.

Depreciation: An allowance made for a loss in value of property. The main types of depreciation are declining balance, straight line, and sum of the year's digits.

EEO: Equal Employment Opportunity.

EEOC: Equal Employment Opportunity Commission.

Employee: Person working for another person or an organization for compensation. In certain circumstances, it is difficult to determine whether a person is an employee or an independent contractor.

EPPA: Employee Polygraph Protection Act.

Expense: An expenditure of money; a cost.

Flexible Compensation/Benefit System: One in which each employee has a choice in the form of all or a portion of his/her compensation package.

Flextime: Allows employees to follow different schedules of work each day of the workweek.

FLSA: The US Fair Labor Standards Act (FLSA) governs the payment of overtime compensation. The FLSA states that any employee (non-exempt) who works more than a 40-hour week must be paid

150% of their regular hourly rate for the overtime hours. (Employees whose compensation is exempted from this law are referred to as exempt employees.)

FMLA: The Family and Medical Leave Act (FMLA) states that covered employers must grant an eligible employee up to a total of 12 work weeks of unpaid leave during any 12-month period for one or more of the covered reasons.

Full-Time Equivalent Employee (FTE): An accounting term used to equate an employee or the total number of employees to a full-time equivalent. For example, a part-time employee who works one-half of the time required of a full-time employee would be counted as 1/2 FTE. (The total number of employees, headcount, will always be more than the total FTE if there are part-time employees in the workforce.)

Function: Work than can be distinguished from other work. The kind of action or activity proper to a person, employee, organizational unit, or institution. The primary purpose of a position within an organization.

Hierarchical Management: Traditional functional, or line, management in which areas and sub areas of expertise are created and staffed with human resources. Organizations so established are ongoing in nature.

High-Performance Work Teams: Group of people who work together in an interdependent manner such that their collective performance exceeds that which would be achieved by simply adding together their individual contributions. Characteristics of such a team include strong group identify, collaboration, anticipating and acting on other team members needs, and a laser-like focus on project objectives.

HIPAA: Health Insurance Portability and Accountability Act.

Histogram: A graph of contiguous vertical bars representing a frequency distribution in which the groups of items are marked on the x-axis and the number of items in each class is indicated on the y-axis. The pictorial nature allows people to see patterns that are difficult to see in a table of numbers.

I-9 Form (Federal): Required of all appointees to verify their US citizenship, or, if they are aliens, their eligibility for employment in accordance with the Immigration and Naturalization Act of 1986.

Income Statement: A financial statement that gives operating results for a specific period.

Income: The amount of money or its equivalent received during a period of time in exchange for labor or services, from the sale of goods or property, or as profit from financial investments.

Invoice: (1) Written account or itemized statement addressed to the purchaser of merchandise shipped or services performed with the quality, prices, and charges listed. (2) Contractor's bill or written request for payment for work or services performed under the contract.

Job Specification: The minimum skills, education, and experience necessary for an individual to perform a job.

KISS Model: A pragmatic philosophy of conducting business in which the objective is to keep things, such as procedures, reports, and any other aspect of work, as simple as possible to get the job done. They acronym humorously describes the basic premise of simplicity, which is "keep it simple, stupid."

Liability: A financial obligation, debt, claim, or potential loss.

Objectives: Similar to goals, a good faith effort to meet numerical goals through modifications in employment procedures and practice. Goals and objectives are set after careful external and internal labor analysis.

Foodservice Systems

Menu Development

Menu types

No choice
No choice menus offer the client no opportunity to participate in the selection of meals. This type of menu is appropriate in situations where the client is unable to make a choice, for example, in a nursing home where the residents have dementia. The advantage of no choice menus for the foodservice manager is the increased ability to predict exactly what is needed for each ordering cycle. This type of menu is usually used in conjunction with a cycle planning system, so that the same menu is repeated every month, bimonthly, or seasonally, allowing forecasting to extend farther into the future.

Limited choice
Limited choice menus offer two or three selections for each item; for example, green beans or broccoli as a vegetable. These menus may be static or on a cyclic rotation.

Choice
Choice menus offer a wide variety of selections for each item, which is more likely to meet the food habits and preferences of the client. Static menus with many choices are most common in restaurant settings.

Foodservice operations are constrained by budget in the menu-planning process. Meats, poultry, and fish drive up the menu cost. Reliance on convenience products may lower the need for staff, but also drives food costs up. Complex menus may require the need for the purchase of special equipment or serving ware.

Government regulations provide detailed specifications for the kinds of foods that are served in some settings, such as schools and nursing homes. The USDA provides information and training to foodservice managers on school menu development. The truth-in-menu law protects consumers by requiring that the menu not provide misleading information on nutritional content, serving size, or methods of preparation.

Factors external to the foodservice setting can also influence the menu. Facilities in southern locations may be better able to afford to include fresh produce on their menus in winter. A facility in a small farming community may include more items procured from the local meatpacking plant.

Factors to consider include
Type of menu, Type of facility, Clientele, Nutritional requirements, Income, Age, Region, Production Balance, Layout of Kitchen, Equipment, Personnel, Aesthetics, Taste, Color, Texture, Odor, and Temperature.

Menu Development Evaluation factors
Meets clients nutritional needs
Foods available, within budget

Can be prepared - equipment, personnel
Aesthetics
Repetition
Overall

Assessing the needs of the clientele is the first step to developing a well-conceived menu. Meeting nutritional needs must be balanced with meeting personal preferences. In some settings, such as schools, the nutritional needs will be prespecified. The cultural background of clientele should be considered; facilities that serve a population with a diverse ethnicity would not be well served by a no choice menu. Age is another consideration; children tend to like simple foods they can identify. The menu has a large influence on the facility design. More complex menus require more space and more workstations. Larger menus also demand more dishwashing space to clean the various dishes and utensils that will be used. No choice menus may need fewer but larger pieces of cooking equipment; large choice menus need many types of equipment.
Complex menus usually require more staff, and sometimes require staff with a higher level of training, for example, in the case of a pastry chef.

Menu mix   *high = 70% (+)*   *specific item / all items*

The menu mix is a formula that reveals how popular a menu item is by dividing the number sold of a specific item by the number of all menu items sold. A high menu mix item will contribute to 70% or more of total sales. Low volume sales may result in food waste, and may indicate the need for a menu revision or a more focused menu. The contribution margin reflects the profitability of the menu item. This is calculated by simply subtracting the item's base cost from the price the customer pays. If the item is below the average contribution margin for the entire menu, it is categorized as having a low contribution margin. Good menu engineering involves a balance between profitability and popularity. For example, if an item such as prime rib has a high contribution margin but low sales, the manager may want to remove that item or offer it as an occasional special to avoid costly waste.

contribution = customer cost - item base cost

Customer satisfaction
Utilizing customer satisfaction surveys can help the foodservice manager get customer feedback on new and existing menu items, uncover the reasons behind a customer's disappointing experience, or pinpoint product-related problems. Survey questions can be open-ended, scaled, or scored. The type of survey depends of the nature of the client or customer and what kind of information the manager wishes to gather. Gathering information about the frequency of acceptance is important for managers serving a no choice or short-cycle menu. This refers to how frequently the customer or client would be willing to eat an item. Plate waste refers to the amount of food left on a plate, and has some value in determining whether a menu item was well received. However, if serving sizes are too large, or if the foodservice is in a health care setting where other factors affect appetite, plate waste may not correlate to whether the individual liked the item.

 # item served / total # in category

Popularity index
While the menu mix is used to calculate the actual popularity of a menu item, the popularity index is used as a predictive tool to calculate how much of an item one can expect to sell, and how popular that item is in comparison to other menu items. The formula divides the number of servings of an item by the total number of servings of all items in that category in one day. So, if 10 pieces of cake were served and 100 desserts were served in a day, the popularity index of the cake would be 10%. If one expected to serve 500 customers the next day, 10% of 500 expected servings of cake would be 50 pieces of cake.

menu mix = actual popularity
index = predictive

Benchmarking

Benchmarking evaluates the best practices of the top facility in the foodservice category of interest, and uses those practices or processes as a model for menu planning. If customers have a high level of satisfaction with the menu at Hospital A, the manager at Hospital B may emulate Hospital A's menu engineering strategy.

Menu marketing

A menu is more than just a list of food and beverage items a facility has to offer; a menu can increase sales, educate the client, and showcase special items. Using graphics is an effective way to draw attention to items with high profitability. Graphics and photographs also appeal to children, and can be used to steer children towards healthy choices. The use of symbols can help health-conscious customers identify foods that are low in fat or sodium. Special menu inserts draw the customers' attention to featured menu items and can keep the menu fresh when changed frequently. Menu boards are helpful when specials or other menu items change frequently. Menu boards may be placed outside of a restaurant to draw street traffic.

Institutional meal planning

Cultural and religious considerations

Followers of the Muslim faith adhere to the Halal diet. Pork and all pork products such as bacon, ham, and lard are forbidden. Alcohol is also forbidden. Muslims practice fasting from dawn until dusk during the month of Ramadan, but exceptions are made for sick or pregnant individuals.

Practitioners of the Mormon faith avoid all caffeinated and alcoholic beverages. Mormons also advocate for the limited consumption of meat, although this practice receives less emphasis than the beverage practices.

A traditional belief in the Hispanic population is that meals must be balanced between "hot" and "cold," and eating an unbalanced meal can cause illness. Hispanics enjoy fresh produce, and tend to avoid milk.

Kosher meals refer to those that have been prepared or processed according to strict Jewish laws, and offering foods that are certified Kosher can ensure that these rules have been met. Kosher meals cannot include pork products or shellfish.

Vegetarian diets

Most individuals practicing vegetarianism avoid beef, pork, and chicken, but may include fish, eggs, and/or dairy products to varying degrees. Lacto-vegetarians avoid meat, fish, and eggs but do consume dairy products. Lacto-ovo vegetarians include both dairy products and eggs in their diets. Vegans exclude all foods with animal origins from their diet, including byproducts such as gelatin.

Vegetarian diets tend to be low in iron, although absorption of the non-heme iron present in fortified cereals and vegetables can be facilitated by the vitamin C common in these diets. Vegans are at risk for developing megaloblastic anemia due to the complete lack of vitamin B_{12} in the diet, which is only found in animal sources. Vegans should be counseled about vitamin B_{12} supplementation.

lacto-: dairy
ovo-: egg
vegan-: all animal origins

* iron & B12

[iron + vit C]

Although most vegetarians receive adequate protein in the diet, they should importance of combining complementary proteins to ensure that the essent provided, for example, combining legumes and grains.

Recipe development

Standardized recipes
- <u>Name of Recipe</u> – in addition, the section in the file, card number, and the class... the meal pattern contributions should be included.
- Ingredients – listed in the form of the food used, such as fresh apples or canned cherries, and the order in which they are used in the recipe.
- <u>Weight and Measures</u> – the quantity of each ingredient is given both in weights and volume measures in most recipes. Weighing ingredients is faster, easier, and more accurate.
- <u>Directions</u> – procedures to follow in preparing the recipe, including simple directions for mixing, number and size of pans, cooking temperature and time, and the directions for serving.
- <u>Servings</u> – total yield is given in number of servings or in total volume. Example: 500-1/2 cup servings.
- <u>Cost per serving</u> (optional) – to stay with in the food budget, costing of recipes should be done on a routine basis.

Benefits: Standardized recipes offer many advantages for food service.
- <u>Ensure Product Quality</u> - Provide consistent high-quality food items that have been thoroughly tested and evaluated. If your customers know you always serve good food, your participation may increase.
- <u>Know Projected Portions and Yield</u> - Accurately predict the number of portions from each recipe and clearly define serving size or scoop. This will help to eliminate excessive amounts of leftovers or substitutions because too little was prepared.
- <u>Improve Cost Control</u> - Provide better management of purchasing and storage because standardized recipes specify exact amount of ingredients.
- <u>Support Creativity</u> - Using standardized recipes supports creativity in cooking. Employees should be encouraged to continuously improve recipes. All changes need to be recorded so they can be repeated the next time the recipe is used. As part of recipe development, a recipe should be prepared in smaller quantities for taste-testing, and then tested again in larger quantities to standardize results.

$$[DV = DRV + RDI]$$

Nutritional recommendations
- Daily Values (DVs): a new dietary reference term that will appear on the food label. It is made up of two sets of references, daily reference values (DRVs) and reference daily intakes (RDIs).
- DRVs: a set of dietary references that applies to fat, saturated fat, cholesterol, carbohydrate, protein, fiber, sodium, and potassium.
- RDIs: a set of dietary references based on the Recommended Dietary Allowances for essential vitamins and minerals and, in selected groups, protein. The name "RDI" replaces the term "US RDA." *97 - 98% heathy ppl*
- Recommended Dietary Allowances (RDA): a set of estimated nutrient allowances established by the National Academy of Sciences. It is updated periodically to reflect current scientific knowledge.

AI = no RDA, 50% healthy ppl

- 179 -

control

- Passive Control: Use serving utensil (e.g., glass, bowl, pan).
- Active Control: Need Standardize Recipe, Commitment by Management, and Proper Tools.
- Measuring Weight: Scales (several types).
- Measuring Volume:
  - Scoops to measure "mushy stuff." Number on the scoop = # servings per quart (32 oz) (e.g., #8 scoop = 32 oz / 8 = 4 oz).
  - Ladles - measure liquids.
  - Spoons - portion cheap foods.
- Volume Dispensers: Liquid and semi-liquid foods (e.g., ketchup, soda dispensers).
- Count: Pie, cake, cuts in a pan.

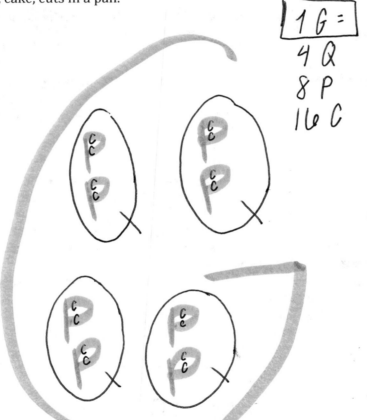

$$1\,G = \\ 4\,Q \\ 8\,P \\ 16\,C$$

$$Scoop = \frac{32\,oz\,(1\,G)}{\#Scoop} = \frac{32}{\#4} = 8\,oz = 1\,C$$

$$\frac{32}{\#16} = 2\,oz = \tfrac{1}{4}\,C$$

Procurement, Production, Distribution, and Service

Ingredient control

Ordering
Getting the amount you want:
- Look at whole menu
- Standardize recipe
- Forecast of needs (count)
- Popularity index

Receiving
Check for quantity and quality. Did you get what you order?
- Put away
- Food safety issues considered
- Rotation of stock
- Track information

Storage
- Know the amount you have
  - Perpetual Inventory
  - Physical Inventory
- Know value of what you have. (Usually, most current price.)
- Know amount you need for smooth F.S.O.
  - Par levels
  - Forecast
  - Inventory Turnover
- Know value you can afford/want for F.S.O.
  - Tight control, less storage cost
  - Tight control might run out of food
  - Inventory value relative to Food Sales/Income

Purchasing

Centralized
Centralized purchasing is usually conducted in larger foodservice establishments that can afford to dedicate an employee or group of employees to make all purchasing decisions. This avoids duplication of effort, and therefore saves time and money. This also gives the vendors a consistent point-of-contact within the organization, which facilitates communication.

Group
Group purchasing involves the cooperation of several discrete but related organizations in the purchasing process. An example would be a group of restaurants under the same umbrella of ownership. The group purchasing power can result in lower prices because of the advantage of volume buying.

Just-in-time

Just-in-time purchasing describes the procurement of items as needed to meet immediate production needs. The items are not stored, but are used as they are received. This type of purchasing may be used for items that are too delicate for storage, or may be used when storage space is very limited.

Methods of purchasing

Informal

Used in small operations when time is a factor; suppliers limited; market stability uncertain.

Formal

Tax-supported institutions, results in a contract between buyer and seller.
Fixed – large quantities; over long period.
- Daily – perishable products; good for few days.

Bids

Line-item bidding

Each bidder bids on each product on the list and who meets the specification at the lowest price is awarded the bid. This method is time consuming and the cost effectiveness is unclear.

All or nothing bidding:

"Bottom line"– Bidder must use best price on complete list (e.g., dairy bids). All bids must be clear about when due, include all appropriate specifications, and duration of the bid. Request contact name and telephone. Be aware of legal considerations.

Types of contracts

Cost-Plus-Award Fee (CPAF) contract

Cost-reimbursement contract that provides for a fee that consists of (1) a base fee (which may be zero) fixed at inception of the contract and (2) an award fee based on periodic judgmental evaluation by the procuring authority. Used to provide motivation for performance in areas such as quality, timeliness, technical ingenuity, and cost-effective management during the contract. In cost-type contracts, the performance risk is borne mostly by the buyer, not the seller.

Cost-Plus-Fixed Fee (CPFF) contract

Type of contract in which the buyer reimburses the contractor for the contractor's allowable costs (as defined by the contract) plus a fixed amount of profit (fee). The fixed fee does not vary with actual cost but may be adjusted if changes occur in the work to be performed under the contract. In cost-type contracts, the performance risk is borne mostly by the buyer, not the seller.

Cost-Plus-Incentive Fee (CPIF) contract

Type of contract in which the buyer reimburses the contractor for the contractor's allowable costs (as defined by the contract) and the seller earns its fee (profit) if it meets defined performance or cost criteria. Specifies a target cost, target fee, minimum fee, maximum fee, and fee adjustment formula.

Cost-Plus-Percentage of Cost (CPPC) Contract

Type of contract that provides reimbursement of allowable cost of services performed plus an agreed-upon percentage of the estimated cost as profits. In cost-type contracts, the performance risk is borne mostly by the buyer, not the seller.

Purchasing records

- Requisition – products needed.
- Purchase order – products ordered – Number of copies varies with size of operation.
- Invoice – products received – Compare to purchase order immediately:
    - Check product description.
    - Check product amounts.
    - Check product prices – Beware of substitutions, outages, and errors.

Procurement

Product specifications

Written specifications are used by foodservice managers to clearly specify the features of the product they wish to procure. The more detailed the manager can be in his requirements of the item, the more the product will meet the needs of the establishment. Specifications are written in measurable terms, avoiding such loosely defined quality measures like "high quality" or "low quality." Specifications help the manager procure the right product for its intended use; for example, a manager might buy grade B eggs for use in baking and grade A eggs for use as a breakfast item. A written specification for an item might be as long as several pages. For example, in the case of apples, quantity, variety, grade, size, and packaging method should be specified. If brand name products are desired, that should be in the spec, but managers should not pay more for a brand name if a generic product will do, unless the brand is specified on the menu, in which case truth-in-menu law applies.

Edible portion

When a foodservice manager or purchasing agent makes procurement decisions, the amount of food that can actually be consumed must be calculated. Meats and poultry contain bones and fat; produce contains stems, seeds, and peels. The edible portion may be included in the written specifications and/or should be information the vendor is able to share about the product. Most vendors can provide the edible portion information for all of their products in a chart form to help buyers make decisions about how much to buy. For example, a chart may list that the edible portion of the oranges they provide is 70%, which makes the net edible portion 135 grams per unit of sale. The amount that should be purchased is calculated by dividing the edible portion by the percent yielded per pound. Determining the edible portion is also important in figuring out how much money each portion size will cost the facility.

edible portion / % yield per lb

Shrinkage

Foods that are cooked lose volume in the preparation process, and the purchasing agent or foodservice manager must account for these losses when determining how much product to purchase in order to meet the needs of the establishment. If a foodservice kitchen uses products that have already been trimmed, such as pre-cut steaks, the shrinkage will be less but the savings might be lost by paying a premium for the convenience built into a pre-cut meat product. The actual cost per pound of finished product needs to be determined in order to calculate precise food costs. Multiplying the percentage of shrinkage by the raw weight reveals how many pounds are lost in preparation.

Raw weight x % shrinkage

Economic order quantity

The economic order quantity model uses a calculation that helps the purchasing agent decide between frequent ordering, which has the advantage of maintaining smaller inventories, and infrequent ordering, which lowers the fixed costs associated with ordering such as paperwork. The formula reveals the best quantity that will keep both inventory and ordering costs down.

Receiving

The receiving dock of a foodservice operation must be designed so that large delivery trucks can access the area, and so that large boxes and heavy crates can be moved easily to production or storage areas. Although the receiving task may be assigned to whoever is available at the time, a close inspection of the goods is important to ensure that the quality and quantity of goods matches the purchase order. An invoice will accompany the order and will list the weight or size of the items and the cost of each item. A scale is helpful to allow the receiving clerk to verify the weights of foods purchased by the pound.

Quality inspection should ensure that foods are delivered at their proper holding temperatures, and frozen foods that have been allowed to thaw should be rejected. A policy should be in place to allow for brand or item substitutions on out of stock items.

The following elements are key to a well-functioning receiving department:
- Competent and trained personnel.
- Facilities and equipment– space, size, and location– Equipment – large and small.
- Specifications.
- Critical Control Point in Receiving.
- Sanitation – delivery truck and receiving area.
- Adequate supervision – by management.
- Scheduled hours – buyer's schedule.
- Security – loss and theft prevention; tampering.

Purchasing records

Requisition – products needed
Purchase order – products ordered – Number of copies varies with size of operation
Invoice – products received – Compare to purchase order immediately
Check product description
Check product amounts
Check product prices – Beware of substitutions, outages, and errors.

Inventory Control Tools
ABC Method – resources for inventory control allocated based on value; time management
A – 15% to 20% of inventory; 75% to 80% value
B – 20% to 25% of inventory; 10% to 15% value
C – 60% to 65% of inventory; 5% to 10% value
Minimum-Maximum Method
Safety stock – the backup supply – Lead time – requisition and receipt – Usage rate

Inventory valuation

Inventory Valuation
Actual purchase price – each item $
Weighted average
FIFO – "first in, first out" – current cost
LIFO – "last in, first out" – minimized inventory value
Latest purchase price – simple, fast

Inventory systems

Perpetual
Perpetual inventory means that the actual amount of stock in the facility is recorded each time an item is removed for production or added from the receiving dock. This method is desirable when dealing with an item for which scarcity is a problem. Maintaining a perpetual inventory is labor-intensive but it may be helpful to use temporarily to uncover theft or other unexplained losses of stock.

Physical
Physical inventory involves counting each item in stock at the end of each accounting cycle or other designated time period. The inventory must be conducted at a time that falls between delivery cycles, and during a time that does not interrupt the production process.

Fixed order quantity
Fixed order quantity inventory systems provide the manager with a formula that determines when a product should be ordered based on daily usage, delivery lead time, and the minimum amount of stock always kept on hand.

Inventory management tools

Par stock method
The par stock method ensures that a minimum amount of an item is kept on hand at all times. Each time an order is placed, the items are replenished to bring the stock up to the specified level. For example, if a foodservice manager keeps a par of eight dozen eggs, and the stock levels are down to five dozen, then three dozen will be ordered.

FIFO
FIFO is an acronym for "first in, first out." This is a way of arranging inventory so that the products that were purchased first will be used first in the production process. FIFO reduces the chances that food will be discarded because of spoilage that occurred when an item was pushed repeatedly to the back of the shelf.

Mini-maxi stock method
The mini-maxi stock method means that a minimum and maximum level of product will be kept on inventory. Ordering takes place when the minimum amount of product is reached, and the amount of product ordered will bring the stock back to the maximum level.

Determining value of inventory

Actual purchase price
Purchase price inventory value calculating is the straightforward method of counting all the products in the inventory and adding their actual price.

Weighted average
Weighted average purchase price calculates the average price paid for all items in inventory over the time of the accounting period.

FIFO
The FIFO, or first-in, first–out, method of inventory accounting means that the first products that were brought into the stockroom will be the first ones that will be used in production. For example, on January 20, 10 cases of peaches were purchased for $20 a case, and on January 27, 10 cases of peaches were purchased for $22 a case. At the end of January, 10 cases of peaches remained. Assuming FIFO, the $20 cases were used, so the inventory value of the remaining peaches is $220.

LIFO
LIFO, or last-in, first-out, assumes that the most recently purchased product will be used first, so inventory is calculated accordingly.

Economic order quantity formula
The total cost of inventories is the summation of these rising and declining costs, or the total costs curve. It has been shown that, under reasonable assumptions, the minimum point on the total costs curve can be found by an equation called the EOQ formula:
$$EOQ = \sqrt{2FS/CP}$$
*Where: EOQ is the economic ordering quantity, or the optimum quantity to be ordered each time an order is placed.
F = fixed costs of placing and receiving an order
S = sales or usage in units/yr
C = carrying cost expressed as a percentage of inventory value
P = purchase price per unit of inventory

Managing food production

Foodservice managers may design a spreadsheet to create a daily work production schedule so that each employee knows exactly what his or her duties will be for the shift. Food preparation, cleaning, and equipment checks may be initialed by the responsible employee upon completion to ensure all tasks are carried out. Gantt progress charts are used to ensure that the production is completed in a timely manner.

Standardized recipes are used by many foodservice operations to ensure consistency in the product, improve forecasting, and reduce inventory waste. Measurements and preparation methods are specified, and the number of servings is known in advance. Quantity control is also achieved through the use of numbered scoops or other standardized serving tools. The server should use the tool specified in the recipe. As scoop size increases, the serving size amount decreases. For example, a #6 scoop yields a 5 ounce serving, and a #30 scoop yields a 1 ounce serving.

Measuring quality objectively

A penetrometer is a tool that measures the firmness or tenderness of select food products. The device can be used on fruits to check for ripeness, or on custards to check the firmness of the gel structure. The value is then compared to a chart that suggests desirable levels of firmness or tenderness for the product.

A viscosimeter measures the thickness of a liquid or semi-soft product, such as batter or peanut butter. It is used more in food manufacturing than in kitchens.

Specific gravity examines how much air has been incorporated into a batter or foam, which indicates the volume of the product. This measurement can be assessed without the use of special tools. The weight of the batter or foam is divided by an equal amount of water to determine the specific gravity. The foodservice manager may observe how much mixing was required to reach the desired specific gravity, and incorporate this into a standardized recipe.

Measuring quality subjectively

A triangle test is used to compare subtle differences between similar products. Three products are sampled, and two are identical. This is useful in evaluating a product that has been refined or improved.

Ranking or scaling compares a number of similar products, but does not specify the degree to which one product is preferred over another.

In hedonic rating, a number of products are sampled, and the volunteer must rate each one on a scale that varies from "strongly dislike" to "strongly like." The ratings are then assigned scores so that a researcher can conduct statistical analyses on the testing session.

Paired preference testing compares two products to determine which is preferred, but the method does not determine the degree of preference.

The flavor profile method depends on experts to analyze the attributes of interest in a product under evaluation. The attributes of the product can be broken down into specific categories, so that a product is not just categorized as "spicy," but that hints of allspice and cumin are present.

Hedonic scale method: This rating scale method measures the level of the liking of foods, or any other product where an affective tone is necessary. This test relies on a person's ability to communicate his or her feelings of like or dislike. Hedonic testing is popular because it may be used with untrained people as well as with experienced panel members. A minimum amount of verbal ability is necessary for reliable results.

In Hedonic testing, samples are presented in succession and the subject is told to decide how much he likes or dislikes the product and to mark the scales accordingly. The nature of this test is its relative simplicity. The instructions to the panelist are restricted to procedures, and no attempt is made at direct response. The subject is allowed, however, to make his own inferences about the meaning of the scale categories and determine for himself how he will apply them to the samples. A separate scale is provided for each sample in a test session.

Descriptive flavor analysis panel: DFAP helps identify and quantify specific flavor attributes. It is comprised of a panel of experts.

Food production stages

Production stage:
The production stage includes making plans for a production line to manufacture the product. Do not arrange a full-scale production line until after successfully test marketing a new product. Many entrepreneurs will have their products co-packed by an existing plant for test marketing. The production line should be set up according to a blueprint of its layout. Keep in mind drainage, ventilation, waste disposal, lighting, equipment size and flow, energy conservation, safety, sanitation, ease of cleaning, storage area, and compliance with government regulations.

Packaging stage:
This stage is especially important because the package often sells a new product. Consumers want colorful, attractive, conveniently packaged forms. Packaging should not impart flavor to the product or react chemically with the food. It should be lightweight, economical, and resistant to tearing.

Shelf-life stage
The shelf-life stage is extremely important because a processor must know how long a new product will keep under a variety of temperatures and other environmental conditions. Shelf-life loss may be due to chemical or microbial (bacteria, mold, and yeast) spoilage. Small firms normally have to contract with independent or consulting laboratories to have accelerated shelf-life studies performed on new products. The studies are done by raising the temperature of the packaged product above normal storage conditions (110° to 120°F). Although this is not as good as a prolonged shelf-life study at normal temperatures (75° to 80°F), it does give some indication of product shelf life. Lot codes for recall and product liability are based on these studies.

Food labels

Food labeling was originally designed by the government to protect consumers from fraud. Recent surveys indicate that consumers use labels to identify and avoid perceived health hazards rather than to seek and obtain benefits (does the product contain preservatives, fats, cholesterol?). A label consists of the "principal display panel," used to attract consumers, and the "information panel," placed immediately to the right of the principal display panel.

Information that is mandatory on food labels includes:
- Statement of identity/product name, Net weight (in ounces and grams), Name/address of manufacturer.
- Ingredient listing, Manufacturing code.
- Nutritional labeling (some exemptions apply).

Information that is voluntary but if included must be worded according to regulations includes:
- Grades.
- Labeling for special dietary use.

Optional information includes:
- Universal product code.
- Open dating.
- Registered trademarks/symbols.

Foodservice systems

Some major foodservice systems are: Conventional, Cook/chill, Cook/freeze, Commissary, and Assembly-serve.

Conventional food service system

Conventional foodservice systems prepare all foods on the premises. This is expensive, both because of the skilled labor needed, and also because of the investment in equipment that is required. It is also time-consuming; however, there are lulls in production that occur between mealtimes in which staff is not being utilized efficiently. The increased food handling that occurs in the production process means that extra care must be taken to avoid unsanitary or unsafe food-handling practices that could increase the risk of introducing food borne illness to the client.

Advantages include the high degree of control in the production process, which may translate into increased quality. However, quality may vary because of inconsistencies in the skill of the staff. There is flexibility in the way food can be prepared, so individual differences can be accommodated. The food is not transported across large distances, so holding times are minimized and freshness is emphasized.

Cook-chill and cook-freeze systems

Ready prepared production systems include the cook-chill and cook-freeze methods, which involve preparing the foods on the premises and then refrigerating or freezing them for service at a later time.

This system is flexible in that foods can be prepared any time, allowing for third-shift employees to take part in the preparation of foods that will be served during the day. Another advantage is the preparation of foods in bulk, so that if chicken noodle soup is on the menu every Friday, the entire batch may be prepared at once and then heated and served as needed. Limitations include the types of food that remain palatable after freezing or chilling and reheating. A higher initial investment for large freezer lockers or cold storage units may or may not be offset by long-term savings in labor costs. Special care must be taken to cool bulk foods rapidly and reheat without allowing foods to be held at unsafe temperatures.

Assembly-serve systems

Assembly-serve systems are also referred to as total convenience systems, because the food preparation work is done outside of the foodservice operation. The facility needs only to reheat and portion the food for service. Because the foods purchased are fully prepared, the facility will pay a premium for the convenience and processing involved. High food costs will be offset by lower labor costs, as no skilled work is required to prepare foods from scratch. Initial investment in equipment is lower as well; the only equipment needed is that which will be used to store the food and reheat it. Disadvantages include the limited variety of prepared foods available for purchase. Foodservice managers may come to rely on select favorites, only to find the vendor has discontinued these products. Quality for prepared, processed foods is usually below that of foods prepared from scratch.

Commissary food service system

Satellite facilities receive transported food that may be:

- Chilled
- Frozen
- Hot bulk
- Individual portions

This type of food service system is often used in airlines, chain restaurants, large school districts, and vending.

Market Analysis

A market analysis can help foodservice facility planners determine the best ways to generate sales and profits from their new venture. One of the first steps in a market study is to determine where the facility will be located and what population it will serve.

Demographic data in the community can identify target market segments; people with large disposable incomes spend more on dining out. Market strategies match the strengths of the facility to the needs of the target population. Facilities located in areas with high pedestrian traffic or automobile traffic benefit from their location. A competitive analysis can identify competing facilities in the area to determine if the niche is overpopulated.

Conservative marketing objectives may include the projected sales for the facility, which factors in projected customer counts and estimated average check. Deciding on the best product mix requires the consideration of trends, customer desires, and efficient use of labor and inventory.

Food purchase

Managers of small foodservice operations may find it more efficient or economical to use an open market style of procurement. This informal method of purchasing involves the buyer seeking quotes from several vendors on the products of interest. The purchasing decision will usually be made based on the vendor who can provide the product at the lowest price, but vendors who provide extra customer service measures such as specialized delivery schedules may win the business of the facility.

Informal purchasing methods may also be used by large-scale operations that need a special product their normal vendor is unable to provide.

Competitive bid buying is the procurement norm for large-scale foodservice institutions such as hospitals or school systems. The purchasing agent must provide accurate specifications on all of the products needed. The institution makes a public announcement through standard channels to invite all potential vendors to submit their best price, or bid. The bids are opened at the same time, and the vendor with the lowest price gets the contract.

Forecasting models

The causal model of forecasting works by analyzing the reasons that individual products sell or do not sell. For example, variables such as the cost of a menu item are to used determine how much of the item will be sold in the future. The model is complicated, and includes methods such as regression analysis, which reveal the pattern of association between variables. Inexperienced managers may not be able to discern which variables are causal and which are extraneous.

The subjective model of forecasting relies heavily on the expertise of the foodservice manager, and may be articulated as a form of making an "educated guess." This model may be necessary when insufficient data exist that would make other statistical analyses based on past observations impossible, for example, in the first year of an operation.

ABC inventory

The ABC inventory system is a method of ranking the products according to what percentage of the purchasing dollar they compose. The items in the "A" category are the most expensive items, such as meats, fish, poultry, and dairy products, which account for 70% to 80% of the food budget. The items in the "B" category account for 15% to 20% of the food budget, and the "C" category accounts for the remaining percentage. The items in the "A" class have the greatest value and may be subject to more accurate forecasting calculations or more intensive checks at the receiving dock in an effort to control costs.

A limitation of the ABC inventory system is that the value of an item is based on its cost, and not the frequency of use on the production line. If flour is categorized as a "C" but the foodservice does a great deal of in-house baking, the manager should consider this when taking inventory.

Commissary production system

Commissary production systems use a centralized kitchen to prepare all menu items, which are then either transported hot to the place of service or chilled and transported to the point of service, where reheating takes place. School systems and airlines commonly use commissary systems. This mode of production can be economical for several reasons. The large volume of food purchased in order to serve all the satellite kitchens mean savings from bulk purchases will be realized. Foods are usually prepared from scratch, so expensive processed and pre-prepared foods are not necessary. Controls over ingredients and inventory are organized and tend to be superior in commissary systems.

Ingredient rooms where staff pre-measure foods for standardized recipes reduce waste. Expensive pieces of equipment need only be purchased for one facility, and that facility may be located in a part of town where real estate is cheaper.

Disadvantages include the cost of transporting the foods by special truck or van, and the need for a large skilled labor force.

Cooking principles

Heat transfer methods

Conduction: Conduction heating methods occurs when fast-moving molecules transfer their kinetic energy to adjacent slow-moving molecules as the particles collide. If one uses a cooking vessel with a high thermal conductivity, then the heat will be transferred quickly from the burner to the product. Copper, aluminum, and cast iron cookware heat up rapidly, and allow the cook to sear foods to seal in juices. Glass and stainless steel conduct heat poorly, so may be appropriate in slow cooking applications.

Convection: Convection occurs when a mass of heated molecules transfer their heat to adjacent molecules, as opposed to one particle at a time in conduction. This occurs in convection ovens, as currents of hot air are moved by a fan to cool regions, the cool air is displaced and sinks to the bottom, where it is heated and pushed to the top again. The even heat in a convection oven results in faster cooking and the elimination of hot and cold spots in the oven.

Induction: Whereas conduction and convection cooking methods transfer heat to a cooking vessel, which then transfers heat to the food, cooking by induction makes the cooking vessel the original source of heat. The cooking appliance uses electromagnetic technology to transfer energy to the cooking vessel. The cooking appliance, such as a range top, stays cool, but the energy that has been transferred to the cooking vessel creates a current that is manifested as heat. Because of its reliance on magnetic technology, this mode of cooking requires all cooking vessels be made of a metal that is affected by magnetic fields. Iron cookware can be used, but aluminum and glass cookware are unaffected by induction technology. This limitation makes it expensive to retrofit a kitchen with an induction appliance, as new cookware may need to be purchased. Advantages include cool cooktops, resulting in cooler production areas.

Radiation: Radiation cooking methods include those that transfer infrared waves from a heat source such as a grill or toaster, and microwave ovens. Microwaves generate radio waves that are readily absorbed by fats, sugars, and liquids. This in turn causes the molecules to vibrate, and the kinetic energy is manifested as heat. The waves have a limited ability to penetrate thick foods, which can result in uneven heating. When the microwave oven is turned off, residual heating occurs through conduction as the heat is transferred through the product. The cooking time is usually too brief to achieve the browning that gives foods desirable taste, texture, and appearance. Microwaves have a limited utility in foodservice operations because of their limited capacity, but they may have some usefulness in small reheating applications.

Non-enzymatic browning   [Sugar + Protein]

Features of Maillard Reaction: Presence of reducing sugars and amino compounds (proteins, amino acids). It requires dry heat and high temp – baking, frying, toasting. This occurs rapidly at pH> 7, and slower at pH < 6.

Color: colorless yellow brown dark brown.

Advantages: contributors to flavors in soy sauce, bread crusts, milk chocolates, caramels, fudges, toffees (reducing sugars react with milk proteins), broiled and fried meat.

Disadvantages: loss of essential amino acids (i.e., lysine), formation of mutagenic heterocyclic amines during cooking of protein-rich foods.

Caramelization: Sucrose and reducing sugars heated with and without NH4 salts. It is used to make caramel color for soft drinks, beer, baked goods, syrups, and candies.

Food preservation

Canning process

The canning process involves placing foods in jars and heating them to a temperature that destroys microorganisms that could be a health hazard or cause the food to spoil. Canning also inactivates enzymes that could cause the food to spoil. Air is driven from the jar during heating, and as it cools, a vacuum seal is formed. The vacuum seal prevents air from getting back into the product, bringing with it microorganisms to recontaminate the food. The *Clostridium botulinum* microorganism is the main reason why pressure canning is necessary. Though the bacterial cells are killed at boiling temperatures, they can form spores that can withstand these temperatures. The spores grow well in low-acid foods, in the absence of air, such as in canned low acid foods (vegetables and meats). When the spores begin to grow, they produce the deadly botulinum toxins (poisons). These spores can be destroyed by canning the food at a temperature of 240°F or above for the correct length of time. This temperature is above the boiling point of water so it can only be reached in a pressure canner.

Boiling water bath method: The boiling water bath method is safe for fruits, tomatoes, and pickles, as well as jam, jellies, and other preserves. In this method, jars of food are heated by being completely covered with boiling water (212°F at sea level). High-acid foods contain enough acid (pH of 4.6 or less) so that the *Clostridium botulinum* spores cannot grow and produce their deadly toxin. High-acid foods include fruits and properly pickled vegetables. These foods can be safely canned at boiling temperatures in a boiling water bath. Tomatoes and figs have pH values close to 4.6. To can these in a boiling water bath, acid in the form of lemon juice or citric acid must be added to them.

boiling water bath = low PH

Benefits: Canning relies on sterilization by heat and the exclusion of air to destroy the microorganisms that cause food spoilage. Commercial canning operations use pressure canning methods in order to bring the temperatures above the boiling point and reduce the amount of time the product has to be exposed to the heat. The acidity of the food being processed is one of the determining factors in deciding what canning method should be used. High-acid foods, such as pickles and rhubarb, do not foster the growth of heat-resistant bacteria. A boiling water bath may be suitable for foods with a low pH. Low-acid, high-pH foods are likely to encourage the growth of anaerobic, heat-resistant bacteria, and must be canned under pressure. Aseptic canning uses rapid heating and cooling to sterilize the product before it is placed into a sterile container. Canned goods lose quality over time, and foodservice operations should honor the "use-by date" and utilize FIFO to maintain quality.

pressure = high PH

high pH (alkaline) = > 4.6 pH

Pressure Canning Methods

Pressure canning is the only safe method of canning low-acid foods (those with a pH of more than 4.6). These include all vegetables, meats, poultry, and seafood. Because of the danger of botulism, these foods must be canned in a pressure canner. Jars of food are placed in 2 to 3 inches of water in a pressure canner and then heated to a temperature of at least 240°F. This temperature can only be reached in a pressure canner.

Freezing

Freezing provides a way to preserve food so that most of the flavor, texture, and nutrients are retained. Freezing is a way to preserve foods that cannot be preserved by other methods such as canning. It is important to note that the microorganisms that cause food spoilage are not destroyed in the freezing process; they are simply rendered inactive. Proper cooking procedures must be observed for frozen items to destroy any pathogens. Frozen food cannot be kept indefinitely, and foods lose quality at temperatures above 0°F. Packaging used for frozen foods should resist moisture in order to keep moisture in the product and prevent freezer burn.

Products that are quick frozen at or below -20°F will form smaller ice crystals, which results in a higher quality of texture. Frozen foods should be thawed under refrigeration or under running cold water; never on the counter.

Freezers:

Upright freezers

These appliances have the same general shape and appearance as home refrigerators. They have one or two outside doors and from three to seven shelves for storing food. Freezers of this type are popular because of their convenience, the small floor space they require, and the ease with which food may be put in or removed. However, more cold air escapes each time the door is opened.

Chest freezers

Freezers of this type require more floor area than the uprights but are more economical to buy and operate. These freezers lose less cold air each time they are opened. Make sure this type of freezer is equipped with sliding or lift-out baskets to permit easy loading and removal of food.

Refrigerator-freezer combination

This is a single appliance with one or two doors. It has one compartment for frozen foods and another for refrigerated foods. The freezing compartments may be above, below, or to one side of the refrigerated area. If selecting this type, be certain that the freezer is a true freezer (will maintain 0°F or less) and not just a freezing compartment.

Defrosting freezers

Manual-defrost freezers need defrosting at least once a year or when there is more than one-fourth inch of frost over a large area of the freezer. Defrosting should be scheduled when the food inventory is relatively low and defrosting can be completed within one to two hours. A manual-defrost model should be disconnected from the electrical supply before defrosting. Frozen packages should then be placed in large cardboard cartons or insulated ice chests. With a cardboard carton, several layers of newspapers may be used for extra insulation. Clean the freezer as quickly as possible, following your manufacturer's instructions. A few manufactures recommend placing pans of hot water in the freezer and closing it. Then, remove the frost as it loosens and replace the water as it cools. Make sure the freezer is completely cool before restarting it. Other manufactures do not recommend using pans of hot water because in their freezers, refrigerator pressure could build up in the evaporator, making restarting the freezer difficult. These manufactures recommend allowing the frost to thaw naturally or with the aid of a fan. Place towels in the bottom of the freezer to catch water and frost.

Food storage

Guidelines
- Store all potentially hazardous foods (e.g., eggs, milk or milk products, meat, poultry, fish) at 41°F or below. The Danger Zone is 41°F to 140°F.
- Check food temperature with a clean, calibrated food thermometer before serving.
- Potentially hazardous food(s) should not be kept at room temperature.
- Store raw meat and poultry products on the bottom shelf of the refrigerator.
- Keep food products away from cleaning products, medicine, and animal food.
- Do not put cooked food in the same container or on the same unwashed container, platter, or cutting board that was used for uncooked meat or poultry.
- Use a food thermometer to make sure you have achieved an internal temperature of 155°F. Cook raw hamburger thoroughly until juices run clear.

Beef/pork = 140°F   ground = 160°F   poultry = 165°F

<u>Types of Storage</u>
Dry storage – Facility
Floors and Walls
Windows/doors
Locks – key and who has them
Equipment
Shelving and pallets
Food - safe storage containers
Storeroom diagram – Label and date – Monitoring process
Low Temperature – refrigerators, tempering boxes and freezers
Monitoring equipment – thermometers, alarms
Energy conservation
Access/Accountability – Label and date products
Critical control point in storage

<u>Ingredient Control-Storage</u>
Know the amount you have.
Perpetual Inventory
Physical Inventory
Know value of what you have.
Usually, most current price
Know amount you need for smooth F.S.O.
Par levels
Forecast
Inventory Turnover
Know value you can afford/want for F.S.O.
Tight control, less storage cost
Tight control might run out of food
Inventory value relative to Food Sales/Income

<u>Food storage areas</u>

Dry storage:
Dry storage areas should be well ventilated, dry, and easy to clean. Easy access to production areas and refrigerated storage is important to allow personnel to work efficiently. Large doors allow deliveries on hand trucks to be made, but the area must be secured to prevent theft. Cleaning supplies must be kept in a separate area to avoid accidental contamination of food. The temperature of the area should be maintained between 50° and 70°F to ensure an adequate shelf life. Food should be elevated at least six inches from the floor and two feet from the ceiling to avoid high temperatures at ceiling level. Humidity should be maintained between 50% and 60%, and ventilation systems should be designed so that exhaust does not contaminate foods or production areas.

Frozen and refrigerated storage:
The size of the freezer needed will depend on how many menu items are prepared from frozen products and how frequently deliveries are made. Most frozen items are shipped in rectangular boxes, so the shelving and height of the freezer are important considerations. The freezer should be maintained at a temperature of zero to 10°F, and freezer temperatures should be monitored and recorded every shift. Refrigerated storage areas must be kept between 35° and 41°F, and temperatures should be monitored and recorded regularly. Proper food storage procedures should

be followed to avoid the possibility of contamination. For example, raw meats should be stored on the lower shelves, and foods should be covered. Food should be dated, and unlabeled foods should be thrown away.

Foodservice should follow standard storage times for foods or "use by dates" instead of relying on smell and appearance to determine the freshness of the product.

Types of storage
- Dry storage – Facility
- Floors and Walls
- Windows/doors
- Locks – key and who has them

Equipment
- Shelving and pallets
- Food - safe storage containers
- Monitoring process: would include a storeroom diagram and a process to label and date food
- Low Temperature: refrigerators, tempering boxes and freezers
- Monitoring equipment: thermometers, alarms
- Energy conservation

Dispersion systems

Food dispersions are the result of solids, liquids, or gases being suspended in various mediums, resulting in a product whose consistency can vary from a liquid, like gravy, to a solid, like angel food cake. The dispersed particles may be small, such as the sugar and water solution of simple syrup, or large, such as the cooked starch in gravies. Foams result when gas is suspended in liquid, such as meringues. Emulsions result from a liquid being dispersed in a liquid, such as the fat in whole milk. A sol is a solid dispersed in liquid, such as gravy. A gel is a liquid suspended in a solid, such as pudding. Dispersions can stabilize or break down in the presence of heat or mechanical manipulations. For example, the gas bubbles that contribute to the volume of a meringue are held in place when beating denatures the protein of the egg white and incorporates air bubbles. The application of heat stabilizes the foam by coagulating the egg protein.

Cause-and-Effect Diagram
A tool developed by Kaoru Ishikawa for analyzing process dispersion. It illustrates the main causes and subcauses leading to an effect or symptom. It is sometimes referred to as a fishbone chart because it resembles a fish skeleton.

Sanitation and Safety

National Sanitation Foundation

National Sanitation Foundation (NSF) International, The Public Health and Safety Company™, a not-for-profit, non-governmental organization, is the world leader in standards development, product certification, education, and risk-management for public health and safety. NSF develops national standards, provides learning opportunities through its Center for Public Health Education, and provides third-party conformity assessment services while representing the interests of all stakeholders. Its professional staff includes engineers, chemists, toxicologists, and environmental health professionals with broad experience both in public and private organizations. Organizations have voluntary participation and can receive a seal of approval.

Reasonable Certainty of No Harm

The Food Quality Protection Act (FQPA) requires that tolerances be "safe," defined as "a reasonable certainty that no harm will result from aggregate exposure," including all exposure through the diet and other non-occupational exposures, including drinking water, for which there is reliable information. It also distinguishes between cancer and non-cancer effects, consistent with Environmental Protection Agency (EPA) practice. The new law establishes a single, health-based standard for all pesticide residues in all types of food, replacing the sometimes conflicting standards in the old law (Delaney clause). There are no differences in the standards applicable to tolerances set for raw and processed foods.

Delaney clause

The Delaney clause is a law that prohibits the use of any food additives in processed foods that may cause cancer in humans. Before the Food Quality Protection Act (FQPA), pesticides had been considered food additives and been subjected to the Delaney clause. Although a well-intentioned law, there were significant problems of applying the Delaney clause to pesticide residues. If a pesticide that causes cancer in humans or laboratory animals concentrated in ready-to-eat processed food at a level greater than the tolerance for the raw agricultural commodity, then the Delaney clause prohibited the setting of a tolerance. This had paradoxical effects in terms of food safety, since alternative pesticides could pose higher (non-cancer) risks and the EPA allowed the same pesticide in other foods based on a determination that the risk was negligible.

Additives exempt from testing

Prior sanctioned substances were approved for use by the FDA or the US Department of Agriculture prior to the 1958 Food Additives Amendment. GRAS (generally recognized as safe) additives are exempt because their extensive use in the past has produced no known harmful effects. Since 1969 the FDA has been systematically reviewing GRAS substances and reclassifying them into five categories indicating their degree of safety. As of yet, no firm evidence exists to prove that aspartame actually causes as many adverse reactions as consumers claim it does. FDA has banned the use of sulfites on raw fruits and vegetables and on commercially marketed fresh potatoes while continuing to monitor sulfite use on other foods. What can individuals do when they are concerned about food additives? All of us have a right to be conscientious consumers—to ask questions and demand accountability.

Food borne illnesses

S. aureus lives in nasal passages and in cuts on the skin. Food is infected when individuals sneeze or cough on food or handle food with uncovered cuts. Common foods affected include egg products, milk, seafood, cheese, and cream-filled pastries. These foods should be held below 40°F or above 140°F to prevent the growth of the bacteria. Good worker sanitation procedures and the use of sneeze guards also prevent the microbes from entering foods. Symptoms of S. aureus illness develop within 2 to 6 hours of eating contaminated foods, and include nausea, vomiting, diarrhea, and headache.

C. botulinum is an anaerobic bacterium that is common in the environment. The bacteria release a toxin that can cause fatal food poisoning. Symptoms present within 12 to 36 hours and include vomiting, dizziness, and respiratory distress. The bacteria thrive in home-canned, low-acid foods. Cans that bulge or contain milky fluid should be discarded.

Several different Salmonella bacteria cause food poisoning. The bacteria are found in feces and can contaminate food through cutting boards, cracked eggs, or infected water. Ingesting live bacteria causes illness within 5 to 72 hours, with symptoms including nausea, diarrhea, abdominal cramps, and headache.

Consuming undercooked poultry, eggs, meat, or dairy products increases the risk of Salmonella poisoning. Foods should not be held between 41° and 135°F, and separate cutting boards should be used for produce and raw meat.

Listeria bacteria are resistant to cold, heat, and acid. Unlike other microbes, it can grow in refrigerated conditions below 40°F. Unpasteurized cheeses, deli meats, and hot dogs have caused Listeria outbreaks in the past. Symptoms develop 7 to 30 days after exposure, and include fever, headache, and vomiting.

Pregnant women and newborns can suffer life-threatening complications from listeriosis, and are advised to avoid unpasteurized dairy products and deli meats, unless heated to steaming.

Center for Food Safety and Applied Nutrition

The Center for Food Safety and Applied Nutrition (CFSAN) is one of six product-oriented centers, in addition to a nationwide field force, that carries out the mission of the Food and Drug Administration (FDA). FDA is a scientific regulatory agency responsible for the safety of the nation's domestically produced and imported foods, cosmetics, drugs, biologics, medical devices, and radiological products. It is one of the oldest federal agencies whose primary function is consumer protection. The agency touches and directly influences the lives of everyone in the United States. FDA is recognized internationally as the leading food and drug regulatory agency in the world. Many foreign nations seek and receive FDA's help in improving and monitoring the safety of their products. FDA is part of the executive branch of the United States' government within the Department of Health and Human Services (DHHS) and the Public Health Service (PHS).

FDA= packaged food
shelled eggs
seafood
game meat

USDA= meat
poultry
processed eggproducts
catfish

Food, Drug, and Cosmetic Act

- Prohibits adulteration
- Prohibits misbranded information
- Regulates food additives/generally recognized as safe (GRAS)
- Monitors carcinogenic effects
- Calls for extensive testing

* Does not cover fish, meat, poultry, and eggs.
* Does monitor shellfish transport with interstate regulations.

Food Safety and Inspection Service

The Food Safety and Inspection Service (FSIS) is the public health agency in the US Department of Agriculture responsible for ensuring that the nation's commercial supply of meat, poultry, and egg products is safe, wholesome, and correctly labeled and packaged.

Federal Meat Inspection Act
Under the Federal Meat Inspection Act (FMIA), FSIS provides inspection for all meat products sold in interstate commerce, and reinspects imported products to ensure that they meet US food safety standards.

Poultry Products Inspection Act
Under the Poultry Products Inspection Act (PPIA), FSIS provides inspection for all poultry products sold in interstate commerce, and reinspects imported products to ensure that they meet US food safety standards.

Egg Products Inspection Act
Under the Egg Products Inspection Act (EPIA), FSIS inspects egg products sold in interstate commerce, and reinspects imported products to ensure that they meet US food safety standards. In egg processing plants, inspection involves examining, before and after breaking, eggs intended for further processing and use as food.

National Marine Fisheries

National Oceanic and Atmospheric Administration (NOAA) Fisheries is the federal agency, a division of the Department of Commerce, responsible for the stewardship of the nation's living marine resources and their habitat. NOAA Fisheries is responsible for the management, conservation and protection of living marine resources within the United States' Exclusive Economic Zone (water 3 to 200 miles offshore). Using the tools provided by the Magnuson-Stevens Act, NOAA Fisheries assesses and predicts the status of fish stocks, ensures compliance with fisheries regulations, and works to reduce wasteful fishing practices. Under the Marine Mammal Protection Act and the Endangered Species Act, NOAA Fisheries recovers protected marine species (e.g., whales, turtles) without unnecessarily impeding economic and recreational opportunities. With the help of the six regional offices and eight councils, NOAA Fisheries is able to work with communities on fishery management issues. NOAA Fisheries works to promote sustainable fisheries and to prevent lost economic potential associated with over fishing, declining species, and degraded habitats. NOAA Fisheries strives to balance competing public needs and interest in the use and enjoyment of our oceans' resources.

OSHA

The Occupational Safety and Health Administration (OSHA) enforces standards of safety that focus on reducing accidents and illness in the workplace. If an accident resulting in an injury occurs in a foodservice operation, the manager should fill out a report and may need to report the incident to OSHA. An investigation may ensue to determine the cause of the accident and to make adjustments to prevent future accidents.

Related to foodborne disease, OSHA requires that food be prepared and handled in a way that prevents spoilage or contamination. OSHA is mostly concerned with foodborne illness as it may affect food processors or servers.

OSHA requires that material safety data sheets be kept for each hazardous chemical on the premises, and the information should include the identity of the chemical, the potential physical and health hazards of the chemical, precautions for safe handling, and first-aid measures for someone affected by the chemical.

Nutrition Labeling and Education Act

The FDA and the USDA require that food labels list the following mandatory information, and in the following order: total calories, calories from fat, total fat, saturated fat, trans fat, cholesterol, sodium, total carbohydrate, dietary fiber, sugars protein, vitamin A, vitamin C, calcium, and iron. The nutrients are expressed as a percentage of the daily recommended value, which helps consumers to understand how a chosen food fits into their daily diet. If the product claims to be "light" or "high fiber," the product must fit into the guideline's definition for light or high fiber. This ensures that the terms are used consistently between products. If a health claim is made about a food, it must be evaluated and approved by the FDA or the product must include a disclaimer. Most foods sold in grocery stores must carry the label. Exempt products include foods intended for immediate consumption, food prepared on premises such as bakery items, and food shipped in bulk.

Nutrition information

To meet the FDA guidelines, point-of-purchase nutrition information for raw fruits, vegetables and fish must include the following:
- Name of the fruit, vegetable, or fish that has been identified by FDA as being one of the 20 most commonly eaten in the United States.
- Serving size.
- Calories per serving.
- Amount of protein, total carbohydrates, total fat, and sodium per serving.
- Percent of the US Recommended Daily Allowances for iron, calcium, and vitamins A and C per serving.

This information is required because FDA believes it is important for consumers to know which foods will increase one's intake of nutrients and which will not.

Standards for food safety

The USDA's Labeling and Consumer Protection division develops policies and procedures that ensure safe meat, poultry, and egg products. Meat and poultry is inspected at the time of slaughter, and egg processing facilities are inspected during production.

The US Department of Commerce is concerned with the safety of seafood processing plants via inspection by the National Marine Fisheries Service.

The Public Health Service (PHS) and the Centers for Disease Control are both focused on investigating and preventing foodborne illness. The PHS oversees the requirement for the pasteurization of milk, and also focuses on vending machines and restaurants as a source for foodborne illness.

The Food and Drug Administration (FDA) prohibits the adulteration and misbranding of food products. The FDA also mandates standards of identity, so that a product with a familiar name must meet certain ingredient requirements; standards of quality; and standards of fill, so that cans, bags, and boxes may not appear to contain more product than they do.

Standards of identity

Standards of identity define what a given food product is, its name, and the ingredients that must be used, or may be used in the manufacture of the food.
Standards of quality are minimum standards only and establish specifications for quality requirements.
Fill-of-container standards define how full the container must be and how this is measured. FDA standards are based on the assumption that the food is properly prepared from clean, sound materials.

Standards for foodservice equipment

Equipment manufactured for the foodservice industry must meet safety standards provided by organizations such as the National Sanitation Foundation (NSF) and Underwriters Laboratories (UL).

The standards set forth by the NSF are particularly salient to foodservice operations because they ensure that equipment meets safety and sanitation guidelines. The NSF is a nonprofit organization whose mission it is to improve public health. If an equipment manufacturer wishes to obtain the NSF seal of approval, they must pay a fee to have a representative conduct a voluntary inspection and test of the equipment. If the equipment meets the NSF safety standards for design, materials, construction, and performance, the manufacturer can display the NSF certified seal of approval. Custom-made equipment can follow NSF handbooks detailing safety standards.

UL conducts voluntary inspection of electrical and fire extinguishing equipment to ensure that safety standards are met according to the more than 800 guidelines the nonprofit organization has developed.

Standards for fire extinguishers and cooking supplies

Fires are categorized as type A, B, C, or D. Special fire extinguishers must be present in foodservice operations to prepare for the possibility of these different fires. Type A fires involve ordinary flammable materials such as wood, paper, or cloth. The green triangle symbol is used to designate extinguishers used in type A fires. Type B fires involve flammable liquids, such as grease, oil, or gas. A red square is used to designate extinguishers for type B fires. Type C fires refer to live electrical fires. The extinguishing agent used in this type of fire does not conduct electricity, and the extinguisher is marked with a blue circle. Type D fires involve combustible metals and are not a concern to foodservice operations.

Chemical cleaning supply usage is regulated by the Environmental Protection Agency. The EPA specifies the solution strength of the common sanitizing agents, including chlorine, iodine, and quaternary ammonia.

Use of appliances

Deck ovens consist of two or more units stacked on top of each other. They take up a large amount of space, making them impractical for small kitchens, but their large interior makes them ideal for some applications, like pizza.

Convection ovens are popular because of their efficient energy usage, small footprint, and the reduced cooking time that results from hot air being forced over the food. Convection ovens are useful in the preparation of many foods, including meats, potatoes, and bakery products.

Rotary ovens increase the flow of hot air over foods, but they do this by moving the food through the oven instead of forcing the air over the food with a fan.

The tilting skillet can be used for grilling, stewing, steaming, braising, and sautéing. The tall sides mean a large volume of food can be accommodated, and the tilting feature makes pouring and cleaning easy.

Molds and food spoilage

Molds are widely distributed in the environment and may occur as part of a food's normal flora, on inadequately sanitized food processing equipment, or as airborne contaminants. Since molds are poor competitors and grow slowly, their growth is often a problem under conditions that are unfavorable to bacterial growth. Foods with low pH, low moisture, high salt or sugar concentrations, and those stored at refrigeration temperatures are susceptible to mold spoilage.

Preventing food spoilage

Some molds are desirable in foods such as blue cheese, and mold spores are found to some degree in most foods. Mold needs a warm environment to produce the threads commonly associated with the visible fuzzy mold that may be observed on food. Molds are able to survive freezing temperatures, but molds do not start to grow until temperatures exceed the freezing point. Rapid growth takes place between 50° and 100°F, and temperatures above 140°F kill molds.

Like molds, yeasts grow from spores and are desirable in some foods, like sauerkraut and beer. Yeasts can produce off flavors or musty flavors in other foods. Yeasts are inactive in cold temperatures, grow readily between 50° and 100°F, and are destroyed at temperatures above 140°F.

Enzymes can enhance the quality of food or detract from it. Enzymes lend sweetness to fruits during the ripening process, but the enzymatic browning that takes place when an apple is sliced detracts from the quality of the product. Enzymes are inactive in cold temperatures and active at temperatures between 85° and 120°F. Enzymes are destroyed at temperatures above 140°F.

Of the three microorganisms responsible for food spoilage, bacteria are more resilient to variations in temperature, and bacteria (or the substances they produce) can produce the most serious health effects. In fact, the spores of Clostridium botulinum can survive several hours of continuous boiling. Bacteria can be classified as aerobic or anaerobic, depending on whether the microorganism requires oxygen to grow. In addition to botulinum, Staphylococcus aureus is another thermophilic bacterium that survives many hours of boiling, which provides a rationale for canning under pressure in order to reach temperatures of 240°F or more.

Safe food temperatures

Frozen foods should be maintained at temperatures ranging from zero to -10°F. Generally, every a 10-degree rise in temperature above zero reduces storage life by half. Cooked foods should be cooled to 70°F within 2 hours, and should be cooled to 41°F or below within 6 hours. Bulky foods should be cooled in shallow pans or placed in an ice water bath to speed the chilling process. Foods that cannot be placed in shallow pans should be divided into smaller portions and/or subjected to blast chillers to enhance cooling. Foods held for serving should be greater than or equal to 135°F. Foods reheated from a chilled state should be brought to a temperature of 165°F within 2 hours after thaw. Holding potentially hazardous foods between 41° and 135°F invites pathogen growth and development.

Equipment and Facility Planning

Foodservice facility design

Program evaluation and review technique

PERT is an acronym for program evaluation and review technique. This planning tool allows the foodservice manager to break down a complex system, such as designing a new foodservice facility, into workable phases. A sequencing rationale is developed for each phase, and the expected duration of each phase is calculated. Each phase or step is illustrated graphically in the PERT diagram, which includes estimated time and necessary preceding steps. The possibility of completing any steps simultaneously is considered.

Critical path method

The critical path method (CPM) looks at the plan holistically, and estimates the minimum time needed for project completion if the slowest possible progression through the phases takes place. Roughly, the development of a new foodservice facility will involve concept development, design development and analysis, oversight of construction, equipment and inventory procurement, and employee hiring and training.

Designing a foodservice facility

A feasibility study is conducted to determine the potential profitability of a foodservice operation. The market feasibility considers factors such as community demographics to determine if enough traffic will be generated to turn a profit. The financial feasibility analyzes whether the projected net income will be sufficient to meet the owner's expectations for profit.

Before a new foodservice facility is constructed, the planning team develops a prospectus that summarizes the proposed design sequence of the project. The planning team may include the owner, foodservice manager, builder, architect, and equipment vendors. The prospectus may include floor plans showing the location of equipment, utility plans showing electrical and plumbing outlets, a list of equipment to be purchased, the specifications of materials to be used, and a description of the way the installation is to proceed.

The menu will drive such design features as the amount of kitchen space required, the types of equipment needed, the size of cold and dry storage areas needed, and number and required skill level of employees.

Planning a work environment

Ergonomic features

Ergonomics considers how the work environment will affect worker efficiency, safety, and satisfaction. When planning sufficient workspace, the planning team must consider the number of people working in the area, the size and amount of clearance the equipment requires, and what kinds of movement the workers will routinely engage in (standing, lifting, stooping, etc.). Work surfaces should be at a standard height and width to accommodate the average worker without causing excessive stooping or reaching. Standard work surfaces accommodate a 30 inch reach and a working height of 35 to 37 inches. Appropriate tools and equipment should be purchased to reduce the possibility of injury and fatigue. Hand trucks, carts, and ramps facilitate the movement of heavy boxes and crates. High noise levels are common in food preparation levels, contributing to worker fatigue and irritability. The use of acoustic ceiling tiles and carpeting in the dining room can reduce noise, as can separating the dish room from the production area in the kitchen.

Interior finishes

The materials used in the floors, walls, and ceilings of a foodservice kitchen are determined by budgetary considerations, as well as ease of cleaning and durability. Floors should be easy to clean, slip-resistant, and impervious to grease. Quarry tiles are commonly used in the food production and dishwashing areas, as they are slip-resistant and nonporous.

A common choice for walls is glazed ceramic tile, which is expensive but durable and easy to clean. Painted surfaces should be avoided in production and dishwashing areas, as the heat and moisture causes the paint to flake off. Concrete blocks with epoxy paint may be appropriate in dry storage and receiving areas.

Ceilings include the structural component of the building, and the aesthetic false ceiling, which hides ductwork. Acoustical ceilings are inexpensive and noise reducing, and some are manufactured specifically for kitchen use. Aluminum panel ceilings are easy to clean and may even be run through the dishwasher.

Ventilation and lighting

A well-conceived kitchen ventilation system must capture and remove large quantities of moisture and grease-laden hot air from cooking and dishwasher areas. The grease must be removed from the air before it is exhausted outside, and the air must be replenished with air from outside and/or from other parts of the building. Filters or extractors in the hood canopy capture the grease, and must be cleaned regularly. The exhaust requirements are usually determined by building codes. Foodservice kitchens are rarely air-conditioned, so a good ventilation system is also essential to the comfort of the employees.

Providing proper illumination is necessary to reduce worker strain, fatigue, and error level. Ideal foot candle levels vary from 35 to 70 in dining and standard food prep areas, while workers performing detailed tasks may need up to 150 foot candles. Storage rooms, receiving areas, and restrooms usually require between 10 and 30 foot candles of light.

Aisle space requirements

Determining proper aisle clearance is important in the planning phase of the foodservice operation, as it cannot be changed easily after the facility is complete. If the aisles are too narrow, the employees will be too cramped to work comfortably. If the aisles are too wide, employees will get fatigued. A single aisle with limited equipment and limited traffic may need a width of 36 inches. A double aisle with limited equipment or a single aisle with protruding equipment may need a width of at least 42 inches.

Production area layout

The production area includes the pre-prep, hot-prep, cold-prep, and final prep areas. Sinks and chopping appliances are useful in the pre-prep area, where washing, peeling, and chopping of produce takes place. The hot-prep area needs to be large enough to accommodate the range and the ventilation system. The cold-prep area should be close to the refrigerator. The final prep area is used to prepare foods that cannot be held for extended periods, such as fried eggs.

Materials used in foodservice equipment

Stainless steel is an expensive but durable material commonly used in items that will receive heavy usage and wear in the foodservice kitchen, such as tabletops, sinks, and shelving that will need to support heavy weight. Lower gauge items have a greater thickness, and are therefore more expensive. High gauge steel may be used where strength is not important, such as paneling or door covers.

Galvanized iron or sheet metal is used when cost is an issue, and it may be chosen for the same applications as stainless steel. Disadvantages include unattractiveness and that it is more difficult to clean than steel.

Aluminum is used where strength needs to be balanced with a lighter weight than steel. Aluminum may be a good choice for mobile equipment such as carts and shelving on wheels.

Dishwashers

Dishwashing equipment is one of the most expensive pieces of equipment to operate in the foodservice facility. The machine and dish tables represent an expensive investment, and the water, electricity, detergent, maintenance, and labor costs are ongoing. Investing in a larger dishwasher may reduce operating costs, as larger machines use water and detergent more efficiently than small machines, and labor costs should be lower for machines that can quickly handle large loads.

Dishwashers first dispense a spray of hot water and detergent to loosen grease and remove large food particles. The final rinse water must be at least 180°F to sanitize the dishes, or a chemical sanitizing agent may be used.

Single-tank door machines are suitable for facilities serving less than 250 meals per hour. A flight-type dishwasher consists of separate tanks for pre-wash, wash, and rinse cycles; a conveyor belt moves the dishes through the machine. The flight machine is found in facilities that serve more than 600 meals per hour.

Commercial dishwashers
Much larger heavy-duty dishwashers with a high output are available for use in catering and commercial establishments where a large number of dishes are to be washed and sanitized. Commercial machines are capable of washing a rack of dishes in just a few minutes or less using a wash water temperature of usually 110° to 120°F for a low temperature sanitizing machine or 150 minimum wash temp for a hot water sanitizing machine. NSF sets the standards for wash and rinse time along with proper water temperature for chemical or hot water sanitizing methods. Hot water sanitizing requires a rinse temperature of at least 170°F. There are many types of commercial dishwashers, including undercounter, single tank, conveyor, flight type, and carousel machines.

Sterilization
Domestic dishwashers do not sterilize the utensils, as proper sterilization requires autoclaving at 121°C with pressurized wet steam for at least 15 minutes. Dishwashers (even commercial ones used in restaurants) do not do this. Commercial dishwashers can use one of two types of sanitization methods. One is to use hot water sanitizing, using final rinse water at a temperature of

at least 83°C (180°F). The other method is a chemical sanitization method, which many commercial low temperature machines use, using chlorine injected in the final rinse water.

Ovens

Microwave ovens:
A microwave oven (or microwave) is a kitchen appliance employing microwave radiation primarily to cook or heat food. This is type of oven saves time.

Convection ovens:
Convection ovens use heated air that is forced into the oven by fans located in the back of the oven, generally for cooking food. By moving heated air past the food, convection ovens operate at a lower temperature than a standard conventional oven and they can cook food more quickly. They are mostly used in industrial and commercial applications, but can be purchased for the home as well. With a convection oven there will be about a 25% to 30% decrease in cooking temperature and a 20% decrease in cooking time as compared to a conventional oven.

Deck ovens:
A deck oven essentially consists of 1) a bake chamber that contains a hearth or deck, 2) a fire chamber beneath the bake chamber, which contains a gas burner, 3) a thermostat for regulating the amount of flame, and 4) a flue or stack for venting combustion gases. Deck ovens are often used as a pizza oven.

Rotary ovens
Rotary ovens increase the flow of hot air over foods, but they do this by moving the food through the oven instead of forcing the air over the food with a fan.

Tilting skillet
The tilting skillet can be used for grilling, stewing, steaming, braising, and sautéing. The tall sides mean a large volume of food can be accommodated, and the tilting feature makes pouring and cleaning easy.

Steamers

There are several types of steamers: pressureless or convection, low pressure, high pressure, and pressure/pressureless. A steamer is categorized by the pounds of pressure per square inch (psi) in the cooking chamber. The steamer's cooking temperature is directly affected by its cooking cavity operating pressure. Pressureless steamers operate at zero psi, which corresponds to a cooking temperature of 212°F. Low pressure steamers have a psi range from five to ten and cook at temperatures from 228° to 240°F. High pressure steamers cook at 15 psi and a temperature of 250°F. All steamers can use direct steam or a steam boiler. The gas- or electric- powered steam boiler is usually self-contained and located in the cabinet below the steamer. The self-contained steamer requires a water source to fill the boiler in order to produce steam. In pressureless or convection steamers, the heat transfer is accomplished by forced convection. Pressureless steamers are well suited for a wide variety of food types, from fresh vegetables to loose pack frozen or frozen block vegetables. The advantage of the pressureless steamer is the ability to open the door during the cooking process, which cannot be done with either the low-pressure or high-pressure steamers.

Steam-jacketed kettles

Steam-jacketed kettles are often used to rapidly and uniformly heat food and agricultural products to processing temperatures. Steam is injected into a thin jacket that surrounds the bowl of the kettle. The steam condenses on the product-surface of the kettle jacket and transfers its latent heat of vaporization to the product. Condensed steam (condensate or water) is removed from the jacket of the kettle to allow more steam to enter and continue the heating process. Most steam-jacketed kettles used in food and agricultural processes are operated in the range of 5 to 60 psi steam pressure. The temperature of steam at these pressures is 227° to 307°F. The two main types of kettles are fixed, gravity drained and tilting, siphon drained. The food does not touch the steam and these kettles are very energy efficient.

High-pressure steamers

High-pressure steamers are appropriate for preparing foods just before or during the mealtime, when a reduction in holding times is desired. They can quickly prepare vegetables for immediate service, resulting in a higher quality product. No-pressure steamers can handle large quantities of vegetables, eggs, or seafood, and are more compact than high-pressure models.

Fire extinguishers

Class A extinguishers

These will put out fires in ordinary combustibles, such as wood and paper. The numerical rating for this class of fire extinguisher refers to the amount of water the fire extinguisher holds and the amount of fire it will extinguish.

Class B extinguishers

These should be used on fires involving flammable liquids, such as grease, gasoline, or oil. The numerical rating for this class of fire extinguisher states the approximate number of square feet of a flammable liquid fire that a non-expert person can expect to extinguish.

Class C extinguishers

These are suitable for use on electrically energized fires. This class of fire extinguishers does not have a numerical rating. The presence of the letter "C" indicates that the extinguishing agent is non-conductive.

Class D extinguishers

These are designed for use on flammable metals and are often specific for the type of metal in question. There is no picture designator for Class D extinguishers. These extinguishers generally have no rating nor are they given a multi-purpose rating for use on other types of fires.

Important terms

Brokers – Contract with manufacturers, processors, or prime source producers to both sell and market products; Represent a variety of products; Provide a variety of services including marketing and menu planning.

Cost center - The purchasing department at a cost center is responsible for managing the expenses of the foodservice establishment in such a way that profit is emphasized and maximized. The purchasing departments of cost centers manage expenses, but are not responsible for generating a profit, as in the case of public schools.

Full or broadline – food, equipment, furniture.

Future contracts - Future contracts are used when the foodservice manager wants to buy goods at a fixed price, but wants them delivered at a future date. This allows the manager to avoid the potential for a rise in product cost.

Manufacturers' Representatives – Represent fewer and more specialized lines.

Prime vending - Prime vending is defined by a relationship between the foodservice establishment and vendor in which the vendor seeks to provide most of the product. The vendor may offer pricing incentives, special credit lines, or premium customer service to entice the foodservice management.

Procurement - Procurement refers to the process of obtaining the food and supplies the foodservice establishment needs to operate at the lowest cost.

Special breed – chain customers.

Specialty – particular product (dairy, bread).

Wholesale club – cost effectiveness.

Wholesalers – purchase from various manufacturers/processors; store, sell and deliver products to suppliers.

Sustainability

Examples of sources of information on sustainability

Seafood
According to Seafood Watch, a program offered by the Monterey Bay Aquarium, the most sustainable seafood choices to buy are caught or farmed using methods that do the least possible harm to other wildlife or habitats, and are well managed. Good alternatives are those that may be caught or farmed in less than ideal ways, but can consider buying with some additional information about how they were obtained. Those to avoid are caught or farmed in ways that are harmful to the environment or other marine life forms, or are overfished, which can threaten species extinction. For example, spiny lobster from Mexico is a best choice. Lobster from the United States and the Bahamas is a good alternative. Spiny lobster from Belize, Brazil, Honduras, and Nicaragua should be avoided. Alaskan and New Zealand salmon are best choices. Canadian, California, Oregon, and Washington wild-caught salmon are good alternatives. Farmed Atlantic salmon should be avoided.

Tap water quality
The Environmental Working Group (EWG) has compiled a database of tap water quality throughout the United States. For cities with populations above 250,000, EWG rated water utilities according to three criteria: (1) total number of chemicals identified over the past five years, (2) percentage of chemicals detected in city water tested, and (3) the largest average amount of each individual pollutant compared to national averages or legal limits. Among pollutants tested, the three most common are arsenic, nitrate, and disinfection byproducts.

Sustainable foodservice products

Plastics
The complexity of plastic foodservice products is related to considerations of toxicity in manufacturing and disposal, and plastics variety. The universal recycling symbol (three folded arrows forming the three corners of a triangle) typically indicates something is recyclable; however, the number inside that symbol from 1-7 differentiates plastics' recycling desirability. Generally, plastics with numbers 1, 2, 4, and 5 are recyclable, while those with numbers 3, 6, and 7 are undesirable to recycling companies, and are rarely recycled. The following are the substances indicated by each number:
1: polyethylene terephthalate (PET or PETE)
2: other polyethylenes (PE) including acrylonitrile butadiene styrene (ABS), polycarbonates (PC), polystyrene (PS), polyurethanes (PU), and acrylic
3: polyvinyl chloride (PVC)
4: polypropylene (PP) and ethylene vinyl acetate (EVA)
5: bio-based polymers
6: Styrofoam
7: polycarbonate and other various plastics
Numbers 3, 6, and 7 may create hazardous byproducts during manufacturing and disposal, leach toxic chemicals into food, or contain known carcinogens. These carcinogens include flame-retardants, lead, cadmium, Bisphenol A, phthalates, and other hormone disrupters.

Paper
Most disposable paper foodservice products are not biodegradable, and none are recyclable. However, several brands manufacture these using recycled content. Two organizations certifying

these are EcoLogo and Green Seal. Both require chlorine-free manufacturing. EcoLogo has a greater focus on manufacturing process standards, while Green Seal tends to emphasize using recycled content. While most takeout containers typically contain no recycled content, the Bio-Plus Earth Container from the Fold-Pak company does. Solo, prominent maker of drinking cups, has introduced its *Bare* brand of cups, which are made with recycled content.

Sustainable kitchen equipment

The biggest proportion of most restaurants' energy expenses is food preparation, which accounts for around 30% of energy costs. In addition, roughly 15% is attributed to refrigeration costs. These, combined with HVAC systems, water heaters, and exhaust hoods, make up the majority of energy that foodservice facilities use. These high expenses in energy and water costs can be lowered significantly by using commercial kitchen equipment designed to be energy- or water-efficient. Such equipment is often designated by Energy Star labels, or rated highly energy-efficient by the Food Service Technology Center (FSTC), Consortium for Energy Efficiency (CEE), or other reputable research organizations.

Several local utilities and US states have initiated tax credit and rebate programs as incentives for foodservices to buy energy- and water-efficient equipment. Links to rebate programs are available online at www.sustainablefoodservice.com. Refrigeration equipment especially, combined with state rebates, can give foodservices paybacks almost immediately. FSTC has tested, listed, and reported the performance of specific models of cooking equipment for energy efficiency. Steam cookers, holding cabinets, and fryers are among Energy Star cooking equipment. Steam cookers and convection ovens are naturally more energy-efficient.

Energy efficient products

Turbo Pot, made by Eneron, is one example of a line of cooking supplies that saves substantial energy. These pots move more energy to themselves and their contents by having fins that act as heat sinks. The Food Service Technology Center (FSTC) has tested the Turbo Pots, finding they boiled water in half the usual time, shortening total cooking time, and enabling chefs to maintain steady temperatures with lower stovetop flames, saving energy and money. Both FSTC and Energy Star rate refrigerators and ice machines for energy and water efficiency. Although water-cooled ice machines can use half the electricity as air-cooled ones, they use ten times the water, doubling to quadrupling their lifetime costs through water use. A link to an ice machine cost calculator from Texas water expert Bill Hoffman is available at www.sustainablefoodservice.com. Foodservices can install new, high-efficiency walk-in freezers and coolers and plan ahead with refrigeration repair services to procure high-efficiency compressors and motors, since repair companies sometimes stock only inexpensive, standard low-efficiency models.

Responsible food storage

In the same way that individual consumer households want to preserve leftovers to eat another time, foodservice operations that prepare large quantities of foods daily must store unused amounts properly if they are to serve them again. This is imperative for minimizing waste, as well as preventing economic loss from purchasing food that will go uneaten. Also like individual consumers, foodservices are advised by environmental experts to eliminate or at least substantially decrease the amounts of plastic they use for food storage.

Glass is far longer-lasting and environmentally safer than plastic. It is typically oven-safe, freezer-safe, and dishwasher-safe. Dual-purpose glass Mason jars for canning and freezing are designed specially to tolerate boiling and freezing temperatures. They are excellent for storage and attractive. Weck canning jars sealed with rubber rings held with stainless steel clips are becoming popular, offering quick, easy, secure storage. Airtight stainless steel containers are excellent and come in all sizes. Reusing plastic containers, freezing appetizers or small portions in muffin tins, and using eco-friendly freezer paper or wrap are additional options.

Water efficiency

Water conservation by foodservice operations is generally inadequate. Just a few examples among the hundreds of ways foodservices can save water include:
- keeping boiling water covered during slow periods
- maintaining pasta cookers not at rolling boils but simmer levels
- keeping running water, when required, at minimum flow rates
- using efficient faucet aerators and flow control valves on sinks
- cleaning floors with brooms and mops or pressurizing waterbrooms rather than hoses
- melting ice by placing it in dish or mop sinks instead of running water on it
- following best practices for handling grease, oil, and fat
- serving guests water by request instead of automatically
- requesting the local water utility to conduct a water audit

In landscaping, planting water-efficient native plants is paramount. Additional practices include efficient watering techniques and irrigation systems, rainwater collection, and organic gardening methods.

Waste reduction practices

In today's landfills, 75% of materials are compostable or recyclable. In foodservice operations, 50-70% of garbage weight is made up of compostable food matter. While the other 30-50% of garbage weight comes from food packaging, these packaging materials make up about 70% of foodservice trash volume. Not producing waste in the first place is the best way to decrease it; this is called source reduction or precycling. Precycling includes selecting bulk food supplies, vendors who reuse packaging, beer kegs instead of bottles, other products that use minimal or no packaging, and products packaged in recyclable containers, such as cardboard or other materials that are more recyclable than plastics. Restaurants can begin reducing waste by conducting a waste audit; www.sustainablefoodservice.com offers a waste audit how-to. They should also train employees in sorting and recycling and post visual graphic recycling guides. They can also implement new programs, such as worm bins, composting, and replacing disposables with reusable, durable, or compostable goods.

In the foodservice industry, disposable products are often undesirable, yet necessary for health or practical reasons. However, more sustainable disposable choices are available today, including products that are biodegradable, reusable, or use recycled content. Foodservices should first reduce the amount of disposable products they use, eliminating any unneeded disposables, and use devices like the Xpressnap paper napkin dispenser to control how many customers take. They can also encourage customers to bring their own coffee cups and adopt reusable takeout containers, such as the Eco-Clamshell.

As an example, some college cafeterias have experienced success with Eco-Clamshells. At the beginning of the year, they charge students a small deposit for this reusable container, which students exchange every time they order to-go meals. Cafeterias not only save money from not having to purchase single-use containers, but also, since they sell so much takeout food, they enjoy very brief payback times.

Practice Test

1. All of the following are **TRUE** about essential fatty acids **EXCEPT:**
   a. Good sources of essential fatty acids include fatty fish such as salmon and tuna.
   b. They are available mainly through diet but the human body is able to make a limited supply.
   c. Essential fatty acid deficiency can affect growth, wound healing, and vision and cause a scaly skin rash.
   d. Alpha-linoleic acid and linoleic acid cannot be synthesized by the human body.

2. Which of the following enzymes assist in the digestion of protein?
   a. Lipase and amylase
   b. Ptyalin and maltase
   c. Sucrase and dextrinase
   d. Pepsin and trypsin

3. The primary role of the large intestine is:
   a. Water and sodium resorption
   b. Water and sodium excretion
   c. Fatty acid digestion
   d. Performs the majority of the digestive processes

4. If an average adult consumed 20 kcal/kg per day, what do you think the consequence would be?
   a. Weight gain
   b. Weight loss
   c. Weight maintenance
   d. Depends upon how much exercise the person gets

5. Beriberi is a deficiency caused by:
   a. Niacin
   b. Riboflavin
   c. Thiamin
   d. Biotin

6. Which of the following is **NOT** a potential consequence of hypercalcemia:
   a. Soft tissue calcification
   b. Interference with the absorption of iron and zinc
   c. Nausea, vomiting, constipation
   d. Vitamin D toxicity

7. What are the estimated daily maintenance fluid requirements for a 30-year-old female weighing 130 pounds?
   a. 1,500 mL
   b. 2,100 mL
   c. 3,000 mL
   d. 3,600 mL

8. When following a recipe, the term "fold" refers to:
   a. Layering wet and dry ingredients
   b. Rapidly combining fat and sugar in order to incorporate air
   c. Using a spatula or large spoon to add an ingredient such as whipped cream to other ingredients, using a gentle turning motion
   d. Gently stirring ingredients together to form a batter

9. The most appropriate method of cooking a chuck roast is:
   a. Braising
   b. Grilling
   c. Broiling
   d. Roasting

10. Which of the following would increase the risk of *Clostridium botulinum* in the canning process?
    a. Leaving an inch of headspace for canned vegetables
    b. Processing canned foods in a pressure canner
    c. Allowing the canner to cool to room temperature on its own (i.e., not running it under cool water to speed the process)
    d. a low-acid, moist environment

11. A client is requesting information on meatless meals. You suggest using tofu, which the client has never heard of. All of the following are benefits of using tofu **EXCEPT**:
    a. Tofu contains high biological value protein.
    b. Tofu is high in soluble fiber and is relatively easy to digest.
    c. Tofu can help to lower LDL cholesterol.
    d. Tofu is a good source of calcium and B vitamins.

12. Which of the following would **LEAST LIKELY** be considered an example of functional foods?
    a. Orange juice
    b. Garlic
    c. Iodized salt
    d. Tomatoes

13. Which of the following terms refers to the circulation of hot air to evenly distribute heat?
    a. Convection
    b. Conduction
    c. Radiant
    d. Conventional

14. A cookie recipe calls for cake flour but none is available. Bread flour is substituted. What could be a possible consequence of this substitution on the end product?
    a. The cookies rise too high.
    b. The cookies are over-caramelized.
    c. The cookies do not spread enough.
    d. The cookies spread too much.

15. Which of the following individuals is **LEAST LIKELY** to require magnesium supplementation?
    a. An individual taking long-term furosemide
    b. A breastfed infant
    c. An individual with chronic alcoholism
    d. An older adult

16. What is the primary purpose of nutrition screening?
    a. To identify patients who need nutrition education
    b. To identify patients with factors that place them at risk for malnutrition or nutritional issues
    c. To identify patients who are obese
    d. To identify patients who need to be considered for government food programs

17. Which of the following parameters would most reliably indicate nutritional risk?
    a. Unintentional weight loss of 12% in 6 months
    b. Low serum albumin
    c. Weight loss of 5% over 3 months
    d. Lactose intolerance

18. Which of the following would be considered the most appropriate time frame in which to complete a nutritional screening of an adult patient admitted to an acute care hospital?
    a. 14 days
    b. 48 hours
    c. 12 hours
    d. 24 hours

19. Which of the following is the acronym used by the Nutrition Screening Initiative (NSI) to help measure an older individual's nutrition risk?
    a. DEPENDABLE
    b. COMPETENT
    c. DETERMINE
    d. DEFENSE

20. Which of the following would be considered an advantage of using food frequency to obtain dietary information?
    a. Food frequency allows for the recording of actual intake throughout the day.
    b. Food frequency provides information on how food is prepared.
    c. Food frequency does not require the individual responding to be able to estimate portion sizes.
    d. Food frequency can be very useful when it is used in conjunction with other methods of obtaining dietary information.

21. The statement that best describes a nutrient intake analysis is:
    a. A tool used to obtain dietary information by recording an individual's actual intake over a 72-hour period
    b. A tool used to obtain dietary information from the previous 72 hours based on an individual's memory recall
    c. A tool that utilizes a questionnaire to determine how often certain foods are consumed
    d. A tool that offers a comprehensive and accurate measurement of an individual's dietary intake over 48-72 hours

22. The term kwashiorkor refers to:
    a. A form of protein-calorie malnutrition characterized by severe weight loss and protein depletion
    b. A form of malnutrition where protein deficiency causes edema and depletion of visceral protein
    c. A mild form of malnutrition commonly seen in developing countries
    d. A form of malnutrition rarely seen because of improved food supply and access to food

23. During a nutrition-focused physical assessment of an infant, the RD notices a yellowish tinge to the infant's skin. What nutrient might this be associated with?
    a. Excessive intake of vitamin A
    b. Deficiency of vitamin A
    c. Deficiency of vitamin E
    d. Excessive intake of vitamin E

24. All of the following are leading health indicators for Healthy People 2020 **EXCEPT:**
    a. Physical Activity
    b. Obesity
    c. Diabetes Mellitus
    d. Substance Abuse

25. Using the Hamwi method, calculate the ideal body weight for a 47-year-old male with a height of 6'2" and a weight of 175 pounds.
    a. 171-190 pounds
    b. 171-209 pounds
    c. 190-209 pounds
    d. 180-200 pounds

26. What is the name of the data source through the Centers for Disease Control and Prevention (CDC) that obtains information from individuals in the form of interviews and physical examinations in order to assess the overall nutritional and health status of the United States?
    a. Dietary Guidelines for Americans
    b. National Health and Nutrition Examination Survey
    c. Nationwide Food Consumption Survey
    d. Nutrition Screening Initiative

27. What is the main goal of the Dietary Guidelines for Americans?
    a. To reduce the incidence of diabetes mellitus
    b. To teach parents how to feed their children appropriately
    c. To provide a sample 2,000-calorie meal plan for the majority of Americans to follow in order to lose weight
    d. To try to reduce the overall risk for developing certain chronic diseases through improvement of diet and physical activity

28. All of the following are **TRUE** about Dietary Reference Intake (DRI) **EXCEPT:**
    a. The DRIs take into account both gender and age.
    b. Recommended Dietary Allowances (RDAs), Adequate Intake (AI), and guidelines for safer upper limits all fall under the umbrella of the DRI.
    c. The DRIs are updated every 5 years.
    d. The DRIs were originally written as RDAs to help prevent nutrient deficiencies.

29. What three components comprise a nutrition diagnosis statement?
    a. Problem-Etiology-Signs/Symptoms (PES)
    b. Diagnosis-Etiology-Treatment (DET)
    c. Issue-Cause-Symptoms (ICS)
    d. Problem-Origin-Signs/Symptoms (POS)

30. All of the following are domains within classifications of nutrition diagnoses **EXCEPT:**
    a. Medical
    b. Intake
    c. Behavioral-Environmental
    d. Clinical

31. How does a nutrition diagnosis differ from a medical diagnosis?
    a. They are essentially the same except the nutrition diagnosis is written by the dietitian.
    b. A nutrition diagnosis is a problem or issue that can be addressed through the nutrition intervention of a dietitian or other dietetics professional.
    c. A dietitian cannot diagnose medical conditions. Therefore, a nutrition diagnosis must be substituted.
    d. A nutrition diagnosis enables the dietitian to bill for services rendered.

32. A 30-year-old man is admitted to the hospital with a flare of his Crohn's disease. He is 6' tall and his usual weight is 170 pounds, which he weighed 1 month ago. His weight on admission is 160 pounds. His BMI is 21.7 kg/m². He has not been eating well due to abdominal pain that has been worsening over the past month. Which of the following might be a potential PES statement for this patient?
    a. Increased energy requirements related to decreased intestinal function due to Crohn's disease as evidenced by unintentional weight loss of 10% in the past month
    b. Increased energy requirements related to decreased intestinal function due to Crohn's disease as evidenced by unintentional weight loss of 6% in the past month
    c. Increased energy requirements related to decreased intestinal function due to Crohn's disease as evidenced by loss of muscle mass
    d. Increased energy requirements related to decreased intestinal function due to Crohn's disease as evidenced by a BMI of 21.7 kg/m²

33. You have identified "excessive fat intake" as a problem for one of your clients and "food and nutrition-related knowledge deficit" as the etiology. Which of the following would be most appropriate to use as signs/symptoms?
    a. Decreased serum amylase
    b. HDL cholesterol level of 45 mg/dL
    c. Observation of client eating an order of French fries prior to counseling session
    d. Serum cholesterol level of 260 mg/dL

- 218 -

34. A client is referred to you after being diagnosed with Type 2 diabetes. The client is visibly overweight, reeks of cigarette smoke, and is drinking a bottle of regular soda. As you begin to interview the client, he is sitting with his arms crossed and keeps staring out the window. You learn this is the second time he has been referred to a dietitian. The first time was for assistance with weight loss and blood glucose levels borderline for diabetes, but he did not follow up. You assess one problem to be "not ready for diet/lifestyle change." Based on this information, which is the best choice for a PES statement?

    a. Not ready for diet/lifestyle change related to lack of interest as evidenced by negative body language and failure to engage in counseling

    b. Not ready for diet/lifestyle change related to new diagnosis of diabetes as evidenced by elevated serum blood glucose levels

    c. Not ready for diet/lifestyle change related to failure to engage in counseling as evidenced by negative body language

    d. Not ready for diet/lifestyle change related to failure to keep appointments as evidenced by new medical diagnosis

35. What is the form of documentation that was developed with the Nutrition Care Process in mind?
    a. SOAP
    b. PES
    c. ADIME
    d. PIE

36. Which of the following statements does **NOT** reflect the goals or objectives of nutrition intervention as part of the Nutrition Care Process?
    a. Goals and objectives must be reasonably attainable.
    b. The dietitian should set the most appropriate goals and objectives for the client or patient.
    c. Goals and objectives must be able to be quantified.
    d. Goals and objectives should be centered on the patient or client.

37. Which of the following would be the **MOST IMPORTANT** nutrition intervention for a person identified as having pre-diabetes with a BMI of 27 kg/m²?
    a. Reduction of total fat intake
    b. Moderate weight loss
    c. Reduction of sodium intake
    d. Elimination of concentrated sweets

38. Which of the following foods would **NOT** be allowed on a gluten-free diet?
    a. Canned pears
    b. Cream of rice cereal
    c. Beer
    d. Cottage cheese

39. What factor has the most significant impact on the course of Short Bowel Syndrome (SBS)?
    a. Resection of the jejunum
    b. Age at time of surgery
    c. Resection of the distal ileum
    d. Resection of the duodenum

40. What is the daily protein requirement for a patient with uncomplicated cirrhosis without encephalopathy?
    a. 0.4-0.6 grams/kg
    b. 0.8-1.0 grams/kg
    c. 1.3-1.5 grams/kg
    d. 1.5-2.0 grams/kg

41. What would be an appropriate substitution for a formula-fed infant who has just been diagnosed with a cow's milk protein allergy?
    a. Enfamil
    b. Neosure
    c. Nutramigen
    d. Neocate

42. A 32-year-old female who is 24 weeks pregnant has a random glucose test of 215 mg/dL. She has a pregravid BMI of 31 kg/m². A fasting blood glucose done the next day is 110 mg/dL. She is referred to your office for management of gestational diabetes. What would be an appropriate first step in your nutrition intervention for this woman?
    a. Initiate counseling to reduce carbohydrate intake to 35-40% of total calories
    b. Initiate counseling to reduce carbohydrate intake to 50-60% of total calories
    c. Recommend additional blood glucose testing in the form of a fasting glucose level or an oral glucose tolerance test
    d. Recommend the initiation of insulin or oral hypoglycemic agents to optimize blood glucose control

43. You are beginning to counsel the woman in the previous question on her meal plan. What would be the most appropriate strategy for counseling?
    a. Provide a week's worth of preplanned menus
    b. Teach a No Concentrated Sweets diet
    c. Provide a meal plan using the diabetic exchange system
    d. Provide a meal plan using carbohydrate counting

44. When evaluating an adolescent female for the possibility of an eating disorder, what clinical signs may indicate a diagnosis of bulimia nervosa instead of anorexia nervosa?
    a. Irregular menstrual periods
    b. Hypokalemia
    c. Erosion of the enamel of the teeth
    d. weakness and delayed gastric emptying

45. All of the following are ways that schools are working towards implementing the Dietary Guidelines for Americans **EXCEPT:**
    a. Using a la carte items to supplement calories to meet guidelines
    b. Using standardized recipes to incorporate commodity foods into meal plans
    c. Adjusting portion sizes to meet requirements for various age groups
    d. Voluntary participation in the National School Lunch Program (NSLP)

46. Which of the following is **NOT** an example of ways that the Dietary Guidelines for Americans are utilized?
    a. Development of educational materials and tools based on the guidelines
    b. Placement of information from the guidelines on food labels and the Nutrition Facts Panel
    c. Programs such as the Elderly Nutrition Program, national child nutrition programs, and SNAP
    d. Development of laws such as the Dietary Supplement Health and Education Act

47. How does the Senior Farmers' Market Nutrition Program benefit older adults?
    a. It provides coupons for use by qualified low-income seniors to purchase fresh produce, herbs, and honey at locally sponsored farmers' markets, roadside farm stands, or other community-based agriculture programs.
    b. It provides direct delivery of fresh produce to low-income seniors.
    c. It provides coupons for use by low-income seniors to purchase fresh produce in supermarkets.
    d. It provides assistance with the purchase of locally grown fresh produce, herbs, or honey at farmers' markets and other community-supported farm programs based on a sliding scale for income.

48. Which of the following are the 4 modifiable risk factors that have been identified as key in the prevention and control of high blood pressure?
    a. Weight, sodium, potassium, and physical activity
    b. Weight, sodium, physical activity, and alcohol
    c. Physical activity, alcohol, sodium, and potassium
    d. Sodium, calcium, weight, and physical activity

49. Which of the following is the best initial nutrition prescription for a patient with gastroparesis?
    a. Liquid or puree meals that are high-calorie, high-protein, and low-fat
    b. Small, frequent meals that are high-fiber and moderate-fat plus a minimum of 30 minutes of physical activity per day
    c. Jejunostomy tube placement for enteral nutrition
    d. Small, frequent meals that are low-fiber and low-fat followed by mild exercise such as a walk

50. Which of the following is **TRUE** about the nutrition prescription?
    a. It is the nutrition treatment that is deemed correct for a certain nutrition diagnosis.
    b. It is written prior to the PES.
    c. It is the equivalent of the physician diet order.
    d. It is based on the nutrition and diet history along with the admitting diagnosis.

51. The final step of the Nutrition Care Process is Monitoring/Evaluation. Which of the following domains would **NOT** be the most appropriate starting point in choosing the nutrition outcome indicators?
    a. Nutrition-Focused Physical Findings
    b. Comparative Standards
    c. Client History
    d. Knowledge/Beliefs/Attitudes

52. As the RD for the dialysis clinic, you are following a 54-year-old male patient with end-stage renal disease who started hemodialysis 4 months ago. He has reportedly received diet instruction at his previous dialysis clinic but seems to have trouble adjusting his potassium intake. You have identified the nutrition diagnosis as "Excessive intake of potassium as evidenced by food and nutrition-related knowledge deficit related to elevated serum potassium of 5.5 and frequent consumption of high-potassium foods such as banana and orange juice." The planned nutrition intervention was comprehensive nutrition education on a potassium-modified diet including appropriate food substitutions that are lower in potassium. Which of the following is the best choice for monitoring/evaluation of this patient?

   a. Urine volume and specific gravity (Biochemical data, medical tests, and procedures domain) and level of food and nutrition knowledge (Food/nutrition-related history domain)
   b. Serum potassium (Biochemical data, medical tests, and procedures domain), food/meal selections, and self-reported adherence (Food/Nutrition-related history domain)
   c. Amount of food, types of food/meals, and food variety (Food/Nutrition-related history domain)
   d. Comparison to estimated potassium needs (Comparative standards domain) and serum potassium (Biochemical data, medical tests, and procedures domain)

53. You have a client with a nutrition diagnosis of overweight/obesity and a family history of coronary heart disease and diabetes. The client needs help with weight reduction. All of the following may be appropriate monitoring/evaluation plans for this client **EXCEPT:**

   a. Readiness to change, level of knowledge, physical activity, and total energy intake
   b. Fat and cholesterol intake, total fiber intake, BMI
   c. Lipid profile, fasting blood glucose, triglyceride and cortisol levels
   d. Percentage of usual body weight or ideal body weight, waist circumference, BMI, percent weight change

54. A patient with ovarian cancer and malnutrition is being started on total parenteral nutrition (TPN). What are the **MOST** important lab values to monitor upon initiation of TPN?

   a. Serum phosphorus, potassium, glucose
   b. Serum phosphorus, renal function, glucose
   c. Serum potassium, glucose, triglycerides
   d. Serum sodium, potassium, liver function

55. An 80-year-old female is admitted to the hospital with a stage 2 pressure ulcer on her coccyx. She weighs 100 pounds on admission with a height of 5'2". She has a body mass index of 18.3 and a serum albumin level of 2.2 g/dL. She needs at least 1,500 calories and 68 grams of protein per day. She is able to eat and has been prescribed a high-protein, high-calorie diet with supplements Bld. What is the best way to measure her response to nutritional intervention?

   a. Daily weights
   b. Monitoring for increases in serum albumin and her serum zinc level
   c. Monitoring her protein intake as well as her intake of vitamins and minerals
   d. Consulting with the skin care nurse on progress with healing of the pressure ulcer

56. What is the appropriate action for a patient who does not have a nutrition diagnosis?
    a. If the patient has potential for a nutrition diagnosis or is at risk for developing a nutrition diagnosis, this should be documented.
    b. No nutrition diagnosis should be documented at this time but a plan for reassessment should be documented in the Monitoring/Evaluation step.
    c. No documentation is required.
    d. All patients will have some sort of nutrition diagnosis. You will need to delve further to determine one.

57. Which of the following best describes the labs that would normally be obtained when monitoring liver function?
    a. Bilirubin (direct and indirect), BUN, creatinine, CHEM-7
    b. Alkaline phosphatase, PT/PTT, ferritin
    c. ALT, AST, bilirubin, LDH, ammonia
    d. Ceruloplasmin, zinc, ALT, AST

58. The best choice for measuring long-term glucose control would be:
    a. Fasting glucose
    b. Pre-prandial capillary plasma glucose
    c. Glucose tolerance test
    d. HbA1c

59. All of the following are **TRUE** about documentation of step 4 of the Nutrition Care Process (Monitoring/Evaluation) **EXCEPT:**
    a. The schedule for the frequency of monitoring is based solely on departmental policy and procedures.
    b. It requires a definitive plan of action rather than just "watching" or "following."
    c. Components of this step include monitoring progress, measuring outcomes, and evaluating outcomes.
    d. Progress toward nutrition goals could be more objectively measured on a numerical scale such as 1-5.

60. All of the following are appropriate reasons for discontinuation of care by the dietitian **EXCEPT:**
    a. The patient has met goals for nutrition intervention.
    b. The patient is discharged from the hospital.
    c. The client is not ready to make the necessary changes to meet intervention goals at this time.
    d. No further change in nutrition diagnosis is expected and reasons for lack of progress are documented.

61. In performing a nutrition-focused physical assessment in the area of the mouth, you notice bleeding, spongy gums. What vitamin or mineral may be deficient?
    a. Vitamin A
    b. Vitamin C
    c. Iron
    d. Zinc

62. Which of the following would **NOT** be an appropriate use of nutrition outcome measures in quality improvement?
     a. Evaluation of the healthcare savings associated with a reduced length of stay for certain types of patients
     b. Evaluation of the effectiveness of nutrition care
     c. Evaluation of progress towards national obesity goals
     d. Evaluation of patient-centered outcomes such as quality of life or self-management skills

63. Which of the following most accurately describes the Healthy Diet Goals of the American Heart Association (AHA)?
     a. Consume less than 2,300 mg of sodium, less than 300 mg of cholesterol, 4-5 servings of fruits and vegetables per day, and reduce sugar consumption.
     b. Consume less than 1,500 mg of sodium, less than 200 mg of cholesterol, 5-10 servings of fruits and vegetables per day, reduce sugar consumption, and limit alcohol to 1 drink per day for both men and women.
     c. Consume less than 2,300 mg of sodium per day, increase consumption of soy, eat fish twice per week, and reduce cholesterol intake to less than 300 mg per day.
     d. Consume less than 1,500 mg of sodium, less than 300 mg of cholesterol, 8-10 servings of fruits and vegetables per day, limit alcohol to 1 drink per day for women and 2 per day for men, and reduce consumption of sugar.

64. Which of the following best describes the American Cancer Society's nutrition recommendations for cancer prevention?
     a. Achieve and maintain a healthy weight, increase physical activity to at least 30 minutes per day, increase consumption of fruits and vegetables, choose whole grains, reduce consumption of red meat, limit alcohol intake.
     b. Try to reach ideal body weight, limit alcohol intake, eat 3-5 servings of fruits and vegetables per day, increase exercise to 60 minutes per day.
     c. Achieve and maintain a healthy weight, increase intake of antioxidants through nutrition supplements or foods, avoid aspartame.
     d. Try to reach ideal body weight, reduce fat intake, reduce intake of processed foods, and increase activity to 60 minutes per day 3 times per week.

65. A client enters your office for his initial counseling session for management of hypertension. The physician has asked you to help this man with weight loss, reducing sodium intake, and overall risk reduction. The client sits down, immediately begins to frown, arms are crossed over his chest, and he does not make any eye contact when you initiate conversation. What are the non-verbal clues telling you about this client?
     a. The client is relaxed, ready to listen.
     b. The client is feeling defensive, cold towards you or the situation.
     c. The client is bored or not interested.
     d. The client is anxious about his medical condition.

66. A client is telling you how difficult it is for her to eat healthy when she travels with close friends who are not following the same diet modifications. Which of the following is an example of reflection on the part of the dietitian?

a. "You find it difficult to make healthy food choices while traveling so perhaps we need to rethink these vacation plans so you do not lose ground."

b. "I understand. When I travel, I eat what I want then try twice as hard when I get back."

c. "You feel ashamed that you need to diet while all your friends can eat whatever they want."

d. "You find it difficult to make healthy food choices while on vacation because all your friends are able to eat whatever they want and you find that frustrating."

67. All of the following would be examples of appropriate behavior modification that may be used for children for weight control **EXCEPT:**

a. Limiting TV and computer time to 2 hours max and providing a food reward if goal is met

b. Substituting water for soda or sweetened beverages

c. Eating at the table with family instead of in front of the television

d. Eating a healthy breakfast every morning that is low in sugar, contains fiber and protein, and is low in fat

68. According to the Transtheoretical Model, at which stage of change would an individual be most ready to make nutritional changes?

a. Precontemplation

b. Contemplation

c. Preparation

d. Action

69. All of the following are important communication skills necessary in the facilitation of changes in behavior by the nutrition professional **EXCEPT:**

a. Avoidance of putting the client on the defensive

b. Helping the client to develop discrepancy

c. Confrontation

d. Expression of empathy

70. A 19-year-old female was diagnosed with Type 1 diabetes 4 months ago. She has been doing fairly well trying to implement all the recommendations that have been given to her. She is a late sleeper and often does not have time in the morning to eat breakfast, which leads to issues with hypoglycemia. What would be the **MOST** appropriate intervention to help her make time for breakfast so she can avoid hypoglycemia?

a. Help her come up with healthful breakfast ideas that are easy to eat quickly in the morning.

b. Explain to her the dangers of skipping breakfast and insist that she wake up 1 hour earlier in order to eat a healthy breakfast.

c. Advise her to keep snacks on hand to help prevent hypoglycemia.

d. Acknowledge her difficulty waking up and encourage her to pick up breakfast on the way to school or work to ensure she gets her meal in even if it is not the most healthful.

71. A financial services company has been experiencing an increasing number of absences by employees. Many of the sick days are related to chronic health conditions. The company decides to implement a voluntary nutrition education program that involves seminars on healthy eating, weight loss, increasing physical activity, and managing chronic health conditions such as diabetes. After a period of 9 months of participation, the company wants to evaluate the effectiveness of the program. Which of the following would be the best choice?
    a. Provide a detailed questionnaire to the employees about participation and sick day use.
    b. Determine a baseline for the average amount of sick time used per employee over a period of time and reassess at predetermined intervals.
    c. Compare use of sick time for each employee before and after attending seminars.
    d. Ask employee health services to release information on employees with chronic diseases and determine if use of sick time has declined after participation in the seminars.

72. At the local community center, you are starting a nutrition education series on Heart Healthy Cooking and Eating. What would be a way to evaluate the effectiveness of the program?
    a. At the last session, ask each participant open-ended questions to determine comprehension.
    b. Assess for changes in BMI or serum cholesterol level.
    c. After the series is completed, send participants home with a survey asking for feedback.
    d. Test participants' knowledge before and after they attend the series, then compare the results.

73. The National Institutes of Health initiated the Women's Health Initiative (WHI) in 1991. This was the largest prevention research study done to date. This study is an example of what type of research design?
    a. Epidemiological study
    b. Randomized controlled clinical trial
    c. Cohort study
    d. Phase I trial

74. What was the name of the largest randomized controlled study to date that looked at the effects of dietary protein restriction on how renal disease progresses?
    a. The Effect of Dietary Protein Restriction on the Progression of Renal Disease
    b. Protein Restriction and End Stage Renal Disease
    c. The Modification of Diet in Renal Disease (MDRD)
    d. Dietary Protein and its Effect on the Progression of Renal Disease (DPPRD)

75. What is the definition of a cohort study?
    a. Subjects with the same condition or using the same treatment are followed and observed over time, then compared to subjects without the condition or treatment.
    b. Subjects with the same condition or using the same treatment are paired up with controls to track progress.
    c. Subjects with the same condition are divided into groups and given different treatments, then followed over time to determine best practice. The subjects are not aware of exactly what treatment they are receiving.
    d. A retrospective review of subjects with the same disease

76. For Evidence-Based Practice (EBP), which of the following resources would **NOT** be a primary source of information?
a. Databases such as MEDLINE or Cochrane Library
b. ACP Journal Club
c. Clinical Evidence or eMedicine
d. Wikipedia or Medpedia

77. Which response best describes the purpose of websites such as www.uptodate.com, www.acpmedicine.com, or www.clinicalevidence.com?
a. Websites available for use by the general population
b. A subscription-based source of medical information and recommendations based on current medical research
c. A source of medical information and recommendations based on current medical research available free of charge
d. Database portals allowing access to search medical literature

78. Because hospital stays are becoming increasingly shorter, many hospital food service departments are changing the type of menu used to:
a. Selective
b. Semi-selective
c. Non-selective
d. Static

79. The use of a pre-selective menu would be **MOST** appropriate for:
a. An acute care pediatric inpatient ward
b. A hospital cafeteria
c. A maternity ward at a local hospital
d. A catering function

80. When beginning the menu development process for a 3-week cycle menu, which of the following is the first step in the process:
a. Planning the soups
b. Planning the side dishes
c. Planning the entrees
d. Planning the dinner meals

81. All of the following are part of the menu evaluation. Which is the most important for a long-term care food service operation?
a. Attractiveness of the menu (color, contrast, textures, flavors)
b. Repetition of food items throughout the cycle
c. Determining if the workload is manageable with the available staff and equipment
d. Determining if the menu meets nutritional guidelines

82. Once a menu is established for a long-term care facility, how are therapeutic and modified-consistency diets accommodated?
    a. Modified menu extensions are written by the RD based on the master and are used in conjunction with the institution's diet manual.
    b. A separate menu is written as needed based on physician order.
    c. Menu cycles are written for modified-consistency diets and the most common therapeutic diets.
    d. The menu is served as written and items are substituted as necessary based on diet order.

83. All of the following are steps in the purchasing process. Which step is the first?
    a. Desired quantity is determined and inventory is taken for each item.
    b. Purchase orders are written.
    c. Needs are identified based on the master menu for the operation.
    d. Negotiate with vendors.

84. As the purchasing agent for a local food service operation, you are ordering meat from a vendor located in a neighboring state. Any meat purchased and shipped between states must meet requirements set forth by which of the following government agencies:
    a. U.S. Department of Agriculture
    b. Environmental Protection Agency
    c. Food and Drug Administration
    d. Department of Health and Human Services

85. The type of purchasing method that involves a submission of bids by vendors followed by a formal contract agreement that states the agreed-upon vendor will supply the majority of items needed such as meat, poultry, produce, and dairy is called:
    a. Blanket purchase agreement
    b. Prime vending agreement
    c. Cost-Plus purchase agreement
    d. Competitive agreement

86. All of the following would be an acceptable inventory method for food service **EXCEPT:**
    a. Physical inventory
    b. LIFO
    c. Mini-max system
    d. Par stock system

87. The delivery truck is met at the loading dock for delivery of the dairy order. The employee chats with his coworker as the order is unloaded. The temperatures are quickly checked and recorded. The employee then begins to chat with the driver for a few minutes before he loads up the order and puts it away within 30 minutes of delivery. What important step was missing from this process?
    a. Putting the inventory away
    b. The employee did not check the actual delivery against the purchase order to make sure the delivery was accurate.
    c. The employee did not open all the crates and boxes to check the quality of each item.
    d. The employee did not check the actual delivery against the purchase order and then against the invoice for accuracy.

88. All of the following are important in quantity food production. Which of the following is the **MOST** important factor?
    a. Quality food is the end result
    b. To promote the maximum retention of nutrients through appropriate preparation
    c. To maximize production schedules for the most efficient use of staff and equipment
    d. The use of standardized recipes to help control costs and provide consistent products

89. What would be the easiest way to increase the number of muffins prepared from a small-scale recipe from 1 dozen to 10 dozen?
    a. Use the forecasting method
    b. Use the percentage method
    c. Use the factor method
    d. Conduct a recipe yield evaluation

90. All of the following are advantages to a conventional food service system **EXCEPT:**
    a. This type of system lends itself well to incorporating regional food items and ethnic recipes.
    b. Menus can be easily adapted to incorporate seasonal food items such as fresh produce or to alter the menu based on price fluctuations.
    c. There are less freezer space requirements because food is made from scratch instead of pre-purchased food items.
    d. The production schedule is more predictable and utilization of employee productive time is maximized.

91. If a case of food-borne illness is suspected, the first step would be to contact:
    a. The local health department (city or county)
    b. The state health department
    c. The Centers for Disease Control and Prevention
    d. The National Outbreak Reporting System

92. All of the following foods are on the Food and Drug Administration's "Potentially Hazardous Food" list **EXCEPT:**
    a. Sliced cantaloupe
    b. Peanut butter
    c. Sliced tomatoes
    d. Cooked pinto beans

93. Food-borne illness caused by *Staphylococcus aureus* has an incubation period of:
    a. 6-48 hours
    b. 1/2-6 hours
    c. 8-22 hours
    d. 18-36 hours

94. Which of the following has the most dangerous implications for pregnant women?
    a. Staphylococcus aureus
    b. Bacillus cereus
    c. Listeria monocytogenes
    d. Campylobacter jejuni

95. In order for chlorine to be effectively used as a sanitizer in a food service operation, the pH level must be:
 a. Below 8
 b. Below 5
 c. Above 8
 d. Above 5

96. The maximum temperature that the water in a multi-temperature dish machine should reach is:
 a. 170°
 b. 165°
 c. 212°
 d. 194°

97. Important factors in planning the facilities for a university food service with multiple dormitories and a large commuter population would include all of the following **EXCEPT:**
 a. A first floor location near the main hallway
 b. A state-of-the-art ventilation system to prevent odors from the kitchen from reaching public spaces such as classrooms
 c. Avoiding duplicate purchases of large pieces of food service equipment to cut down on costs
 d. Planning for a cook/chill or cook/freeze system in order to reduce the amount of cooking equipment needed

98. In a facilities design project, which of the following would best describe the information contained in the prospectus?
 a. Project rationale, physical operations and characteristics, necessary regulatory data such as safety features, noise control, and energy use
 b. Members of the planning committee, architectural features, budget considerations
 c. Feasibility study, determination of the food service system to be implemented, spatial considerations
 d. Preliminary design plan, menu analysis, feasibility study

99. Which of the following best describes the characteristics of a bake shop or dessert preparation area within a food service department?
 a. It should be located close to the main production or preparation areas.
 b. It should be laid out in a counterclockwise configuration to increase efficiency, with the final product finishing closest to where it will be served or transported.
 c. It should be laid out in a typical triangle configuration for maximum efficiency.
 d. It can be located within the main food preparation area.

100. A large tertiary care hospital utilizes a cook/chill food service system. Food is prepared in the main preparation area. Trays are prepared on the tray line and then transported to galleys located on the inpatient units, where they are reheated later at meal time to serve to the patients. This type of distribution system is known as:
 a. Centralized
 b. Decentralized
 c. Patient-Centered
 d. Cafeteria style

101. A hospital has an open position for an entry level clinical dietitian. What would be the **LEAST** effective recruiting tool?
   a. Advertising at local area hospitals or colleges with internship programs
   b. Web-based recruiting such as Monster.com or indeed.com
   c. The help wanted section of the local Sunday newspaper
   d. The American Dietetic Association's career center or state affiliate job bank

102. Which of the following is the best way to obtain information during an interview about a potential applicant's experience with managing a large-scale cafeteria?
   a. "Are you able to handle managing a busy cafeteria?"
   b. "Give me an example of a day where staffing levels were short, the cafeteria was busy, and how you handled it."
   c. Describe a situation that has occurred in the cafeteria recently. Ask the applicant if this has ever happened to them.
   d. Call the applicant's references on the spot and ask the same question of them.

103. An employee fired recently due to excessive absenteeism has given your name as a reference for a new job he is applying for. Which of the following would be the **LEAST** appropriate response?
   a. Agree to give the reference but only provide information on dates of employment and job assignment.
   b. Call the former employee and let him know you will not be able to provide a good reference for him.
   c. Refuse to give a reference.
   d. Provide general information to the potential employer about why you think the employee was absent so much and whether the situation has changed enough to merit them hiring this individual.

104. When preparing a performance review, the most important aspects to cover would be:
   a. Employee goals for the coming year
   b. Your goals for the employee for the coming year
   c. Describing the employee's strengths, areas that need improvement, and an action plan for addressing areas that need to change
   d. Determining training needs for the coming year

105. You have prepared a performance appraisal for an employee who has difficulty getting to work on time. The past week has been especially difficult because other employees have had vacation and you needed this employee to get to work on time to start the day. The performance review with the employee takes a long time because you keep focusing on your frustrations. The employee points out that, aside from her tardiness, she does a good job but the performance appraisal does not appear to reflect that. This is known as:
   a. The Halo Effect
   b. The Devil Effect
   c. The Delusional Effect
   d. The Glory Effect

106. The method of budgeting that uses the information from the previous year's budget and then makes adjustments based on predicted changes in revenue and expenses is called:
    a. Level budgeting
    b. Incremental budgeting
    c. Zero-based budgeting
    d. Performance budgeting

107. All of the following are included on a balance sheet **EXCEPT:**
    a. Assets such as cash on hand, petty cash, and accounts receivable
    b. Liabilities such as accounts payable, salaries, and sales tax owed
    c. Assets such as money due from state or federal funds and purchased food and supplies
    d. Liabilities such as equipment or furniture

108. In school food service operations, the unit measure most often used to quantify the effectiveness of the program is:
    a. A la carte items
    b. Student reimbursable breakfast
    c. Student reimbursable lunch
    d. All student reimbursable meals

109. Which of the flowing is **NOT** an example of an essential report used for financial accountability in food service?
    a. Year End Summary
    b. Profit and Loss Statement
    c. Daily Food Cost Report
    d. Daily Beverage Report

110. The Factor Method of menu pricing is commonly used. Which of the following is **TRUE** about the Factor Pricing Method?
    a. The same factor is used with the raw food cost to determine all menu prices taking into account supplies, labor, and profit.
    b. The same factor is used with the total cost of food and labor for each menu item to determine price.
    c. This method often predicts prices that are reasonable for all menu items.
    d. A separate factor for low, medium, and high labor-intensity food items can be used with the raw food cost to determine appropriate pricing.

111. All of the following are ratios used to analyze worker productivity in food service **EXCEPT:**
    a. Total food cost per labor hour
    b. Meals per labor hour
    c. Meals per FTE
    d. Labor minutes per meal

112. A fast food restaurant is considering setting up an operation in a foreign country where people do not eat beef for religious reasons. There are also many more vegetarians in this foreign country than in the United States. Which would **NOT** be an effective marketing tool for this fast food restaurant to employ in order to be successful?

  a. Develop a more extensive vegetarian menu to meet the needs of the majority of the population.
  b. Remove all beef from the menu in order to show respect for the religious beliefs of the area.
  c. Maintain separate work areas that are designated for vegetarian items and non-vegetarian items.
  d. Implement the same menu used in the United States.

113. As a restaurant manager, you are trying to market to "Generation Y." Which of the following would be the **LEAST** effective marketing strategy for this age group?

  a. Set up Facebook, Twitter, or Evite accounts.
  b. Maintain an interesting and informative website.
  c. Play background music from classical selections.
  d. Host entertainment-type events such as karaoke, trivia games, or live music to attract your target audience.

114. Which of the following individuals is known as the "Father of Scientific Management?"
  a. Henry Gantt
  b. Frank Gilbreth
  c. Max Weber
  d. Frederick Taylor

115. Which of the following best describes the primary principles of the Classical Theory of Management?

  a. The highest level of authority within the organization is the one who makes the decisions and distributes instructions. Employees instinctively divide themselves into groups within the organization.
  b. There is a chain of command that starts at the top with the CEO. Disciplinary action is used to improve performance of employees. Mathematical tools and models are used to help managers make decisions.
  c. There is a defined division of work with only one person giving orders. There should be a chain of command starting with the lowest level employee all the way up to the top. Teamwork is the basis for success of the organization. Employees derive great motivation from salary and raises.
  d. Managers must adapt their leadership to the needs to the employee. The motivating factor for each employee must be determined and used to effectively enhance productivity and efficiency.

116. Which of the following skills would be considered the most desirable for an upper-level manager to have?
  a. Human skills
  b. Conceptual skills
  c. Technical skills
  d. Negotiating skills

117. What is the following an example of?

Payroll title: Nutrition Assistant

Department: Patient Services

Supervised by: Trayline Manager

Job Summary: Assists patients in receiving the appropriate modified and therapeutic diet in accordance with hospital policy and procedures. Assists with the setup of the trayline at designated times and participates in cleaning activities when the trayline is finished.

Educational Requirements: Minimum high school diploma or equivalent. Must read and write English. Must be able to communicate effectively in English.

Experience Required: 6 months experience in a hospital or nursing home.

Physical Requirements: Must be able to stand for long periods of time (2 hours) and lift 30 pounds.

Personal Requirements: Must be neat, clean, and have good personal hygiene.

Salary Code: level 4

Opportunities for Advancement: Food Service Supervisor
   a. Job specification
   b. Job description
   c. Work schedule
   d. Job posting

118. An RD moves to a new state and applies for a job as a clinical dietitian. Which of the following would be considered a breach of the American Dietetic Association Professional Code of Ethics?
   a. The dietitian is licensed in her home state but has not yet applied for licensure in the new state of residence.
   b. The dietitian has a side business selling nutritional supplements geared to helping patients with cancer improve their nutritional status.
   c. The dietitian uses the credential of CSR (Certified Specialist in Renal Nutrition) even though she let the credential lapse and did not retake the exam before the deadline.
   d. The dietitian took a break from practice in between jobs to work on an alcohol dependency issue.

119. Which of the following is **NOT** included on the Joint Commission on Accreditation of Healthcare Organizations (JCAHO) official "Do Not Use" List?
   a. IV
   b. IU
   c. Q.D.
   d. @

120. The physician in the hospital has written an order for 10U of regular insulin. The order is transcribed as 100U and given to the patient. Within minutes, the patient begins to have a severe hypoglycemic reaction with a blood glucose level of 15 mg/dL and is transferred to the ICU for management. According to the JCAHO, this would be known as:
   a. Medical Error
   b. Sentinel Event
   c. Adverse Event
   d. Root Cause Analysis

121. Which of the following is **TRUE** regarding the Hand Hygiene recommendations from the JCAHO for individuals passing trays to patients in a hospital?
 a. Artificial nails are acceptable if scrubbed well before serving.
 b. The person serving the trays should stop and wash their hands with soap and water after each tray is delivered.
 c. The person should put on a pair of gloves at the beginning of tray delivery then remove them when trays have been completely passed.
 d. The person passing the food tray should practice proper hand hygiene if direct contact is made with the patient while delivering the tray.

122. Total Quality Management (TQM) is based on which of the following assumptions?
 a. Most employees do not have an innate desire to do their job well and in fact require substantial extrinsic motivators such as salary or bonuses.
 b. A management approach that encourages independent thinking and competition within the workplace to get the best results possible.
 c. Most employees have self-motivation, an innate desire to do their job well, and a desire to learn and improve themselves within their job.
 d. A management approach that focuses on the end result, which is the product.

123. What is the TQM problem-solving tool that illustrates the cause and effect of a specific problem?
 a. Fish diagram
 b. Pareto chart
 c. Process chart
 d. Scatter diagram

124. All of the following agencies help to regulate food safety **EXCEPT:**
 a. USDA
 b. FDA
 c. EPA
 d. CSPI

125. All of the following would fall under the regulation of OSHA **EXCEPT:**
 a. The right to receive training on the chemicals you may be exposed to in the workplace
 b. The right to file a discrimination complaint for refusing to work in an unsafe environment
 c. The right to reasonable accommodations in the workplace for a disability
 d. The right to request that safety hazards be addressed even if they are not in violation of OSAH standards

Answers and Explanations

1. B: Alpha-linoleic acid and linoleic acid are essential fatty acids (EFAs) that cannot be synthesized in the human body and must be consumed through the diet. Alpha-linoleic acid is a precursor to eicosapentaenoic acid and docosahexaenoic acid. Linoleic acid is the precursor for arachidonic acid. EFAs have a wide range of functions and many are still under investigation. These acids have a role in vision and brain development, may also play a role in reducing cardiovascular risk, and may act as anti-inflammatory agents. EFAs may also play a role in the treatment of certain neurologic and mental disorders such as Alzheimer's disease and bipolar disorder. The research is ongoing regarding the benefits of EFAs. Fatty fish are a great source of EFAs and so are certain types of vegetable oil such as safflower, sunflower, and flaxseed oil.

2. D: The enzyme pepsin is present in gastric juice and works to hydrolyze peptide bonds into polypeptides and amino acids. Trypsin is found in exocrine secretions from the pancreas and works to hydrolyze peptide bonds as well. Other enzymes that have a role in protein digestion include chymotrypsin, carboxypeptidase, aminopeptidase, and dipeptidase. Protein digestion begins in the stomach primarily by the action of pepsin. Pepsin requires the presence of hydrochloric acid in order to be converted from its inactive form called pepsinogen. The end product of protein digestion is amino acids.

3. A: The large intestine is also known as the colon. The large intestine is made up of the cecum, ascending colon, transverse colon, descending colon, and sigmoid colon. The primary role of the large intestine is water and sodium resorption. As much as 10 liters of water derived from food and secretions enter the large intestine throughout the day. Most of this water is reabsorbed in the colon. Any alteration in this process can lead to massive diarrhea and dehydration. The large intestine also absorbs vitamin K produced by bacteria found in the colon. The majority of the digestion and absorption of food has already occurred once the food reaches the large intestine. The remnants of the digestion process continue to move through the large intestine in the form of waste until it is ultimately excreted.

4. B: The average adult without any major stresses will typically require approximately 30-35 kcal/kg daily. If this same person becomes stressed with an injury, infection, or other insult, daily calorie requirements may increase to above 35 kcal/kg. A range of 20-25 kcal/kg per day is typically used to promote weight loss. These are just quick rules of thumb and there are alternative ways to estimate energy requirements. The Harris Benedict equation calculates basal energy expenditure. Activity and/or stress factors are added to the equation to get an estimation of calorie requirements. Calorie requirements can also be measured by indirect calorimetry, which measures the resting metabolic rate. That rate is about 10-20% higher than the basal metabolic rate.

5. C: Beriberi is caused by a thiamin deficiency. Beriberi is a type of neuropathy with symptoms of mental confusion, difficulty with speech, difficulty ambulating, loss of sensation in hands and feet, tingling sensations, and erratic eye movements. It is a rare disorder because many foods are now fortified with a variety of nutrients, including thiamin. People with chronic alcohol abuse have a greater risk of developing beriberi because of poor nutrition and poor absorption of thiamin related to the alcohol abuse. There is also a genetic form of beriberi. Food sources of thiamin include enriched whole grains, lean meats such as pork, fish, and dried beans. People with chronic alcohol abuse should take a thiamin supplement.

6. D: Hypercalcemia can result from persistently high intakes of calcium (greater than 200 mg per day). Excessive calcium consumption is especially dangerous when it occurs in conjunction with high doses of vitamin D, which can further elevate serum calcium levels. Hypercalcemia does not cause vitamin D toxicity. Soft tissue calcification in areas such as the kidneys is a potential consequence. Hypercalcemia can interfere with the absorption of iron, zinc, and manganese. It can have an adverse effect on GI function (by causing a decline in the autonomic nervous system) and may increase gastric acid secretion, which can lead to nausea and vomiting. Constipation is a potential result of hypercalcemia-related dehydration. Hypercalcemia can also cause secondary bone fractures, have a negative effect on muscle strength, and interfere with contractions of the heart. Hypercalcemia is very dangerous and should be treated and corrected immediately.

7. B: There are many different ways to calculate maintenance fluid requirements. A quick rule of thumb is 35 mL/kg for adults, 50-60 mL/kg for children, and 150 mL/kg for infants. The Holliday-Segar Formula is based on weight as well. For weights of 0-10 kg, fluid requirements are 100 mL/kg. For weights of 11-20 kg, fluid requirements are 1,000 mL + 50 mL/kg for each kg above 10 kg. For weights greater than 20 kg, fluid requirements are 1,500 mL + 20 mL/kg for each kg above 20 kg. In the above example, the 30-year-old woman weighs 130 pounds or 59 kg. Her fluid requirements using the first equation would be 2,065 mL of fluid. Using the Holliday-Segar Formula, her fluid requirements would be (1,500 mL) + (20 mL x 39 kg) = 2,280 mL. The best answer would be 2,100 mL per day.

8. C: The term "folding" refers to a gentle turning motion to incorporate one ingredient such as whipped cream into another. The purpose of folding is to keep the air distributed throughout the ingredients, not to eliminate it. The end product should be light and fluffy. A recipe that has been folded too much will not rise as well because the air has escaped. If a recipe calls for folding in dry ingredients, the result will be a much tenderer product because the gluten will not be overdeveloped. Folding is typically done at the end of a recipe after the main ingredients have been added.

9. A: Any cut of meat that comes from an area on the animal that gets a lot of exercise will be less tender. A chuck roast is a less tender cut of meat. This cut comes from the shoulder area and needs a moist method of cooking in order to soften the meat and tenderize. Braising usually involves quickly browning the roast in hot fat such as oil then simmered in liquid in a covered pot. This method typically lasts several hours to produce a tender roast. The purpose of braising less tender cuts of meat is to allow time for the tougher connective tissue to break down and turn into gelatin. The liquid that is left at the end of braising can be used to make a gravy or sauce. Other cuts of beef such as eye of round can handle either a moist method of cooking, such as braising or being cooked in a slow cooker or a dry method such as roasting.

10. D: Proper canning procedures for various types of food can greatly reduce the risk for *Clostridium botulinum*. This bacterium can cause death and needs to be taken seriously. Ideal growing conditions for *C. botulinum* spores include a low-acid, moist environment, improper canning temperature (i.e., between 40° and 120° F), and oxygen content less that 2%. Low-acid foods have a pH of 4.6 or higher and include seafood, meats, dairy, and all fresh vegetables except tomatoes. Allowing proper head space is important. For a low-acid food, proper head space would be 1-1.25". Any low-acid food should be sterilized to a minimum of 240° F. Pressure canners are recommended for all low-acid foods and the canner should be allowed to return to room temperature on its own.

11. B: Tofu is also known as soya curd. It is generally a bland tasting protein alternative that comes in firm, soft, and silken textures. Tofu is an excellent source of high quality protein and is a good source of calcium and B vitamins. Tofu itself is low in fiber because the fiber is removed in the processing of the soybean. Tofu contains isoflavones, which may help to reduce the risk for certain types of cancer. Tofu can also help to reduce the overall cardiac risk by lowering LDL cholesterol. Other reported health benefits include reduction in menopausal symptoms (due to the presence of phytoestrogens) and in the risk for osteoporosis.

12. C: The American Dietetic Association defines a functional food as any food that may reduce the risk for developing certain diseases and/or promote the best possible health status. Categories of functional foods include conventional foods such as garlic for its antioxidant properties or tomatoes for their potential cancer-fighting properties due to their lycopene content. Another category is modified foods with subcategories of fortified foods such as calcium-fortified orange juice, enriched foods such as folate-enriched to bread to help reduce the risk of neural tube defects, and enhanced foods such as energy bars and beverages with vitamins or protein. Medical foods such as tube-feeding products also fall under the umbrella of functional foods. So do foods that are intended for special dietary use such as gluten-free or lactose-free foods.

13. A: Convection cooking is similar to using a conventional oven except that a convection oven has a fan that circulates hot air throughout. This reduces the amount of time required to cook, promotes more even cooking, and helps the oven to work more efficiently by eliminating hot spots. A convection oven enables the baking of multiple cookie sheets without the risk of overcooking the sheet closest to the heating element. Meats or poultry that are cooked in a convection oven will be browned all over rather than just on the top.

14. C: The type of flour used in a recipe is very important. Flour contains protein and upon contact with liquid, becomes gluten. Gluten is what provides the elasticity to baked goods. The different types of flour contain differing amounts of protein. All-purpose flour typically contains 10-12% protein whereas cake flour contains only 6-8%, making for a tenderer product. Bread flour contains more protein at 12-14%. If cake flour is not available, a better substitution would be all-purpose flour rather than bread flour. The use of bread flour may not allow for proper spread while baking.

15. B: Magnesium deficiency is rare in the United States. Symptoms may include nausea, vomiting, poor appetite, tingling sensation, muscle cramps, and abnormal rhythms of the heart. Of the individuals listed, a breast-fed infant will least likely require magnesium supplementation. The only vitamin or mineral a breast-fed infant may need is iron or vitamin D. Certain medications such as diuretics or antibiotics may increase magnesium excretion. Individuals with chronic alcohol abuse are at risk for magnesium deficiency typically related to overall poor quality of diet because food is often replaced with alcohol. Individuals with conditions that cause chronic diarrhea such as regional enteritis, Crohn's disease, ulcerative colitis, or malabsorption are at risk for magnesium deficiency. Older adults are also at risk because as the aging process occurs, magnesium absorption rates decrease. This coupled with a possible reduced magnesium intake can lead to deficiency.

16. B: Nutrition screening is the first step in the process of nutrition assessment. The main goal is to identify individuals who have risk factors placing them at risk for malnutrition. Another goal is to identify the individual who may need a more in-depth nutrition assessment by an RD. The nutrition screening process involves a healthcare professional such as an RD, dietetic technician, nurse, or doctor who administers a questionnaire to the individual. The information that is obtained relates to weight history, diagnoses, prior use of a modified diet, use of parenteral or enteral nutrition, certain laboratory data, medication use, and status of the individual's gastrointestinal tract such as

the presence of nausea, vomiting, or diarrhea. All of this information is evaluated for triggers and the individual is referred to the RD as needed for further assessment.

17. A: There are many parameters that are often used to identify nutritional risk. These parameters include unintentional weight loss, change in appetite, decreased ability to chew, certain food allergies, BMI, certain laboratory data, and diet modifications. Only two of these parameters have actually been validated, unintentional weight change and change in appetite or food intake. Generally, an unplanned weight loss of 5% or more in 1 month or 10% or more over 6 months is considered to be a risk factor. Insufficient intake for a period greater than 1 week is also considered to be a risk factor. Albumin and other serum proteins have frequently been used to screen for nutritional risk. But there are so many variables that can affect those values that they are not always the most reliable screening parameters for malnutrition.

18. D: An adult who is admitted to an acute care hospital should receive nutritional screening within 24 hours. This is a realistic time frame to identify those individuals at risk for malnutrition and it is also a requirement of the JCAHO. For a long-term care facility, 14 days is acceptable. A patient receiving home care services should be screened at the initial nursing visit. If a patient is indentified as being at risk, a referral is made for a full assessment by the RD including a detailed nutrition history, review of weight and other anthropometric data, and a review of the medical history and status. If the patient is not at nutritional risk, a plan should be made to rescreen after a predetermined period or to rescreen if the patient's condition changes and could potentially affect nutritional status.

19. C: The NSI was developed collaboratively by the American Dietetic Association, American Academy of Family Physicians, and National Council on the Aging to help more effectively screen older adults for nutrition issues. A questionnaire was developed using the acronym DETERMINE. This stands for **D**isease, **E**ating Poorly, **T**ooth Loss or Mouth Pain, **E**conomic Hardship, **R**educed Social Contact, **M**ultiple Medicines, **I**nvoluntary Weight Loss or Gain, **N**eeds Assistance in Self-care, and **E**lder Years Above Age 80. This was designed as a tool that would be easy to use by a variety of practitioners or caregivers.

20. D: Food frequency is one method of obtaining information on dietary intake. It is typically in the form of a questionnaire and looks back at how often certain foods are consumed over a period of a day, week, or other time frame; it requires the individual to estimate food portion sizes. Once collected, food consumption data are organized into related categories and can provide insight into the overall quality of an individual's diet. One advantage to using a food frequency questionnaire is that the information obtained can be standardized. Furthermore, when the questionnaire is used in conjunction with another data-gathering method, the information obtained can be even more valuable in determining potential nutrient deficiencies. A disadvantage is that food frequency questionnaires do not give any information about an individual's typical meal patterns.

21. A: A Nutrient Intake Analysis is commonly known as a calorie count or nutrient intake record. It is typically used in a hospital or long-term care facility. Actual intake is recorded over a certain period, usually 72 hours, simply by observing what is left on the individual's tray after meals. Usually a staff member such as the nurse, nursing assistant, or dietary aide will record the information but this is occasionally done by family members as well. One of the disadvantages of a Nutrient Intake Analysis is that it requires the ability to estimate what has been consumed and may leave off food that is consumed at times other than meals.

22. B: Kwashiorkor is a form of malnutrition characterized by preservation of weight but depletion of visceral proteins such as albumin. It is commonly seen in poor countries where the food supply is limited or following natural disasters where the food supply has been impacted. It is also seen in areas where education is limited and people do not have a good understanding of proper nutrition. One of the most common symptoms of kwashiorkor is edema and a protruding abdomen. Other symptoms may include changes in hair, increased infections, skin rash, a reduction in muscle mass, and diarrhea. Stunted growth is common in children with kwashiorkor and long-term stunting will occur if they are left untreated.

23. A: A Nutrition-Focused Physical Assessment is part of the overall nutrition assessment process. Physical signs of malnutrition are identified by systematically reviewing all systems and parts of the body, starting with the head and working to the feet. If non-nutritional causes of yellow skin pigmentation such as jaundice have been ruled out, a nutritional reason may be excessive intake of carotene or vitamin A sources such as carrots or other orange vegetables. Other signs of vitamin A toxicity may include a bulging fontanel or softening of the skull bone, poor appetite, and extreme tiredness. Skin or hair changes may be evident. Women who are pregnant should not take too much vitamin A as it may be harmful to the fetus.

24. C: Healthy People 2020 is a set of national heath objectives to be addressed over the next decade. The overall goals are to increase life expectancy and improve health discrepancies in the population. Leading health indicators are used to address the highest areas of concern and these are further divided into focus areas. The leading health indicators include physical activity, overweight and obesity, use of tobacco, substance abuse, sexual behavior, mental health, violence, quality of the environment, immunizations, and overall access to healthcare. Diabetes is a focus area that is part of several leading health indicators such as physical activity, overweight and obesity, and tobacco use.

25. B: The Hamwi method for calculating ideal body weight was developed by Dr. G.J. Hamwi and published in 1964 in the journal of the American Diabetes Association. This calculation calls for using a different equation for men and women. An adjustment of plus or minus 10% is allowed for differences in body frame size (small, medium, or large). For men, 106 pounds is allotted for the first 5 feet of height and an additional 6 pounds is allotted for each inch over 5 feet. For women, 100 pounds is allotted for the first 5 feet, then 5 pounds for each additional inch. This equation does not take into account age. For a male who is 6'2" inches tall, the ideal body weight for a medium frame would be 190 pounds with a range of 171-209 pounds to encompass small to large frames.

26. B: The National Center for Health Statistics administers the National Health and Nutrition Examination Survey (NHANES) through the CDC. What makes NHANES unique is that information is obtained from individuals in interviews and physical examinations. This program started in the 1960's and has evolved over the years to be an important source of data used to address continually changing health needs. NHANES looks at risk factors such as lifestyle choices, physical activity, and genetic predisposition to certain diseases. The interviews are done in the individual's home and each person must see the study physician for a physical exam. The results of the study are published in various journals and used to plan health programs throughout the nation. One example of how NHANES information is used is in the development of growth charts for children.

27. D: The Dietary Guidelines for Americans were initiated in 1977 in the Senate Select Committee on Nutrition and Human Needs. In 1980, the Department of Health and Human Services (HHS) and the United States Department of Agriculture (USDA) adopted the guidelines, which have been updated every 5 years. The next revision is due in 2010. The main goal is to improve the health of

the nation and reduce the risk of developing chronic diseases through diet and exercise. The guidelines touch on the following areas: weight control, physical activity, eating a variety of foods, increasing fruits and vegetables, reducing fat intake, altering the types of fat consumed, increasing fiber-containing foods, preventing food-borne illness, reducing sodium intake, and reducing alcohol intake. The guidelines were designed for all Americans over the age of 2.

28. C: The RDAs were originally written in 1941 as a way to prevent nutrient deficiencies and the associated diseases and to encourage good nutritional health. The RDAs are revised every 10 years. The terminology changed in 1998 to Dietary Reference Intake (DRI). The DRIs include the RDAs as well as Adequate Intake (AI), Estimated Average Requirement (EAR), and Tolerable Upper Limits (ULs) of certain nutrients for which data is available. The DRIs include guidelines for various age groups, each gender, and for pregnant and lactating women.

29. A: The Nutrition Diagnosis part of the Nutrition Care Process is comprised of 3 parts: the problem or diagnostic label, the etiology or contributing risk factors, and the signs/symptoms or defining characteristics. The acronym PES is used to describe the format for the nutrition diagnostic statement. Words such as increased, decreased, risk of, or altered are used to describe the problem. The purpose of the etiology portion is to help delineate who is responsible for addressing the issue. Sometimes a problem is related to a nutrition issue while others are related to the disease process or other factor. The key is the etiology must link the problem to the cause and is defined by the phrase "as related to." The signs/symptoms are the objective data used to show the problem is real. Words are linked together with the phrase "as evidenced by." This format helps to develop the critical thinking skills of the dietitian in thinking through issues.

30. A: The nutrition diagnoses are divided into 3 domains: Intake, Clinical, and Behavioral-environmental. Each domain is further divided into classes to address all issues. The Intake domain is related to what the individual consumes through an oral diet and through enteral or parenteral nutrition. This would include all nutrients, calories, vitamins, minerals, and fluid. The Clinical domain is all nutritional issues that are related to medical or physical alterations. The Behavioral-Environmental domain encompasses issues related to the environment, knowledge, food-borne illnesses, ability to access food, and any special beliefs regarding food such as religious or cultural.

31. B: A physician is designated as the person who makes a medical diagnosis. A nutrition diagnosis is designed to identify an issue that can be treated with nutrition intervention. The dietitian or other dietetics professional uses the information collected in the assessment phase to label the patient's issue. Special terminology is used to make this diagnosis and can be found at http://www.adaevidencelibrary.com/files/File/Nutrition%20Diagnosis.pdf. Each nutrition diagnosis has a specific definition as well as potential etiologies and signs/symptoms. The nutrition care provided is standardized. Nutrition diagnoses are ranked in order of urgency.

32. B: Using the stated patient scenario, the Intake domain could be utilized with class of nutrients. He has lost 6% of his body weight as compared to usual but his BMI remains within the normal range. In order for BMI to be used, the BMI would need to be less than 18.5 kg/m² indicative of being underweight. One possible PES statement is to comment on his weight loss due to the presence of Crohn's disease. Increased energy requirements (problem) related to decreased intestinal function due to Crohn's disease (etiology) as evidenced by unintentional weight loss of 6% in the past month (signs/symptoms).

33. D: Under the domain of Intake, excessive fat intake is defined as the consumption of higher levels of fat as compared to current recommendations. There are several etiologies that can be used

based on an interview with the client. These could include a knowledge deficit or attitudes related to food or nutrition that may be harmful to overall health (for example, the client may have reported "I am probably going to die early because my father died at age 45 of a heart attack."). Another possible etiology could be that the client does not see the value or merit in changing behavior ("Why does it matter, I am going to need medication anyway?"). Of the signs and symptoms listed, the elevated serum cholesterol is the best defining characteristic for this problem. The HDL level of 45 is protective. An elevated serum amylase would be more indicative of a problem with excessive fat intake. Intake of high-fat foods must be frequent.

34. A: Under the domain of Behavioral-Environmental, the problem of "not ready for diet/lifestyle change" is defined as the client not seeing the value of changing nutrition-related behavior. The client may not be able to see or understand the consequences of current behavior or may exhibit behavior that is the opposite of what is expected of him. Potential etiologies may include denial, absence of a support network to help implement changes, or knowledge deficit that may be harmful in the long term. The most appropriate PES statement would be "Not ready for diet/lifestyle change (problem) related to disinterest in learning information (etiology) as evidenced by negative body language and failure to engage in counseling (signs/symptoms). It is important to differentiate between the root cause of the problem or etiology and the signs/symptoms to define the problem and quantify it. Signs/symptoms would include body language, failure to keep appointments, chronic non-compliance, and overall defensiveness or hostility towards counseling.

35. C: ADIME stands for **A**ssessment, **D**iagnosis, **I**ntervention, **M**onitoring, and **E**valuation. This style of documentation was developed to help facilitate the transition to using the Nutrition Care Process. **A**ssessment includes only the pertinent information used in the assessment such as laboratory data or anthropometrics. **D**iagnosis includes the PES statement. There may be multiple diagnoses but only the ones that will be addressed should be included. **I**ntervention encompasses the plan of action, which could be a change in how a certain nutrient is provided, education, counseling, or referral for additional care. **M**onitoring and **E**valuation include plans for determining if interventions were successful. An example is monitoring for improvement in weight status or a certain lab value.

36. B: In the Nutrition Care Process, nutrition intervention must be client or patient-focused with goals set collaboratively between the patient and nutrition practitioner. The interventions need to be attainable and measurable. Interventions should answer the questions of what, when, where, and how. Standard nutrition intervention terminology is available and can be found at http://www.adancp.com/vault/editor/Docs/IDNT_NI_Terms_Jan09.pdf .

The interventions can encompass food or nutrient delivery such as meals and snacks, supplements, feeding assistance, and the feeding environment. It can also include nutrition education, nutrition counseling, and coordination of nutrition care such as arranging for a team meeting or a referral to community agencies.

37. B: Pre-diabetes is a term that refers to a state of impaired glucose metabolism. A fasting glucose level of 100-125 mg/dL is considered to be pre-diabetes. The American Diabetes Association recommends that all adults over the age of 45 with a BMI greater than 25 kg/m^2 be screened so appropriate intervention can begin. The most important nutrition intervention is counseling on lifestyle and diet changes to achieve moderate weight loss. The goal is to reduce the risk for developing type 2 diabetes and heart disease. This can be achieved with an increase in physical activity and by improving the baseline diet with better and healthier food choices.

38. C: A gluten-free diet is indicated in certain conditions such as celiac disease. Omitting gluten helps the intestinal mucosa heal and return to normal. Grains that are avoided in a gluten-free diet include wheat, rye, barley, and oats. Appropriate substitutions are corn, rice, soybeans, potatoes, tapioca, arrowroot, quinoa, and buckwheat. Labels must be read very carefully to identify any gluten-containing additives as many items containing gluten are added in the processing of certain foods. Beer is typically made from barley and is thus not allowed in a gluten-free diet.

39. C: SBS is a condition of malabsorption of nutrients. It is mainly due to massive resections of the small intestine. If more than 40-60% of the small intestine is removed, severe malabsorption may result. If the jejunum is resected, the ileum will adapt and take over many of the jejunum's functions. Resection of the distal ileum will have the most significant impact on the course of SBS because of its unique functions. One of the main ones is to absorb several liters of fluid throughout the day. The distal ileum is the only site for the absorption of vitamin B12 and bile salts. Bile salt malabsorption leads to an inability to digest fats, which in turn leads to fat malabsorption and deficiencies in the fat-soluble vitamins. Without bile salts entering the colon, the ability of the colon to reabsorb water and salt is reduced, leading to major problems with dehydration and massive diarrhea.

40. B: The amount of protein required in liver disease remains a controversial topic. Many studies have been done over the years; however, changes in nutrition practice are still under review. Current schools of thought suggest that protein restriction occur only during acute hepatic encephalopathy in conjunction with ammonia-lowering medications such as lactulose or neomycin. Once the mental status has cleared, protein intake should advance. A patient with uncomplicated, stable cirrhosis can usually handle at least the RDA for protein. For those patients with malnutrition, an increase to 1.2-1.3 grams/kg/day may be warranted. Those individuals with alcoholic hepatitis or infection may require as much as 1.5 grams/kg of protein daily. The key is close monitoring of protein tolerance.

41. C: As many as 15% of infants develop an allergy to cow's milk protein. One of the first symptoms is the presence of blood in the infant's stool. Various tests are available to diagnose the condition; however, the elimination of the cow's milk protein followed by reintroduction is often the best way to treat the allergy. For breast-fed infants, this would mean removal of all cow's milk protein-containing foods from the maternal diet. For infants who are formula fed, it means a change to a hypoallergenic, extensively hydrolyzed formula such as Nutramigen or Alimentum. Sometimes an amino acid-based formula such as Neocate would be required but is not usually the first step. This is typically tried if the infant is not able to tolerate an extensively hydrolyzed formula.

42. A: The most appropriate initial intervention is counseling by an RD with individualized medical nutrition therapy. Calorie requirements, total weight gain goals, and blood glucose goals should be determined. Approximately 25 kcal/kg daily may be sufficient to achieve these goals. Carbohydrate intake should be calculated to provide 35-40% of total calories. Oral hypoglycemic agents have not been approved for use in pregnant women. Insulin may be required, but a minimum of 2 weeks of medical nutrition therapy should occur first to see where blood glucose levels stabilize. Sometimes insulin is started immediately if the fasting blood glucose level is greater than 115 mg/dL. An oral glucose tolerance test is not required if there is already proof of glucose impairment.

43. D: The most appropriate way to initiate counseling is to control blood glucose levels using carbohydrate counting. Foods that contain carbohydrates should be reviewed with the patient and it should be explained that foods are grouped into serving sizes containing 15 grams of carbohydrate. Serving sizes need to be demonstrated using appropriate tools such as food models

or measuring utensils. Instruction on reading a food label is also important as carbohydrate information can easily be found there. Patients can be provided with generalized food lists that indicate serving sizes within food groups such as starches, fruits, vegetables, sweets, dairy, etc. Discussion of carbohydrate distribution throughout the day is also useful. Other helpful nutrition information to give patients includes sample menus and facts about the importance of lean meats and healthy fats.

44. C: Eating disorders have many potential medical consequences. Among the types of eating disorders are anorexia nervosa and bulimia nervosa. Sometimes the signs and symptoms of these disorders make it difficult to differentiate one disorder from the other. This is especially true for anorexia nervosa because there are 3 subtypes—restricting behavior, bingeing/purging, and a combination. Bulimia nervosa is usually cyclical and is most often due to the need to try to exert control over emotions and to cope with stress. Purging methods include self-induced vomiting, use of laxatives or enemas, fasting, and excessive exercise. An individual who uses vomiting as a way to control intake will eventually exhibit signs of dental erosion. The enamel portion of the teeth will begin to wear off due to the presence of stomach acid. Many of the signs and symptoms are similar to those of anorexia nervosa including weakness, inability to concentrate, menstrual irregularities, constipation, and electrolyte abnormalities.

45. A: The NSLP is a voluntary program through the federal government that aims to assist school districts with cash subsidies, food commodities, and bonus foods for every meal served to children. In 1995, the USDA implemented the School Meals Initiative for Healthy Children with the goal of improving the overall quality of school lunches for children over the age of 2. The meals must contain less than 30% of calories from fat over a week's period and meet a third of the RDAs for protein, iron, vitamins A and C, and calcium. The use of standardized recipes helps to determine how each item served fits into the guidelines. Ensuring that all portions are age-appropriate is another measure taken to meet the guidelines. Generally, the a la carte sales do not meet the requirements for reimbursement and therefore are not part of any measure to improve overall nutrition in schools.

46. D: The Dietary Guidelines for Americans play a role in so many programs and areas. The Guidelines are the basis for many nutrition programs such as the National School Lunch Program, the Elderly Nutrition Program, and the WIC program. The SNAP program, or Supplemental Nutrition Assistance Program formerly known as Food Stamps, now has an educational component known as SNAP-Ed. This is a feature that aims to educate SNAP users on healthy food choices based on the Dietary Guidelines. The Guidelines are also utilized in the development of many educational resources, including the Food Guide Pyramid, and are the basis of the Nutrition Facts panel on food labels. The Guidelines are not a direct basis for the implementation of the Dietary Supplement Health and Education Act, although the federal government does recommend that people try to achieve the Dietary Guidelines using food instead of supplements.

47. A: The Senior Farmers' Market Nutrition Program is funded through the 2008 Farm Bill. The program is administered through the USDA's Food and Nutrition Service. Its goal is to provide locally grown fresh produce, herbs, and honey to low-income seniors. The produce is purchased from local farmers' markets, roadside farm stands, or other local distributors to help the local farmer. The program is income-based and any low-income senior who is over the age of 60 and has an income less than 185% of the federal poverty guidelines is eligible. The program itself lasts as long as the local growing season. Therefore, some areas of the country will have a longer period in which to acquire fresh produce.

48. B: There are many risk factors for the development of hypertension including family history, smoking, high sodium intake, lack of physical activity, and being overweight. Four risk factors have been identified as having the ability to prevent and control hypertension if modified. These risk factors include weight, sodium intake, physical activity, and alcohol intake. Weight loss is especially useful in the prevention of hypertension across the age spectrum. Reducing sodium intake can sometimes cause an immediate reduction in blood pressure in salt-sensitive individuals. As little as 3 alcoholic drinks per day can increase blood pressure, so it is best to limit alcohol intake to less than 2 drinks per day for men. Increasing physical activity can be protective not only against hypertension but also against stroke and heart disease. Other dietary factors that may have an impact on hypertension are potassium, calcium, magnesium, and fat reduction; however, none of these has proven to be useful as a primary method of controlling hypertension.

49. D: Gastroparesis is hypomotility in the stomach that interferes with the normal emptying of the stomach. Symptoms of gastroparesis include nausea, vomiting, bloating, poor appetite, and weight loss. This condition is not curable but can be managed with dietary changes and medications such as ondansetron (Zofran) for nausea or metoclopramide (Reglan) to stimulate the GI muscles. Surgery is sometimes considered as well. Dietary changes involve changing eating patterns to smaller meals eaten more frequently throughout the day. Patients with gastroparesis should select foods that are lower in fiber instead of raw, such as canned or well-cooked vegetables or fruits. Fibrous foods such as celery should also be avoided. Lower-fat foods are a better option for these patients as high-fat foods can delay gastric emptying. Mild exercise after meals is recommended to help stimulate digestion. Individuals with diabetes should make sure that blood glucose levels are well controlled. For more severe cases of gastroparesis that do not respond to medical and dietary interventions, a jejunal feeding tube may be recommended.

50. A: The nutrition prescription is the nutrition treatment plan for a patient based on his or her nutrition diagnosis. The nutrition prescription should reflect assessment findings, the PES statement (Problem-Etiology-Signs/Symptoms), and patient preferences. It is important to remember that each nutrition prescription should be unique to the individual. The nutrition prescription should include both the individualized nutrient requirements and the interventions you will be recommending to address the nutrition diagnosis.

51. C: The fourth and final step in the Nutrition Care Process is Nutrition Monitoring and Evaluation. The purpose of this step is to determine the progress that has been made through nutrition interventions. It is a concrete way to determine if the goals and objectives are being met. Nutrition care indicators are selected using the terminology from International Dietetics & Nutrition Terminology (IDNT) Reference Manual, 2nd edition, copyright 2009, American Dietetic Association. There are 4 Nutrition Monitoring and Evaluation domains—Food/Nutrition Related History; Biochemical Data, Medical Tests, and Procedures; Anthropometric Measurements; and Nutrition Focused Physical Findings. Client History is a domain of the Nutrition Assessment step. Client History cannot be used for monitoring and evaluation because nutrition intervention does not alter any of its subclasses (e.g., gender, past medical history, medical treatment, social history).

52. B: The 54 year-old-man with end-stage renal disease on hemodialysis for 4 months has reportedly received nutrition education. Because he admits consuming high-potassium foods such as bananas and orange juice, it is unclear if he received appropriate education, understood the education, or is exhibiting non-compliant behavior. You have decided that comprehensive nutrition education on potassium modification is indicated along with how to make appropriate food substitutions. Any intervention for hyperkalemia needs to include monitoring of serum potassium because this will have a direct impact on assessing compliance and comprehension. Without

initially telling the patient what his lab results are, you could assess self-reported adherence to the diet and review meal/food selections. Depending upon what the lab value is, you would either reinforce current behavior or encourage strategies to help improve self-care and management.

53. C: There are many potential nutrition diagnoses for an overweight/obese individual. In treating such a client, assisting with weight loss can address a multitude of issues including an increased risk of heart disease, diabetes, and other related diseases. Depending upon what is addressed in the nutrition intervention, there are a multitude of potential ways to monitor/evaluate the effectiveness of the nutrition intervention. They can range from assessing beliefs and attitudes to evaluating food and nutrition knowledge to collecting anthropometric data. All aspects of physical activity can be monitored such as level of intensity, frequency, and duration. Monitoring can also include gathering biochemical data such as lipids or glucose, although cortisol is not a piece of biochemical data that would be monitored. While cortisol may play a role in type 2 diabetes and abdominal obesity, it is not a lab value that can be impacted by nutrition intervention and therefore does not need to be included in the monitoring plan.

54. A: Any patient with malnutrition who is starting any form of aggressive nutrition therapy such as total parenteral nutrition (TPN) is at risk for developing refeeding syndrome. If nutrition therapy is started too aggressively, there may be excessive insulin release that leads to an increase in the uptake of glucose at the cellular level causing metabolic derangement. The metabolic consequences may include hypokalemia, hypophosphatemia, hypomagnesemia, hypoglycemia, and changes in fluid balance. This can be very dangerous and can cause alterations in cardiac function, mental status, and respiratory function. It can even lead to death if not monitored and treated. Normal monitoring of TPN parameters should occur but it is most essential to monitor fluid balance, electrolytes, phosphorus, glucose, and body temperature and to watch for signs of clinical deterioration as TPN begins and advances.

55. D: Older adults are at high risk for the development of pressure ulcers, especially those who are bed bound, use a wheel chair frequently, or have difficulty repositioning themselves on their own. Diabetes, obesity, vascular issues, or other medical issues raise the risk of pressure ulcers even further. Malnutrition is often present, as it is in the woman described in this case. Prevention is the key for pressure ulcers and can be accomplished by monitoring weight, checking skin for breakdown, and monitoring overall nutritional status. If the ulcer does occur, nutrition intervention is key to healing. A high-calorie, high-protein diet is essential and commercial supplements or tube feedings are often required to help meet nutritional requirements. Supplements of vitamin C and zinc are also recommended. The best way of monitoring the response to nutritional care is to determine the progress of ulcer healing, which can be done through consultation with the skin care nurse, staff nurse, or physician.

56. B: The purpose of nutrition diagnosis is to document an actual problem or issue Not every patient in a hospital will have a nutrition diagnosis. In the Nutrition Care Plan format, only actual problems are addressed and documented, not problems that the patient may be at risk for. If it is documented that the patient has no nutrition diagnosis, then a plan for follow-up or reassessment needs to be included in the Monitoring/Evaluation step. The plan could be for re-evaluation weekly or monthly or some other interval depending upon individual standards. Not documenting anything is not acceptable because if nothing is documented, then there is no evidence that the patient was assessed at any time.

57. C: Of the selections listed, monitoring of ALT (alanine aminotransferase), AST (aspartate aminotransferase), bilirubin, LDH (lactate dehydrogenase), and ammonia would be the best choice.

ALT, AST, and LDH are enzymes produced by the liver that would increase with damage to liver cells. Other labs that are frequently monitored for liver function include alkaline phosphatase (ALP), gamma-glutamyl transferase (GGT), and serum ammonia. ALP and GGT are markers for cholestasis. Prothrombin time (PT), partial thromboplastin time (PTT), albumin, and globulin may also be measured as these are all proteins produced in the liver. Serum proteins are not useful markers of nutritional status in individuals with liver disease.

58. D: Constant and consistent glucose monitoring is one of the most important tools for evaluating the effectiveness of diabetes therapy, which typically involves diet, exercise, and medication. Tight glucose control can reduce the risk for developing complications of diabetes such as kidney, heart, and microvascular disease. Hemoglobin A1C (also called HbA1c or glycosylated hemoglobin) is the best way to measure long-term glucose control over a period of 2-3 months. This lab value will typically be checked 1-2 times per year in individuals with diabetes. The fasting blood glucose is useful for day-to-day monitoring. Urine samples can also be monitored for glucose, protein, and ketones as a short-term monitoring tool. An oral glucose tolerance test would not be used for anyone who has an established diagnosis of diabetes.

59. A: Step 4 of the Nutrition Care Process is predetermined follow up of the patient's progress towards the resolution of the nutrition diagnosis. The frequency of follow-up is planned during step 3 based on the overall goals and objectives for the patient's care and the expected outcomes. Follow-up requires an active role in measuring outcomes rather than simply "following" or "watching." Concrete measures are used. The steps involved are **monitoring** progress by obtaining information and data that provide evidence of progress, **measuring** outcomes with relevant indicators, and **evaluating** outcomes by comparing results with goals or reference standards. A numerical scale such as 1-5 may be used as a more objective way to document progress rather than a more vague statement such as "patient making progress."

60. B: The dietitian can make a determination on whether nutrition care is to continue based on the patient's overall progress towards goals. If care is to continue, the RD or DTR can reassess and make a new nutrition diagnosis if necessary. The RD or DTR can also readjust the plan of care to make sure the goals are being addressed. If the patient is discharged from the hospital before he or she has been discharged from nutrition care, the RD or DTR will need to be creative in finding ways to monitor progress such as calling the patient, mailing a survey or questionnaire, or emailing. Patients that require ongoing nutritional care should have post-discharge care arranged with an appropriate professional.

61. C: Many vitamin or mineral deficiencies may be observed in the area of the mouth. Bleeding and spongy gums may indicate a vitamin C deficiency but may also be due to poor oral hygiene, certain medications, or thrombocytopenia. Deficiencies in B vitamins can manifest in the mouth area in a number of ways such as a magenta-colored tongue indicating possible riboflavin deficiency or decreased taste sensation indicating a possible zinc deficiency. Angular stomatitis, which is cracking around the corners of the mouth, may also be caused by riboflavin deficiency or fungal infection. Patches of white or brown on the teeth may indicate an excess of fluoride. It is important to explore all findings to determine if any are nutrition-related.

62. C: Any nutrition outcomes that are measured should have an immediate connection to the nutrition diagnosis and the nutrition goals set in the intervention step. Direct nutrition outcomes can measure changes in behavior, the amount of knowledge the patient has gained, or improvement in the patient's nutritional status. Health outcomes that might be measured include improvement in blood pressure, lowered cardiac risk, or amount of weight lost. Patient-centered outcomes might

determine if quality of life has improved or the patient has gained valuable self-management skills. Measurable costs could be a reduction in the length of stay or decreased medication requirements. Any of these outcomes can be part of a comprehensive quality improvement process. Specific outcomes can be followed and documented using the codes provided in the International Dietetics & Nutrition Terminology (IDNT) Reference Manual, second edition, 2009.

63. D: The AHA updated its nutrition recommendations in 2010. The biggest change was the recommendation to reduce sodium intake from less than 2,300 mg per day to less than 1,500 mg per day specifically for those over the age of 50, for those with hypertension, and for African Americans. AHA recommendations continue to call for consuming less than 300 mg per day of cholesterol and eating a variety of fruits and vegetables with a daily goal of 4-5 servings of each. The recommendations also call for increasing soy intake as a way to replace meat to reduce overall fat intact. Alcohol should be limited to 1 drink per day for women and 2 for men. Whole grains are recommended with 6-8 servings per day as the goal.

64. A: The American Cancer Society revises its nutrition guidelines every 5 years. Its current set of guidelines is from 2006. The main recommendations to help prevent cancer are to:
Achieve and maintain a healthy body weight, especially if obesity is present
Strive for at least 30 minutes per day of moderate exercise 5 days a week, although 45-60 minutes per day is even better (this recommendation applies to adults)
Eat at least 5 servings per day of fruits and vegetables
Select whole grains over refined grains
Reduce intake of processed meats and red meats
Limit alcohol to 1 drink per day for women and 2 for men

65. B: Non-verbal clues from the client suggest that he is feeling defensive or cold towards you or the situation. Crossed arms usually indicate the individual is closed off. If he were sitting relaxed and leaning slightly towards you, it would indicate he is open to conversation. A facial expression of frowning is a subtle form of hostility or anger. Eye contact is important in establishing a relationship and shows interest. Conversely, a lack of eye contact may indicate insecurity. If the client was anxious, he might fidget frequently and smile a lot to try to hide his anxiety. Body language cues that suggest a client is open and listening include eye contact (possibly with eyebrows furrowed to show the client is synthesizing information), slight tilting of the head, and ignoring any distractions that are present. The arms are open, not crossed and legs are usually parallel or stretched slightly apart.

66. D: Reflecting is a way to repeat or summarize what another person has said in order to convey understanding. In the case of counseling, reflecting helps to build a rapport with clients and let them know you are listening and empathizing with them. It also helps to create an environment where change is possible and the client feels valued. Reflection can be accomplished in many ways. Paraphrasing what the client has said is one way. Repeating the words exactly or repeating just the most important words is another. In reflecting, it is important to include the entire subject matter, what it means to clients, and how they feel about it. The last response best fits the definition of reflecting.

67. A: Behavior modification is a way to try to change unhealthy behavior patterns to more healthful ones by repetition of desired behavior and providing positive feedback when results are seen. Although limiting computer or television time to 2 hours or less per day is an appropriate goal, rewarding a child with food when he or she is trying to change eating behaviors would defeat the purpose of behavior modification. A more appropriate reward would be to take the child

somewhere fun like bowling or swimming. Behavior modification is about changing old behaviors that lead to bad habits, such as eating in front of the television leading to unconscious overeating. Having family meals together at the table will help to change the other less desirable behavior. Changing the daily breakfast to one that is healthful will lead to positive changes in food choices over time.

68. D: According to the Transtheoretical Model (also known as the Stages of Change Model), there are 6 independent stages of lifestyle change. The stages are Precontemplation, Contemplation, Preparation, Action, Maintenance, and Relapse. Generally, individuals who are in the Action or Maintenance stage will be ready to implement necessary changes. Those that are in the Precontemplation or Contemplation stage are not yet ready for change. In the Preparation stage, an individual may be ready but needs assistance finding the most appropriate method for implementing change. He or she can either move forward or may fall back into an unreadiness stage. During the Action and Maintenance stages, the goal is to keep the individual motivated in order for change to become habit. If an individual enters the Relapse stage, the process starts again.

69. C: Facilitating change in behavior requires certain communication skills by the nutrition professional. One of the most important is the expression of empathy. This is important in developing a rapport with the client and reflective listening helps to achieve this. Helping the client to develop discrepancy is also important in that it helps the client to recognize the pros and cons of making a behavior change. The nutrition professional should resist confrontation at all costs as this would lead to an adversarial relationship with the client. Putting the client on the defensive will not result in any productive change. The nutrition professional should also be working towards the development of self-efficacy by the client. This means that the client should be able to take full responsibility for making appropriate changes.

70. A: As part of overall diabetes management, it is important for a client to understand the implications of certain actions. Skipping breakfast will inevitably lead to hypoglycemia, poor diabetes control, and, over time, complications. It is important for the RD to ask the woman if she is ready to learn more about the dangers of skipping breakfast and assess her stage of change. Developing quick and easy breakfast ideas that she can eat quickly would be an important step in overcoming this hurdle. While the client can also work on her sleep schedule, it is unlikely that altering her wake-up time and not oversleeping can be an easy or immediate change. The RD can reinforce how much better the patient's diabetes will be controlled if she no longer has to worry about the dangers of hypoglycemia.

71. B: Implementing health and nutrition seminars in the workplace is often a useful way to address general health issues and use of sick time. When use of sick time increases, productivity decreases. A baseline can be determined for how much sick time is used on average per employee related to chronic health conditions such as diabetes. This would need to be done confidentially, however, due to the right to privacy by the employee. The average amount of sick time used per employee can then be reassessed at preset intervals and a comparison can be made based on attendance at the seminars. You would need this type of concrete information in order to evaluate the effectiveness of the program in reducing absenteeism.

72. D: The best way to determine the effectiveness of this nutrition education series is to administer a short test before and after the series. This would help you to ascertain baseline knowledge and compare it with responses after the series has concluded. The second test ideally should be done at the end of the last class. If surveys are mailed home, you may not get a great response rate. Asking open-ended questions is a good way to gauge progress as the series continues along and to make

sure participants comprehend what you are teaching. Comparing changes in BMI or serum cholesterol levels would also be a good evaluation method. However, you would need to get this information at baseline as well. This may be an option at a workshop for clients referred by their physicians as opposed to one attended by the general public for their own information.

73. B: The National Institutes of Health started the Women's Health Initiative (WHI) in 1991 as a way to address health issues common to post-menopausal women. The WHI was a 15-year study that began enrolling participants in 1993 and stopped enrolling in 1998. It was designed mainly as a randomized controlled clinical trial (RCT) but also had components of an observational study to predict disease and look at community approaches to the development of healthful behaviors. The researchers were looking to obtain information regarding osteoporosis, heart disease, breast cancer, and colon cancer. A plethora of information has been obtained from this trial. The RCT portion included hormone therapy, a dietary modification trial, and a calcium/vitamin D trial. Forty clinical research centers across the country were involved and over 161,000 women participated. These women were followed for 8-12 years.

74. C: The randomized controlled trial (RCT) is considered to be the gold standard of research design. The Modification of Diet in Renal Disease (MDRD) is an excellent example of an RCT. The MDRD was initiated in 1998 to look at the effect of protein intake on renal disease. It was made up of 2 studies. One compared 291 subjects following a low-protein diet (0.58 grams/kg per day) to 294 subjects following usual protein intake (1.3 grams/kg per day). The second study compared very low-protein intake (0.29 grams/kg per day) to a low-protein diet (0.58 grams/kg per day). All aspects of the study were tightly controlled. RCT is a way to remove any possible selection bias or other types of bias from research design. In an RCT, subjects are randomly assigned to each study group. This is important for proving if a real effect or difference was seen between the groups.

75. A: A cohort study is a type of research design that is considered to be prospective. It looks at 2 groups of subjects—one group that has a certain condition or is receiving a certain treatment and a second group that does not have the condition or is not getting the treatment. The differences between the 2 groups are observed over a period of time. The Nurse's Health Study is an example of a cohort study. This study looked at nurses over a 30-year period to determine how certain influences such as smoking, exercise, weight, hormones, and many other issues affected their long-term health status. Subjects in a cohort study do not need to be randomized and this type of study is usually less expensive to conduct. The disadvantage is that study results must evolve over time and are not immediately known. Also, subjects may move away or die thus reducing the number of participants.

76. D: In utilizing Evidenced-Based Practice (EBP) or Evidenced-Based Medicine (EBM), the main source of information should be scientific research based on best research practice such as randomized controlled trials. This allows medical professionals to provide the most effective care possible. Reviewing literature can be extremely cumbersome and many sources of appropriate information are available. These include databases such as MEDLINE, which is produced by the U.S. National Library of Medicine, and the Cochrane Library. Other appropriate resources are electronic textbooks such as Harrisons Online or Stat!Ref. eMedicine is an online medical reference that is peer-reviewed and can be used free of charge. ACP Journal Club publishes articles based on a strict set of guidelines and provides commentary by experts in the field. Wikipedia is not an appropriate source as information can be edited by anyone. Medpedia is an informative site but should not be a primary source of information for EBP.

77. B: UpToDate, Clinical Evidence, and ACP Medicine are websites designed to provide clinical information to medical professionals. The information available on these websites is obtained from evidenced-based research, written by experts in the field, and peer-reviewed. Reviews are written on many different topics and are designed to give an overview of a condition or issue along with what to expect, treatment options, and sources of additional information. The formats differ slightly. There is a fee to utilize these types of websites; however, they can be an invaluable source of information for medical professionals who may not have extensive resources available at their fingertips. Patients may also obtain access to this information.

78. B: Traditionally, many hospitals offered a full selective menu to their patients. This type of menu allows for a large variety of choices with the goal of increasing satisfaction. The disadvantage of a selective menu is that it requires a large amount of resources because there are so many choices. Ingredients must be on hand and staff available to prepare the variety of food offered on this menu. Because hospital stays are decreasing, many hospital food service departments have changed to a semi-selective menu. A semi-selective menu offers some selection, but not as much. For example, there may be more than one choice of main entrée but only one option for a side dish or vegetable. This helps to reduce both food and labor costs.

79. C: A pre-selective menu is one that does not offer any choice. It is also referred to as a non-selective menu. This type of menu can be utilized effectively in a maternity ward because the length of stay is often only 24 hours. It may offer a set menu such as cereal, eggs, toast, juice, and coffee for breakfast and a sandwich, soup, dessert, and beverage for lunch. Dinner may be a hot meal of chicken, potatoes, vegetable, salad, dessert, and beverage. Or a pre-selective menu may just offer cold items that are easy to prepare and serve at any given time due to the unpredictability of birth. Typically, a list of write-in items is available for those who are unable to find suitable items on the pre-selected menu. This might include items such as vegetarian choices. A non-selective menu is often used in long-term care facilities, where it is rotated on a cycle to prevent repetition.

80. C: The first step of the menu planning process should be the planning of the entrees. The entrees, whether meat, fish, poultry, or a casserole, are usually the most expensive items on the menu. Careful planning needs to occur in order to spread out the higher-cost items among the lower-cost choices. The next step is typically to plan the sandwich selection, or the soup and sandwich combination if offered, to balance the other entrée choices. The third step is usually planning vegetables and other side dishes that supplement the entrée selections. Next in the planning process is salad followed by desserts. The last part of the planning process involves the planning of breads, beverages, and breakfast selections. Garnishes should also be part of the planning process.

81. D: After the menu has been planned, the evaluation process should take place. The most important piece that needs to be evaluated is whether the menu is meeting nutritional guidelines, especially in the case of a long-term care food service operation because of federal regulations. The menu should be planned according to the RDAs. Other components of the menu to evaluate include the visual appearance of meals, particularly with regard to color, texture, and consistency. The use of garnishes can help add interest to a meal. The balance of flavors should be evaluated to avoid offering too many similar flavors (e.g., very strong or spicy) all at the same meal. The menu should be evaluated for repetition, cost, and use of seasonal produce or other items. The staff and equipment required to prepare meals should also be reviewed to make sure it fits within parameters available. Checklists can help manage this process.

82. A: The master menu is not usually appropriate for all the therapeutic and modified-consistency diets that may be encountered in a long-term care facility. It is a federal requirement that any specialized diet must be provided based on written physician order. A menu extension is typically used to accommodate these diets and is based on the master menu. The menu extensions must be planned, written, and approved by an RD. Additionally, these menus must also meet the nutritional requirements based on the RDAs. An approved diet manual that explains any therapeutic or modified-consistency diet must be available. This diet manual needs to be reviewed and updated every 5 years.

83. C: Purchasing is defined as obtaining goods or services for a facility according to specified standards and costs. The first step in this process is typically identification of needs based on the master menu for the operation. Without this list of identified items, there would be no way to determine what is needed for production. A written set of specifications and standards is determined for each item. This may include quality, grade, etc. The amount of each item needed is determined. The amount needed for purchase is then calculated based on inventory or par levels. Purchase orders are then written. Appropriate vendors are identified for all items needed and negotiation with vendors occurs.

84. A: The government has many agencies and inspectors to check the quality of food for both interstate and intrastate commerce. The inspection process involves looking for signs of diseases, contamination, pests, or anything that would make the food unsafe for consumption. Food purchased and shipped between states must meet all federal requirements whereas intrastate purchases and shipments must meet all state and local requirements if they are at least the same as federal requirements. The U.S. Department of Agriculture (USDA) is responsible for inspecting all meat, poultry, eggs, and certain other processed foods. This is mandatory based on laws such as the Meat Inspection Act. After the item is inspected, a federal stamp is given to indicate the item met high quality standards and was processed in a sanitary environment. The Food and Drug Administration (FDA) is responsible for all other food aside from meat, poultry, and eggs.

85. B: Prime vending is a method of purchasing that involves the submission of vendor bids to receive a contract to provide the majority of needs to the buyer. This could involve food or services. The contract is awarded to one vendor that is able to fulfill the variety of needs such as dairy, meat, poultry, produce, or other items as specified. It may also include chemicals, equipment, pesticide needs, etc. The agreement is made for a set amount of time. The advantage to this method is reduced costs because of the high volume and the reduced amount of time spent in the procurement process. A strong working relationship is soon established with the vendor. A disadvantage is that the prices need to be reviewed periodically, as costs do rise, to make sure the best deal is still being attained. A procedure for reviewing prices should be written into the contract.

86. B: Inventory control is the process by which goods and supplies are monitored to determine when new items need to be reordered taking into account shelf life or expiration date, needs, and cost. Par stock is a system that designates a specific number of each item to be kept on hand and the product is automatically reordered to this level as needed to keep the appropriate number on hand. The Min-max system has both a maximum number to keep on hand as well as a minimum number to prevent an item from being totally depleted. Physical inventory is the actual counting of items and is usually used at predetermined times to verify computerized inventory levels. LIFO is an inventory method that stands for Last In First Out. This would not work for food items because of the expiration dates; items might spoil before they are used. FIFO (First in First Out) would be a better choice.

87. D: All employees who work in purchasing and receiving need to be well-trained in order to help control costs and protect food quality. When a delivery is made, the order must first be checked against the purchase order and then a second time against the invoice. This reconciles the order and the delivery and confirms correct invoicing. Food temperatures should be monitored at the time of delivery and frozen items should be checked to make sure they have not thawed out. Crates or boxes can be randomly checked for accuracy but the entire order does not need to be opened and counted. Monitoring for quality may sometimes occur later when the product is being used. Any deviation in quality after delivery should be reported to the vendor and an agreement for an adjustment made with the vendor.

88. A: Food production itself is a challenge. But when large quantities of food are involved, it becomes even more interesting. The most important factor in quantity food production is the end result, which should be a quality product that is flavorful and is visually appealing. Knowing how to utilize ingredients along with the various types of food service equipment is key in achieving a quality product. Standardized recipes are also important. Knowing the best methods of retaining nutrients is crucial. For example, steaming vegetables is a better method of preparation than boiling or frying. Being able to manage a production schedule is essential in achieving a quality product, too. If a piece of equipment is scheduled to be used at the same day and time for two different recipes, one recipe may suffer in the end. Attention to details such as these leads to improved quality.

89. C: There are two methods of adjusting recipes for a different yield: the factor method and the percentage method. The easiest to use for converting a muffin recipe to a larger yield is the factor method, which involves dividing the desired or end yield by the current yield. For example, if the muffin recipe made 1 dozen and the new desired yield is 10 dozen, divide 10 dozen by 1 dozen to get a factor of 10. Any liquid measurements should be converted to weight, then all ingredients in the recipe should be increased by a factor of 10. Decimals are rounded off. In the percentage method, the weight of the recipe is calculated for all ingredients. The percentage of each ingredient by weight is determined and this becomes the factor for each ingredient to increase the recipe yield. The percentage of each ingredient listed in the recipe should add up to 100%.

90. D: A conventional food service system is one in which all food is purchased in the raw state, prepared, and then served all in the same location. Some food service operations use a modified conventional system in which some of the food is purchased in the ready-to-prepare state such as meats that are precut or produce that is prewashed, already peeled and cut, or frozen. One of the main benefits of a conventional food service system is that the menu can be easily changed to incorporate seasonal produce, ethnic dishes, or regional food items such as shrimp and grits. It can also be changed to remove items that have become prohibitively expensive. Less freezer space is required due to food being purchased mostly in the raw state. The main disadvantage is the schedule. It is difficult to plan because of changing menu selections and there may be quite a bit of downtime where employees are not being fully utilized.

91. A: The first step to take if a food-borne illness is suspected is to call the local health department, which is typically city- or county-based. Each state's department of health can assist with obtaining the appropriate contact information if needed. The local health department is then charged with investigating the incident. The local health departments utilize this information to monitor for outbreaks. An outbreak is considered to be 2 or more individuals experiencing the same symptoms after eating the same food item. The CDC can assist in investigating outbreaks; however, it is not the primary mode of investigation. Its role is to monitor and to provide the information that may be

needed to help with decisions. It is also responsible for a national reference library that logs all food-borne illness-causing pathogens.

92. B: A Potentially Hazardous Food (PHF) is one that can possibly cause food-borne illness if temperature control guidelines are not followed. The Food and Drug Administration's Food Code has identified foods that meet the following criteria for being a PHF: having water activity greater than 0.85, containing protein, and/or having a pH between 4.6 and 7.5, making the food neutral to slightly acidic. These foods include meats, chicken, turkey, fish and shellfish, eggs, dairy products, mushrooms, raw sprouts, baked potatoes, and any cooked plant-based food. Peanut butter is not a PHF because it has low water activity. A citation would not be issued if peanut butter and jelly sandwiches were not refrigerated. Most vegetables are not considered hazardous until they are cut, especially tomatoes. Fruits are also not considered PHFs because they have a low pH until they are cut. It is not required to refrigerate whole fresh fruits and vegetables but it is recommended just to be safe.

93. B: The incubation period for food-borne illness caused by *Staphylococcus aureus* is 30 minutes to 6 hours with a total duration of 24-48 hours. *S. aureus* poisoning may be caused by ham or other cooked meats, dairy products, potato salad, cream-based desserts, or custards. The primary symptoms include nausea, vomiting, and abdominal cramping. It is difficult to distinguish between the various types of food-borne illness since their symptoms are so similar, although their presentations may vary slightly with some also causing headaches or fever. Symptoms of *Clostridium botulinum* poisoning include weakness and difficulty talking, swallowing, and breathing. *E. coli* symptoms include bloody diarrhea and hemolytic uremic syndrome. Incubation periods are often good indicators of the type of illness; the Salmonella and *Bacillus cereus* incubation periods are 6-48 hours and 6-15 hours, respectively. The type of food consumed can be a good indicator, too.

94. C: Pregnant women need to take very special precautions to prevent food-borne illness. Left untreated, any food-borne illness can be dangerous or have complications. The most dangerous one, though, is *Listeria monocytogenes*. This illness starts with flu-like symptoms such as fever, aches, and chills but can rapidly advance to life-threatening meningitis. The infection can seriously harm the fetus by causing miscarriage, preterm birth, and even stillbirth. *Listeria* can be present in soft cheeses such as brie, queso fresco, or feta, ready-to-eat meats such as prepackaged deli meats and hotdogs, and unpasteurized milk and dairy products. These types of food should be avoided during pregnancy.

95. A: In food service, any item that comes in contact with food must be properly cleaned then sanitized. There are 2 ways to sanitize: heat and chemical. Heat sanitizing can be done with a high-temperature dish machine. The minimum temperature necessary to effectively sanitize is 162-165° F. Chemical sanitizing is an alternative method that is often utilized because it can save money on energy usage. Three sanitizers are used—chlorine, iodine, and quaternary ammonium. Items are either dipped completely in the sanitizer for 1 minute or rinsed or sprayed with the sanitizing solution using a machine or by hand. In order for the sanitizer to be effective, the pH level of the water it is mixed with must be at a certain level—7 for quaternary ammonium, below 8 for chlorine, and below 5 for iodine.

96. D: Dish machines have different temperature settings or requirements depending upon the function. Typically, the maximum water temperature that should be reached is 194° F. Readings higher than this may cause problems such as the water turning to vapor and not effectively sanitizing. Or, the pipe carrying the hot water could burst, causing a severe burn if the water came

into contact with a person at such a high temperature. Temperature levels for sanitizing range from 171-180° F, depending upon the type of machine.

97. C: Planning for a university food service is a difficult task. There is no one plan that will fit each institution. The number of dormitories, the types of food service offered, whether a central production kitchen is used, and overall budget are all important aspects to consider. Typically, a first floor location near the main hallway is key. This permits easy access for customers as well as for receiving. The ventilation system must be able to adequately ventilate so odors from cooking do not enter the public spaces. Frequently, a cook/chill or cook/freeze system is desirable because it cuts down on the overall requirements for certain types of cooking equipment. Trying to avoid duplication of large pieces of equipment is not always possible. If more than one food service location is running at the same time, it is impossible to share equipment, especially during peak service hours.

98. A: After preliminary studies are completed on a facilities design project, progress can continue with the development of a prospectus. A prospectus is a written plan that provides detailed information on all aspects of the facility being designed. It is used to communicate during the building and design process. There are 3 main parts to the prospectus. The first is the rationale. This includes information such as the reason for the project, goals, and objectives. It also includes all policies. Part 2 is a description of the physical and operational characteristics of the facility. This includes all architectural designs, information about the menu, the type of food service to be utilized, and information on what type of volume and revenue is expected. Part 3 is regulatory information including energy, electrical, safety, sanitation, and other types of data. After the prospectus is completed, the planning team is organized and a feasibility study is initiated.

99. B: The bake shop or dessert preparation area can be located away from the main preparation and serving area if space allows. It can usually function independently. The optimal layout is in a counterclockwise direction to maximize efficiency. The flow of work moves from one station to the next and employees should not have to cross back and forth to accomplish tasks. All necessary equipment for each step should be located at each station. A typical work triangle would not offer the most efficiency in this case. The last station where the final product is ready should be located close to where it will leave the area to be served or transported. This prevents unnecessary entrance to the bakery area by other employees. If space does not allow, the bakery area can be located near the main preparation area with a baker's table available for preparation.

100. B: There are two main types of distribution or delivery systems—centralized and decentralized. The scenario described above reflects a decentralized system. The trays are assembled and then transported to another site closer to the customer. In a centralized system, the customer is the patient. The galleys located on the patient floors each require their own sets of equipment to heat and serve the trays. Typically, point-of-service items such as toast or coffee can be made right in the galley. Dirty dishes are collected and sent back to the main kitchen for cleaning. In a centralized service, trays are assembled on the tray line at meal service time. The trays leave the area and are delivered directly to the patient for immediate consumption.

101. C: There are many ways to recruit for a position. The least effective is likely the help wanted section of the local Sunday newspaper. Before the internet, the help wanted section was one of the most effective ways to advertise. Now, newspapers are cutting back because more people utilize the internet for this type of activity. Recruiting through local colleges with nutrition or internship programs is a great way to look for entry level dietitians. Web-based recruiting using websites such as Monster.com, indeed.com, or Nutritionjobs.com is also useful. The American Dietetic Association

has a career center for members and most state affiliates also offer some type of job listings for members.

102. B: During an interview, it is best to ask open-ended questions such as "Give me an example of a day where staffing levels were short and the cafeteria was busy and how you handled it." This allows the applicant to think for a moment, then relate a similar situation while providing details that would answer the underlying question. Asking a question that requires a yes or no answer will not yield any information on how the applicant would handle the stress of a situation like this. Calling references in front of the applicant is not usually done. Many times, the person giving the reference is only able to answer basic questions.

103. D: Providing a reference for an employee that has been fired is a challenge. Many times, the policy is only to provide information on dates of employment, the relationship with the former employee, and their former job. If there is no way a good reference can be provided, the former employee should be aware of this. It is helpful for that employee to sign a release allowing information to be given with the promise not to sue based on information provided. It is not a good idea to provide your personal opinion on the employee or to provide personal or medical information about the employee. Confidential information and personal opinions are not to be shared. It is important not to lie to the potential employer and not to say anything that cannot be backed up with written documentation. Also, information that cannot be legally asked for in interview should not be provided during a reference.

104. C: A Performance appraisal, also known as a performance review, is a management tool typically used once or twice a year to give employees feedback on their ability to do their job. The most important aspects to cover are the employee's strengths, areas for improvement, and an action plan to help the employee address any weaknesses. Employees need to hear what they are doing well but also what they are not doing well. Any concrete examples that can be given are helpful to quantify an issue. The overall performance should be taken into account as performance will fluctuate from day to day. An action plan and timeline will give employees an opportunity to address issues through avenues such as training or more on-the-job exposure to skills they need to improve.

105. A: The Halo Effect occurs when a manager's overall perception of an employee is clouded by either unusually bad or good performance in just one area. For example, in this case, the manager is frustrated that the employee does not come to work on time. Although this is the only issue the manager has with the employee, it is influencing all aspects of the performance appraisal. It is difficult to separate issues sometimes, but people can be bad at one thing but good at all the others. It is important for managers to refrain from writing performance evaluations when they are angry or frustrated because this will cloud or impair judgment. It is better to identify the chronic tardiness as an area that needs to be improved and set an immediate timeline for improvement.

106. B: There are 3 main methods of planning a budget—incremental, zero-based, and a combination. Incremental budgeting uses the previous year's budget as the starting point. Adjustments are then made to reflect changes in expenses and revenues. Additionally, any changes being planned for the coming year are built into the new budget. This method does not take as much time as zero-based budgeting, where the budget is started from scratch. Doing this enables a new perspective on the budget process. Each piece of the process is analyzed independently of the previous year's needs, which is why this method takes more time. A combination of the two methods can also be used. Some items from the previous year's budget are incorporated into the new budget along with new estimates on other items.

107. D: The balance sheet is also known as the Statement of Financial Position. The purpose of a balance sheet is to give a snapshot of the financial status of an institution at a point in the budget year. It accomplishes this purpose mainly by listing all assets and liabilities. Assets include the cash balance, money available for expenditures, the value of current inventory, any money due to the operation from state or federal sources, petty cash, and accounts receivable. Equipment and furniture are also considered assets. Liabilities include the cost of salaries and benefits, accounts payable, sales tax owed, and other deferred revenue. There is also the fund balance, which includes money reserved for inventory, money that has not been budgeted, and money that has been invested in capital assets. When all this is calculated, it gives the bottom line for the operation.

108. C: School food service operations most often use meal equivalents to gauge the effectiveness of the program. All meals served are converted to meal equivalents equal to one student-reimbursable lunch. All food that is sold, including breakfast, adult lunches, snacks, and a la carte items, are converted to a meal equivalent. A formula is used to estimate how much of each item or meal served equals one student lunch. For example, the formula for the breakfast equivalent is usually 3 breakfasts equal 2 lunches. A factor of 0.66 is used to convert the number of student breakfasts sold to the meal equivalent of a student lunch.

109. D: Financial accountability is an important aspect of the budgeting process. To achieve it, there must be a system to monitor daily, monthly, and yearly financial and operational data. The data are useful for planning purposes and for understanding an operation's bottom line. Purchasing and receiving records such as invoices and purchase orders, storeroom records, and food production data are all useful information sources. The most essential reports to be generated from the information available are the Daily Food Cost Report, a profit and loss statement that can reflect monthly and yearly progress, and a year-end summary. Typically, the food service manager uses these reports to look for ways to increase revenue or decrease expenditures.

110. A: Two methods commonly used for menu pricing are the factor and prime cost methods. The factor method, also known as fixed-factor or markup, uses one specific factor that incorporates labor, supplies, and profit. This factor is applied to the raw food cost, resulting in the price for the menu item. This method is the easiest to use but it typically results in below-value prices because the amount of labor required to produce each item is not differentiated. Some menu items require low labor while others are high-intensity. The prime cost method uses a unique percentage for both food and labor costs. For example, the food cost may be 42% and the labor cost may be 40%. These factors are applied to the total food and labor costs to determine price. Menu pricing is also possible with a modified method that combines the factor and prime cost methods and reflects the degree of labor intensity.

111. A: Labor costs can be as much as 70% of the expenses in a food service operation. This amount will vary based on the type of operation. For example, a fine dining restaurant will have higher labor costs than a fast food restaurant, but the percentage of labor to total expenses will be similar. One way to make it more feasible to analyze labor costs is to compare them using a ratio such as meals per labor hour, which is calculated by dividing the total number of served meals by the total number of hours needed to produce those meals. Another ratio is meals per FTE (full-time equivalent). This is similar to the previous ratio except the total labor hours needed to produce the meals is converted into FTE. A third ratio is labor minutes per meal. This is calculated by dividing the amount of minutes needed to produce each meal by the number of meals served.

112. D: Any fast food establishment that has a desire to expand beyond the United States will need to employ various marketing strategies in order to be successful. This involves research to get to know your target consumer. In the foreign country being considered, it is obvious that the current menu based in the United States may not meet the needs of the potential clientele due to the major presence of beef offerings. Also, vegetarian selections may be limited. One way to address this would be to revamp the menu to reflect the needs of this clientele. Beef and any food made with beef-containing ingredients should be removed totally from the menu. Development of a more extensive menu will surely attract customers. Keeping separate production and preparation areas for vegetarian and non-vegetarian items will also help with marketing.

113. C: The segment of the population born between 1978 and 2000 is typically known as Generation Y. This generation is technology savvy and tends to favor hip or trendy establishments. Establishing accounts with various social networking sites such as Facebook, Twitter, or Evite is essential when marketing to Generation Y. Using text messaging is also useful. Having a website is not optional as this generation expects to easily access information on the internet. Planning social events that this generation would enjoy is also a good idea; such events could include karaoke nights, trivia contests, or live music on the weekends. The choice of music is important. You will attract a greater number of the Generation Y population by playing alternative rock, classic rock, or pop music rather than classical music.

114. D: The scientific management theory began to evolve in the late 1800s. This theory involves finding the best way to accomplish tasks in order to increase productivity in the most efficient way possible. Frederick Taylor is known as the "Father of Scientific Management." He believed that organizations should spend time examining various tasks and developing procedures to help streamline work flow. Henry Gantt contributed to this theory by developing a type of bar graph to measure progress at each step of production. Frank and Lillian Gilbreth contributed by looking at ways to standardize the motions involved with jobs.

115. C: The Classical Theory of Management involves 14 principles, many of which remain the basis of modern management today. The main principle is a defined division of work. This way, each employee can excel at his or her particular job. The manager has the authority and is ultimately the one responsible for the work done. One person is in charge of giving instructions or orders. More than one creates confusion. However, there is a chain of command that starts with the highest level of authority down to the lowest. Salaries are important and should be fair to both the employee and the organization. Disciplinary action is used when needed to correct less-than-desirable behavior or job performance. Teamwork is important to the success of the organization.

116. B: Robert Katz was responsible for naming the skills that a successful manger should possess. Those skills include technical skills, human skills, and conceptual skills. Technical skills are the ability to carry out specific job functions at an expert level. Human skills are the ability to relate to both individuals and groups and determine what might motivate them. Conceptual skills are the ability to see the big picture based on all areas and functions of the organization. The degree of skill required in each category depends upon the level of manager. Human skills should be required of all managers regardless of their level within the organization. Technical skills are a requirement for lower-level managers because they work directly with the employees performing technical jobs. Conceptual skills are most important for upper-level managers.

117. A: This is an example of a job specification, which is a written document that outlines the minimum standards for a particular job. It usually includes typical job responsibilities, working conditions, and location. It also specifies personal qualities needed, educational requirements, and

preferred experience. A job description is different from a job specification in that it details the specific job responsibilities for a particular position. It is a much more comprehensive document than a job specification and helps to determine which employee or applicant best fits a particular job. Every position within an organization should have its own job description.

118. C: The American Dietetic Association has developed a Professional Code of Ethics for all dietetic practitioners. The code outlines appropriate behavior for all aspects of professional life. It also gives guidance on aspects of the personal life that may be inappropriate if they cross over into the professional realm such as alcohol or drug abuse. In the case described here, the code of ethics violation was the RD using a credential that was not current. The other scenarios do not necessarily constitute a violation, although the potential is there. When moving to a new state, the RD should apply for licensure if the job being applied for requires this. If an RD has a drug or alcohol problem, withdrawing from his or her job to obtain treatment would not be a violation. The RD can sell nutritional supplements as long as it is done in a way that is not misleading or based on unfounded scientific principles.

119. A: In 2004, the JCAHO developed a list of commonly used abbreviations that have safety implications if misinterpreted. This list is called the "Do Not Use" list. It was developed as part of a Sentinel Event Alert initiated in 2001 followed by the implementation of a National Patient Safety Goal in 2002 requiring hospitals to put together a list of abbreviations to avoid within their own institutions. According to the most current list from March 2009, the abbreviation IU (international units) may not be used because it may be confused with IV (intravenous). IV is still an acceptable abbreviation, however. Any of the abbreviations involving the letter Q such as Q.D. or Q.O.D., meaning every day or every other day, can be confused with one another or similar abbreviations such as QID, which means 4 times per day. Drug names should be written out fully to avoid misinterpretation. This list should be reviewed by all practitioners.

120. B: According to the JCAHO, a sentinel event is one in which an unexpected death occurs or there is serious physical or psychological injury that requires immediate attention. JCAHO policy on sentinel events was written to improve patient outcomes and ensure that institutions where such events occur can analyze the events and formulate a plan to prevent reoccurrences. The JCAHO also promotes education and training regarding sentinel events and tries to protect the public through the accreditation process. In this case, the "Do not Use" list was ignored and 10 units was misinterpreted as 100 units, causing harm to the patient. Medication errors caused 547 sentinel events from 1995 through March 2010. Once the root cause is identified and an action plan is created, the changes are implemented. The JCAHO keeps a database of sentinel events.

121. D: To help prevent infection, the JCAHO has introduced another patient safety goal requiring all healthcare workers to follow the hand hygiene guidelines set forth by the CDC. Artificial nails should not be worn at all and natural fingernails should be kept to a maximum length of 1/4 inch beyond the fingertips, although the actual length may be determined by individual institutions. One set of gloves should not be worn throughout the tray passing process. Gloves should be worn if there is a chance of exposure to bodily fluids or blood and then immediately discarded. For those passing trays to multiple patients, proper hand hygiene is required if hands are visibly soiled or have had direct contact with the patient. Otherwise, an alcohol-based hand rub may be used between patients.

122. C: Total Quality Management (TQM) is an approach to management with customer satisfaction as its main goal. Organizations are made up of many different parts but those parts are all interrelated and should have that goal in mind. The principles of TQM assume that most employees

are self-motivated, have an innate desire to do their job well, and want to learn and improve. TQM strives to do each job right the first time, implements systems for continuous improvement, and creates a plan to address deficiencies based on input from all levels of the organization. Teamwork is the cornerstone of TQM. The benefits include lower costs and higher customer satisfaction and retention.

123. A: There are many tools to help illustrate problem solving. One that illustrates cause and effect is called a fish diagram (also known as fishbone). When sketched out, this type of diagram resembles a fish skeleton, with the head on the right of the diagram illustrating effect. Above and below the backbone are bones representing factors contributing to problems such as methods of practice or training issues. A Pareto chart is similar to a bar graph and depicts the reasons for a problem. A process chart helps with logically thinking through an issue by analyzing it a step at a time. A scatter chart uses points on a graph to plot variables on the horizontal and vertical axis. When all points are plotted, the distribution of the data can be observed and possible trends can be determined.

124. D: CSPI is the Center for Science in the Public Interest. It is an advocacy group whose mission is to inform the public about current issues in health and nutrition. It also tries to work with policymakers on improving health and nutrition issues. It does not set any regulations for food service operations. There are many agencies involved in overseeing food safety. The 4 main federal agencies are the Food and Drug Administration (FDA), the United States Department of Agriculture (USDA), the Centers for Disease Control and Prevention (CDC), and the Environmental Protection Agency (EPA). There are also international organizations such as the World Health Organization (WHO), the World Food Safety Organization (WFSO), and the Food and Agriculture Organization of the United Nations (FAO). Actual inspections to ensure compliance with federal regulations occur at the local level such as the County or State Board of Health.

125. C: The Occupational Safety & Health Administration (OSHA) is responsible for keeping American workers safe in the workplace. It is an agency within the U.S. Department of Labor. The Occupational Safety & Health Act of 1970 established many rights for workers including the right to training on any chemicals located within the work environment and to information regarding OSHA standards on injuries or illnesses to workers in the workplace. It also gives employees the right to ask the employer to fix safety issues that may not be in violation of OSHA regulations and to file a complaint without penalty if serious workplace violations exist and are not corrected. The Americans with Disabilities Act (ADA) of 1990 deals with discrimination against disabled individuals in the workplace. It falls within the jurisdiction of the U.S. Equal Employment Opportunity Commission (EEOC). The ADA requires that reasonable workplace accommodations be made for anyone with a disability.

Special Report: Normal Lab Values

Hematologic

Bleeding Time (Template): Less than 10 minutes
Erythrocyte count: 4.2 -5.9 million/cu mm
Erythrocyte sedimentation rate (Westergren): Male- 0-15mm/hr; Female: 0-20mm/hr
Hematocrit, blood: Male- 42-50%; Female: 40-48%
Hemoglobin, blood: Male-13-16 g/dL; Female- 12-15 g/dL
Leukocyte count and differential

- Leukocyte count: 4000-11,000/ cu mm
- 50-70% segmented neutrophils
- 0-5% band forms
- 0-3 % eosinophils
- 0-1% basophils
- 30-45% lymphocytes
- 0-6% monocytes

Mean corpuscular volume: 86-98 fL
Prothrombin time, plasma: 11-13 seconds
Partial thromboplastin time (activated): 30-40 seconds
Platelet count: 150,000-300,000/ cu mm
Reticulocyte count: 0.5-1.5% of red cells

Whole blood, Plasma, serum chemistries

Amylase, serum: 25-125 U/L

Arterial studies, blood (patient breathing room air)

- PO_2 : 75-100 mm Hg
- PCO_2 : 38-42 mm Hg
- Bicarbonate: 23-26 mEq/L
- pH: 7.38-7.44
- Oxygen saturation: 95% or greater

Bilirubin, serum

- Total: 0.3-1.0 mg/dL
- Direct: 0.1-0.3 mg/dL

Comprehensive metabolic panel:

- Bilirubin, serum (total): 0.3-1.0 mg/dL
- Calcium, serum: Male: 9.0-10.5 mg/dL; Female: 8.5-10.2 mg/dL
- Chloride, serum: 98-106 mEq/L

- Cholesterol, serum (total):
  - Desirable: less than 200mg/dL
  - Borderline-high: 200-239 mg/dL (may be high in the presence of coronary artery disease or other risk factors)
  - High: greater than 239 mg/dL
- Creatine, serum: 0.7-1.5 mg/dL
- Glucose, plasma:
  - Normal (fasting)- 70-115 mg/dL
  - Borderline: 115-140 mg/dL
  - Abnormal: greater than 140 mg/dL
- Phosphorus, serum: 3.0-4.5 mg/dL
- Proteins, serum:
  - Pre-Albumin: 0.2-0.4 g/dL
  - Albumin: 3.5-5.5 g/dL
- Urea nitrogen, blood (BUN): 8-20 mg/dL
- Uric acid, serum: 3.0 7.0 mg/dL

High-density lipoprotein: Low- less than 200 mg/dL
Low-density lipoprotein:
- Optimal: less than 100 mg/dL
- Near-optimal: 100-129 mg/dL
- Borderline-high: 130-159 mg/dL (may be high in the presence of coronary artery disease or other risk factors)
- High: 160-189 mg/dL
- Very high: 190 mg/dL and above

Electrolytes, serum:
- Sodium: 136-145 mEq/L
- Potassium: 3.5-5.0 mEq/L
- Chloride: 98-106 mEq/L
- Bicarbonate: 23-28 mEq/L

Follicle-stimulating hormone, serum:
- Male: 2-18 mIU/mL
- Female:
  - 5-20 mIU/mL (follicular or luteal)
  - 30-50 mIU/mL (mid-cycle peak)
  - greater than 50 mIU/mL (postmenopausal)

Lactate dehydrogenase, serum: 140-280 U/L
Osmolality, serum: 280-300 mOsm/kg H_2O
Oxygen saturation, arterial blood: 95 % or greater
Phosphatase (alkaline), serum: 30-120 U/L
Phosphorus, serum: 3.0-4.5 mg/dL
Potassium, serum: 3.5-5.0 mEq/L
Triglycerides, serum (fasting)
- Normal: less than 250 mg/dL
- Borderline: 250-500 mg/dL
- Abnormal: greater than 500 mg/dL

Secret Key #1 - Time is Your Greatest Enemy

Pace Yourself

Wear a watch. At the beginning of the test, check the time (or start a chronometer on your watch to count the minutes), and check the time after every few questions to make sure you are "on schedule."

If you are forced to speed up, do it efficiently. Usually one or more answer choices can be eliminated without too much difficulty. Above all, don't panic. Don't speed up and just begin guessing at random choices. By pacing yourself, and continually monitoring your progress against your watch, you will always know exactly how far ahead or behind you are with your available time. If you find that you are one minute behind on the test, don't skip one question without spending any time on it, just to catch back up. Take 15 fewer seconds on the next four questions, and after four questions you'll have caught back up. Once you catch back up, you can continue working each problem at your normal pace.

Furthermore, don't dwell on the problems that you were rushed on. If a problem was taking up too much time and you made a hurried guess, it must be difficult. The difficult questions are the ones you are most likely to miss anyway, so it isn't a big loss. It is better to end with more time than you need than to run out of time.

Lastly, sometimes it is beneficial to slow down if you are constantly getting ahead of time. You are always more likely to catch a careless mistake by working more slowly than quickly, and among very high-scoring test takers (those who are likely to have lots of time left over), careless errors affect the score more than mastery of material.

Secret Key #2 - Guessing is not Guesswork

You probably know that guessing is a good idea - unlike other standardized tests, there is no penalty for getting a wrong answer. Even if you have no idea about a question, you still have a 20-25% chance of getting it right.

Most test takers do not understand the impact that proper guessing can have on their score. Unless you score extremely high, guessing will significantly contribute to your final score.

Monkeys Take the Test

What most test takers don't realize is that to insure that 20-25% chance, you have to guess randomly. If you put 20 monkeys in a room to take this test, assuming they answered once per question and behaved themselves, on average they would get 20-25% of the questions correct. Put 20 test takers in the room, and the average will be much lower among guessed questions. Why?

1. The test writers intentionally writes deceptive answer choices that "look" right. A test taker has no idea about a question, so picks the "best looking" answer, which is often wrong. The monkey has no idea what looks good and what doesn't, so will consistently be lucky about 20-25% of the time.
2. Test takers will eliminate answer choices from the guessing pool based on a hunch or intuition. Simple but correct answers often get excluded, leaving a 0% chance of being correct. The monkey has no clue, and often gets lucky with the best choice.

This is why the process of elimination endorsed by most test courses is flawed and detrimental to your performance- test takers don't guess, they make an ignorant stab in the dark that is usually worse than random.

$5 Challenge

Let me introduce one of the most valuable ideas of this course- the $5 challenge:

You only mark your "best guess" if you are willing to bet $5 on it.
You only eliminate choices from guessing if you are willing to bet $5 on it.

Why $5? Five dollars is an amount of money that is small yet not insignificant, and can really add up fast (20 questions could cost you $100). Likewise, each answer choice on one question of the test will have a small impact on your overall score, but it can really add up to a lot of points in the end.

The process of elimination IS valuable. The following shows your chance of guessing it right:

If you eliminate wrong answer choices until only this many answer choices remain:	Chance of getting it correct:
1	100%
2	50%
3	33%

However, if you accidentally eliminate the right answer or go on a hunch for an incorrect answer, your chances drop dramatically: to 0%. By guessing among all the answer choices, you are GUARANTEED to have a shot at the right answer.

That's why the $5 test is so valuable- if you give up the advantage and safety of a pure guess, it had better be worth the risk.

What we still haven't covered is how to be sure that whatever guess you make is truly random. Here's the easiest way:

Always pick the first answer choice among those remaining.

Such a technique means that you have decided, **before you see a single test question**, exactly how you are going to guess- and since the order of choices tells you nothing about which one is correct, this guessing technique is perfectly random.

This section is not meant to scare you away from making educated guesses or eliminating choices- you just need to define when a choice is worth eliminating. The $5 test, along with a pre-defined random guessing strategy, is the best way to make sure you reap all of the benefits of guessing.

Secret Key #3 - Practice Smarter, Not Harder

Many test takers delay the test preparation process because they dread the awful amounts of practice time they think necessary to succeed on the test. We have refined an effective method that will take you only a fraction of the time.

There are a number of "obstacles" in your way to succeed. Among these are answering questions, finishing in time, and mastering test-taking strategies. All must be executed on the day of the test at peak performance, or your score will suffer. The test is a mental marathon that has a large impact on your future.

Just like a marathon runner, it is important to work your way up to the full challenge. So first you just worry about questions, and then time, and finally strategy:

Success Strategy

1. Find a good source for practice tests.
2. If you are willing to make a larger time investment, consider using more than one study guide- often the different approaches of multiple authors will help you "get" difficult concepts.
3. Take a practice test with no time constraints, with all study helps "open book." Take your time with questions and focus on applying strategies.
4. Take a practice test with time constraints, with all guides "open book."
5. Take a final practice test with no open material and time limits

If you have time to take more practice tests, just repeat step 5. By gradually exposing yourself to the full rigors of the test environment, you will condition your mind to the stress of test day and maximize your success.

Secret Key #4 - Prepare, Don't Procrastinate

Let me state an obvious fact: if you take the test three times, you will get three different scores. This is due to the way you feel on test day, the level of preparedness you have, and, despite the test writers' claims to the contrary, some tests WILL be easier for you than others.

Since your future depends so much on your score, you should maximize your chances of success. In order to maximize the likelihood of success, you've got to prepare in advance. This means taking practice tests and spending time learning the information and test taking strategies you will need to succeed.

Never take the test as a "practice" test, expecting that you can just take it again if you need to. Feel free to take sample tests on your own, but when you go to take the official test, be prepared, be focused, and do your best the first time!

Secret Key #5 - Test Yourself

Everyone knows that time is money. There is no need to spend too much of your time or too little of your time preparing for the test. You should only spend as much of your precious time preparing as is necessary for you to get the score you need.

Once you have taken a practice test under real conditions of time constraints, then you will know if you are ready for the test or not.

If you have scored extremely high the first time that you take the practice test, then there is not much point in spending countless hours studying. You are already there.

Benchmark your abilities by retaking practice tests and seeing how much you have improved. Once you score high enough to guarantee success, then you are ready.

If you have scored well below where you need, then knuckle down and begin studying in earnest. Check your improvement regularly through the use of practice tests under real conditions. Above all, don't worry, panic, or give up. The key is perseverance!

Then, when you go to take the test, remain confident and remember how well you did on the practice tests. If you can score high enough on a practice test, then you can do the same on the real thing.

General Strategies

The most important thing you can do is to ignore your fears and jump into the test immediately- do not be overwhelmed by any strange-sounding terms. You have to jump into the test like jumping into a pool- all at once is the easiest way.

Make Predictions
As you read and understand the question, try to guess what the answer will be. Remember that several of the answer choices are wrong, and once you begin reading them, your mind will immediately become cluttered with answer choices designed to throw you off. Your mind is typically the most focused immediately after you have read the question and digested its contents. If you can, try to predict what the correct answer will be. You may be surprised at what you can predict.

Quickly scan the choices and see if your prediction is in the listed answer choices. If it is, then you can be quite confident that you have the right answer. It still won't hurt to check the other answer choices, but most of the time, you've got it!

Answer the Question
It may seem obvious to only pick answer choices that answer the question, but the test writers can create some excellent answer choices that are wrong. Don't pick an answer just because it sounds right, or you believe it to be true. It MUST answer the question. Once you've made your selection, always go back and check it against the question and make sure that you didn't misread the question, and the answer choice does answer the question posed.

Benchmark
After you read the first answer choice, decide if you think it sounds correct or not. If it doesn't, move on to the next answer choice. If it does, mentally mark that answer choice. This doesn't mean that you've definitely selected it as your answer choice, it just means that it's the best you've seen thus far. Go ahead and read the next choice. If the next choice is worse than the one you've already selected, keep going to the next answer choice. If the next choice is better than the choice you've already selected, mentally mark the new answer choice as your best guess.

The first answer choice that you select becomes your standard. Every other answer choice must be benchmarked against that standard. That choice is correct until proven otherwise by another answer choice beating it out. Once you've decided that no other answer choice seems as good, do one final check to ensure that your answer choice answers the question posed.

Valid Information
Don't discount any of the information provided in the question. Every piece of information may be necessary to determine the correct answer. None of the information in the question is there to throw you off (while the answer choices will certainly have information to throw you off). If two seemingly unrelated topics are discussed, don't ignore either. You can be confident there is a relationship, or it wouldn't be included in the question, and you are probably going to have to determine what is that relationship to find the answer.

Avoid "Fact Traps"

Don't get distracted by a choice that is factually true. Your search is for the answer that answers the question. Stay focused and don't fall for an answer that is true but incorrect. Always go back to the question and make sure you're choosing an answer that actually answers the question and is not just a true statement. An answer can be factually correct, but it MUST answer the question asked. Additionally, two answers can both be seemingly correct, so be sure to read all of the answer choices, and make sure that you get the one that BEST answers the question.

Milk the Question

Some of the questions may throw you completely off. They might deal with a subject you have not been exposed to, or one that you haven't reviewed in years. While your lack of knowledge about the subject will be a hindrance, the question itself can give you many clues that will help you find the correct answer. Read the question carefully and look for clues. Watch particularly for adjectives and nouns describing difficult terms or words that you don't recognize. Regardless of if you completely understand a word or not, replacing it with a synonym either provided or one you more familiar with may help you to understand what the questions are asking. Rather than wracking your mind about specific detailed information concerning a difficult term or word, try to use mental substitutes that are easier to understand.

The Trap of Familiarity

Don't just choose a word because you recognize it. On difficult questions, you may not recognize a number of words in the answer choices. The test writers don't put "make-believe" words on the test; so don't think that just because you only recognize all the words in one answer choice means that answer choice must be correct. If you only recognize words in one answer choice, then focus on that one. Is it correct? Try your best to determine if it is correct. If it is, that is great, but if it doesn't, eliminate it. Each word and answer choice you eliminate increases your chances of getting the question correct, even if you then have to guess among the unfamiliar choices.

Eliminate Answers

Eliminate choices as soon as you realize they are wrong. But be careful! Make sure you consider all of the possible answer choices. Just because one appears right, doesn't mean that the next one won't be even better! The test writers will usually put more than one good answer choice for every question, so read all of them. Don't worry if you are stuck between two that seem right. By getting down to just two remaining possible choices, your odds are now 50/50. Rather than wasting too much time, play the odds. You are guessing, but guessing wisely, because you've been able to knock out some of the answer choices that you know are wrong. If you are eliminating choices and realize that the last answer choice you are left with is also obviously wrong, don't panic. Start over and consider each choice again. There may easily be something that you missed the first time and will realize on the second pass.

Tough Questions

If you are stumped on a problem or it appears too hard or too difficult, don't waste time. Move on! Remember though, if you can quickly check for obviously incorrect answer choices, your chances of guessing correctly are greatly improved. Before you completely give up, at least try to knock out a couple of possible answers. Eliminate what you can and then guess at the remaining answer choices before moving on.

Brainstorm

If you get stuck on a difficult question, spend a few seconds quickly brainstorming. Run through the complete list of possible answer choices. Look at each choice and ask yourself, "Could this answer

- 270 -

the question satisfactorily?" Go through each answer choice and consider it independently of the other. By systematically going through all possibilities, you may find something that you would otherwise overlook. Remember that when you get stuck, it's important to try to keep moving.

Read Carefully
Understand the problem. Read the question and answer choices carefully. Don't miss the question because you misread the terms. You have plenty of time to read each question thoroughly and make sure you understand what is being asked. Yet a happy medium must be attained, so don't waste too much time. You must read carefully, but efficiently.

Face Value
When in doubt, use common sense. Always accept the situation in the problem at face value. Don't read too much into it. These problems will not require you to make huge leaps of logic. The test writers aren't trying to throw you off with a cheap trick. If you have to go beyond creativity and make a leap of logic in order to have an answer choice answer the question, then you should look at the other answer choices. Don't overcomplicate the problem by creating theoretical relationships or explanations that will warp time or space. These are normal problems rooted in reality. It's just that the applicable relationship or explanation may not be readily apparent and you have to figure things out. Use your common sense to interpret anything that isn't clear.

Prefixes
If you're having trouble with a word in the question or answer choices, try dissecting it. Take advantage of every clue that the word might include. Prefixes and suffixes can be a huge help. Usually they allow you to determine a basic meaning. Pre- means before, post- means after, pro - is positive, de- is negative. From these prefixes and suffixes, you can get an idea of the general meaning of the word and try to put it into context. Beware though of any traps. Just because con is the opposite of pro, doesn't necessarily mean congress is the opposite of progress!

Hedge Phrases
Watch out for critical "hedge" phrases, such as likely, may, can, will often, sometimes, often, almost, mostly, usually, generally, rarely, sometimes. Question writers insert these hedge phrases to cover every possibility. Often an answer choice will be wrong simply because it leaves no room for exception. Avoid answer choices that have definitive words like "exactly," and "always".

Switchback Words
Stay alert for "switchbacks". These are the words and phrases frequently used to alert you to shifts in thought. The most common switchback word is "but". Others include although, however, nevertheless, on the other hand, even though, while, in spite of, despite, regardless of.

New Information
Correct answer choices will rarely have completely new information included. Answer choices typically are straightforward reflections of the material asked about and will directly relate to the question. If a new piece of information is included in an answer choice that doesn't even seem to relate to the topic being asked about, then that answer choice is likely incorrect. All of the information needed to answer the question is usually provided for you, and so you should not have to make guesses that are unsupported or choose answer choices that require unknown information that cannot be reasoned on its own.

Time Management

On technical questions, don't get lost on the technical terms. Don't spend too much time on any one question. If you don't know what a term means, then since you don't have a dictionary, odds are you aren't going to get much further. You should immediately recognize terms as whether or not you know them. If you don't, work with the other clues that you have, the other answer choices and terms provided, but don't waste too much time trying to figure out a difficult term.

Contextual Clues

Look for contextual clues. An answer can be right but not correct. The contextual clues will help you find the answer that is most right and is correct. Understand the context in which a phrase or statement is made. This will help you make important distinctions.

Don't Panic

Panicking will not answer any questions for you. Therefore, it isn't helpful. When you first see the question, if your mind goes blank, take a deep breath. Force yourself to mechanically go through the steps of solving the problem and using the strategies you've learned.

Pace Yourself

Don't get clock fever. It's easy to be overwhelmed when you're looking at a page full of questions, your mind is full of random thoughts and feeling confused, and the clock is ticking down faster than you would like. Calm down and maintain the pace that you have set for yourself. As long as you are on track by monitoring your pace, you are guaranteed to have enough time for yourself. When you get to the last few minutes of the test, it may seem like you won't have enough time left, but if you only have as many questions as you should have left at that point, then you're right on track!

Answer Selection

The best way to pick an answer choice is to eliminate all of those that are wrong, until only one is left and confirm that is the correct answer. Sometimes though, an answer choice may immediately look right. Be careful! Take a second to make sure that the other choices are not equally obvious. Don't make a hasty mistake. There are only two times that you should stop before checking other answers. First is when you are positive that the answer choice you have selected is correct. Second is when time is almost out and you have to make a quick guess!

Check Your Work

Since you will probably not know every term listed and the answer to every question, it is important that you get credit for the ones that you do know. Don't miss any questions through careless mistakes. If at all possible, try to take a second to look back over your answer selection and make sure you've selected the correct answer choice and haven't made a costly careless mistake (such as marking an answer choice that you didn't mean to mark). This double check costs time, but should more than pay for itself.

Beware of Directly Quoted Answers

Sometimes an answer choice will repeat a portion of the question or reference section. However, beware of such exact duplication – it may be a trap! More than likely, the correct choice will paraphrase or summarize a point, rather than being exactly the same wording.

Slang

Scientific answers are better than slang ones. A choice that begins "To compare the outcomes..." is more likely to be correct than "Because some people insisted..."

Extreme Statements

Avoid wild answers that throw out highly controversial ideas that are proclaimed as established fact. An answer choice that states the "process should be used in certain situations, if…" is much more likely to be correct than one that states the "process should be discontinued completely." The first is a calm rational statement and doesn't even make a definitive, uncompromising stance, using a hedge word "if" to provide wiggle room, whereas the second choice is a radical idea and far more extreme.

Answer Choice Families

Two or more answer choices that are direct opposites or parallels usually indication that one of them is the correct answer. Example: one answer choice states "x increases" and another answer choice states "x decreases" or "y increases." Those two or three answer choices are similar in construction and fall into the same family of answer choices. A family of answer choices is when two or three answer choices are similar in construction, and yet often have a directly opposite meaning. Usually the correct answer choice will be in that family of answer choices. The "odd man out" or answer choice that doesn't seem to fit the parallel construction of the other answer choices is more likely to be incorrect.

Additional Bonus Material

Due to our efforts to try to keep this book to a manageable length, we've created a link that will give you access to all of your additional bonus material.

Please visit http://www.mometrix.com/bonus948/rd to access the information.